DISEASE SURVEILLANCE:

Technological Contributions to Global Health Security

Contents

Foreword

Now, more than ever, public health authorities need fast and accurate information about new disease threats. People and their pathogens move quickly, as evidenced by the 2014 Ebola outbreak, the largest in recorded history. Fortunately, we have an array of new technologies, big data sources, and sophisticated analytic approaches. These can serve either to illuminate or to obfuscate disease surveillance data, depending on the appropriateness of the presentation and the understanding of the modern audience. Disease surveillance has changed a lot since Alex Langmuir defined it as "the continued watchfulness over the distribution and trends of incidence through the systematic collection, consolidation and evaluation of morbidity and mortality reports and other relevant data" in 1963, but it remains an essential cornerstone of public health practice. The dramatic changes over the past decade with big data sources and powerful new visualization tools promise to accelerate in the coming decades. In this new textbook, David Blazes and Sheri Lewis have brought together some of the leading thinkers and writers on global health security and disease surveillance.

Disease Surveillance: Technological Contributions to Global Health Security will be a valuable resource for a wide range of readers. New students of public health will benefit from the reviews of electronic disease surveillance and international health regulations policy (Chapters 1 and 2), and experienced health authorities will learn from the comprehensive update on data visualization techniques (Chapter 6) and the detailed review of legal considerations around open source software (Chapter 10). With the expansion of interest and funding for global health security and the rapid technological innovations in surveillance, this new text fills an essential niche.

Scott F. Dowell, MD MPH
Deputy Director for Surveillance and Epidemiology
Vaccine Development, Global Health
Bill and Melinda Gates Foundation
Seattle, Washington

Preface

This book has been a work in evolution over many years as a result of our involvement in the development and implementation of electronic disease surveillance systems around the world, particularly in resource-limited environments. We both come to this topic through our educational and professional experience; however, through working with colleagues from very diverse backgrounds, we have learned a great deal about what makes a successful, sustainable electronic disease surveillance system in an ever-changing technology-driven world.

As recently witnessed in the Ebola crisis in West Africa, the lack of a population-based surveillance system that reaches the broad population, as opposed to just sentinel sites, can have devastating effects. Had there been an effective surveillance system in place, public health professionals may have been alerted sooner to an increase in patients exhibiting high fever and gastrointestinal symptoms. While these types of surveillance systems do not give the user a diagnosis in the earliest stages, they do indicate increases in illness that warrant further investigation.

A great analogy is that an electronic disease surveillance system is like a fire tower looking out over the countryside. When a fire, or in this case a statistical anomaly in disease activity, is spotted, the epidemiologist needs to drill into the data to determine if there really is an epidemiologically significant event taking place. If there is, then other systems, such as the Centers for Disease Control and Prevention's Epi Info™, can take data from the surveillance system to conduct a thorough outbreak investigation. It was this warning system with early event detection analytics that was missing in the Ebola epidemic in West Africa in 2014.

Our experience in electronic disease surveillance has very much been an iterative and learning process. In some cases, we have been amazed at what colleagues have been able to do with very limited resources, while in other cases, we have watched organizations spend vast sums of money on efforts that fail for a variety of reasons, whether for a lack of local support, an unsustainable system, or unrealistic expectations. Historically, public health worldwide is woefully underfunded, but we have learned firsthand that one does not need to have a lot of money to do great things. In fact, limited resources quite often drive innovation.

We have undertaken this book to give a voice to those individuals we have encountered throughout our work in this field who are making significant contributions in the field of global public health and who deserve visibility on the global stage. But even more so, we want to provide a resource to those who may be considering a public health technology project or who are struggling with an existing one. The field of public health has a rich history of sharing lessons learned, both successes and failures, in order to enable the public health community as a whole to grow and collectively move ahead. We hope this book proves useful to public health students who are considering how technology can aid in such a people-intensive field such as disease surveillance, those who are current or aspiring public health authorities who need to make key decisions about how to employ technology in their countries, and global public health professionals worldwide who want to get new ideas or validation for the efforts they have undertaken in this field.

There are many components that make up a successful technology project in the public health sector. These components include (1) understanding the operational environment, (2) using the right tools for the job, (3) incorporating into the existing infrastructure, (4) building the capability from within the organization using a local champion, (5) being flexible to change the system and practices over time, and (6) fostering ongoing collaboration. While each one of these aspects could make an entire book unto themselves, our goal is to highlight successful project principles that will withstand the test of time, despite changing technologies, policies, and personalities.

We feel that while the book can certainly be read from beginning to end, it is meant to also serve as a reference so that the reader can learn about such stand-alone topics as international health policies, challenges surrounding system deployment and implementation, or the strengths and weaknesses of open source software in an increasingly open source world. The contributors to the book are leaders in the public health community; as such, we asked them to draw upon their experiences and describe the challenges facing today's public health workforce and how to effectively deal with these challenges in an increasingly technology-driven environment.

One of the greatest difficulties we encountered as we embarked on creating this book was, ironically, a public health crisis similar to what might be controlled using the very public health technology we chronicle. The Ebola outbreak in West Africa occupied much of 2014–2015 and is very much on the minds of public health professionals today. Many of our colleagues who eagerly agreed to provide insights for the book were personally involved in the ongoing response activities, thereby hindering the efforts to bring this book to completion. However, we think the insights they can now share will make this book even more valuable as we move forward and determine how to be better prepared for future epidemics. The Ebola crisis highlighted many successes and failures of introducing technologies in the midst of an outbreak, information that we hope you, the reader, will be able to translate into your work in global health security.

David L. Blazes
Bethesda, Maryland

Sheri H. Lewis
Laurel, Maryland

Acknowledgments

We are indebted to many people without whom this book would not have been possible. Our colleagues in the field who contributed chapters while responding to a variety of public health threats come foremost, as well as colleagues from the Uniformed Services University (James Mancuso, Patrick Hickey, and Robert DeFraites) and the Johns Hopkins University Applied Physics Laboratory (Kelly Livieratos and the entire Global Health Surveillance Program team). We would also like to thank our spouses (Marian and Rob) and children (Sam, Jack, and Libby, and Gabrielle and Shelby), who tolerated many hours of work after hours to make this book possible.

Finally, this book is dedicated to all those who toil in developing, implementing, troubleshooting, and refining electronic disease surveillance systems globally. Like most things in public health, although one does their job well in this field, nothing beneficial happens; the aim of this book is to call attention to their often under-recognized, constantly made efforts that contribute to global health security.

Contributors

Neil F. Abernethy
Department of Biomedical Informatics and
Medical Education
University of Washington
Seattle, Washington

David Atrubin
Florida Department of Health–Hillsborough
County
Tampa, Florida

Steve Babin
Johns Hopkins University
Applied Physics Laboratory
Laurel, Maryland

David L. Blazes
Department of Preventive Medicine and
Biostatistics
Uniformed Services University of the Health
Sciences
Bethesda, Maryland

David Brett-Major
Infectious Diseases Directorate
Naval Medical Research Center
Silver Spring, Maryland
and
Division of Tropical Public Health
Department of Preventive Medicine and
Biometrics
Uniformed Services University
Bethesda, Maryland

Howard S. Burkom
Johns Hopkins University
Applied Physics Laboratory
Laurel, Maryland

Lauren N. Carroll
Department of Biomedical Informatics and
Medical Education
University of Washington
Seattle, Washington

Obaghe Edeghere
Field Epidemiology Service
and
Real-time Syndromic Surveillance Team
Public Health England
Birmingham, United Kingdom

Alex J. Elliot
Real-time Syndromic Surveillance Team
Public Health England
Birmingham, United Kingdom

Dennis Faix
Department of Deployment Health Research
Naval Health Research Center
San Diego, California

Juliana Perazzo Ferreira
Informatics Center
Centro de Informática da Universidade Federal
de Pernambuco
Recife, Brazil

Julie Fischer
Milken Institute School of Public Health
George Washington University
Washington, DC

Soma Ghoshal
Department of International Health
Johns Hopkins University
Baltimore, Maryland

Erin N. Hahn
Johns Hopkins University
Applied Physics Laboratory
Laurel, Maryland

Ricardo Hora
Biomedical Informatics Department
United States Naval Medical Research Unit No. 6
Callao, Peru

Damian Hoy
Secretariat of the Pacific Community
Noumea, New Caledonia

Rebecca Katz
Milken Institute School of Public Health
George Washington University
Washington, DC

Sarah Kornblet
Milken Institute School of Public Health
George Washington University
Washington, DC

Alain B. Labrique
Department of International Health
Bloomberg School of Public Health
and
Global mHealth Initiative
Johns Hopkins University
Baltimore, Maryland

Onicio B. Leal-Neto
Aggeu Magalhães Research Center
Oswaldo Cruz Foundation
Recife, Brazil

Sheri H. Lewis
Johns Hopkins University
Applied Physics Laboratory
Laurel, Maryland

Brian McCloskey
Global Health
Public Health England
London, United Kingdom

Sasha McGee
District of Columbia Department of Health
Washington, DC

Alize Mercier
Secretariat of the Pacific Community
Noumea, New Caledonia

Carmen C. Mundaca-Shah
Board on Global Health
Institute of Medicine
National Academies of Sciences, Engineering,
and Medicine
Washington, DC

David Muscatello
School of Public Health and Community
Medicine
University of New South Wales
Sydney, New South Wales, Australia

Shraddha Patel
Johns Hopkins University
Applied Physics Laboratory
Laurel, Maryland

Julie A. Pavlin
Infectious Disease Clinical Research Program
Henry M. Jackson Foundation for the
Advancement of Military Medicine, Inc.
Uniformed Services University of the Health
Sciences
Bethesda, Maryland

Christopher L. Perdue
Division of International Health Security
Department of Health and Human Services
Office of Policy and Planning
Washington, DC

Al Romanosky
Office of Preparedness and Response
Maryland Department of Health and Mental
Hygiene
Baltimore, Maryland

Salanieta Saketa
Secretariat of the Pacific Community
Noumea, New Caledonia

Anikah H. Salim
Office of Preparedness and Response
Maryland Department of Health and Mental
Hygiene
Baltimore, Maryland

Karen Saylors
Metabiota, Inc.
San Francisco, California

Gillian Smith
Real-time Syndromic Surveillance Team
Public Health England
Birmingham, United Kingdom

Erin M. Sorrell
Milken Institute School of Public Health
George Washington University
Washington, DC

Claire Standley
Milken Institute School of Public Health
George Washington University
Washington, DC

Dan Todkill
Field Epidemiology Training Programme
and
Field Epidemiology Service
Public Health England
Birmingham, United Kingdom

Lavanya Vasudevan
Center for Health Policy and Inequalities
Research
Duke University
Durham, North Carolina

John Mark Velasco
Department of Virology
United States Medical Component
Armed Forces Research Institute of
Medical Sciences
Bangkok, Thailand

Delphis Vera
Biomedical Informatics Department
United States Naval Medical Research Unit No. 6
Callao, Peru

Richard Wojcik
Johns Hopkins University Applied Physics
Laboratory
Laurel, Maryland

Paul White
Public Health Division
Secretariat of the Pacific Community
Noumea, New Caledonia

PART 1

Disease surveillance concepts

Introduction to electronic disease surveillance

DAVID L. BLAZES AND SHERI H. LEWIS

INTRODUCTION

Disease surveillance has been conducted informally since the dawn of civilization as a means of protecting oneself and ones in-group from infections and other illnesses, mainly through avoidance of high prevalence areas or practices. As human societies became more complex, so did methods for disease surveillance. Increasing interactions between societies, and the resultant interdependence on trade for survival and growth, led to a greater need for more detailed information concerning the spread of disease by people, animals, and trading goods such as food. Unfortunately, medical knowledge of how to treat or prevent illnesses has frequently lagged behind the simple recognition of conditions that are threatening to our health. But it has become conventional wisdom that, in order to fully control a particular disease, an accurate understanding of the epidemiology is required. In today's globalized and fully interconnected world, the potential speed of disease transmission is remarkably fast and often shorter than the incubation period of many infectious diseases. In order to keep pace, rapid disease surveillance methods are required, and simple collection and reporting via traditional paper methods that worked well for many years is no longer considered adequate in an increasingly connected world. Electronic disease surveillance offers numerous benefits to include more rapid transmission of information, more accurate representation of the data, and a greater ability to aggregate individual data streams to provide a more comprehensive understanding of a disease through a big data approach.

MODERN HISTORICAL PERSPECTIVE

Disease surveillance was defined by Langmuir in 1963 as "the continued watchfulness over the distribution and trends of incidence through the systematic collection, consolidation and evaluation of morbidity and mortality reports and other relevant data," with the "…regular dissemination of the basic data and interpretations to all who have contributed and to all others who need to know" (Langmuir 1963). Thacker expanded and refined this definition in 1988 when he wrote, "Public health surveillance is the ongoing systematic collection, analysis and interpretation of outcome-specific data for use in the planning, implementation, and evaluation of public health practice" (Thacker and Berkelman 1988). This linking of public health surveillance with the evaluation of public health practice emphasizes its primary purpose—to direct the expenditure of limited public health resources in a manner that yields the greatest return on investment (Thacker 1994).

Public health surveillance involves clearly defining events of public health interest, counting those events, and then analyzing those events with respect to *person*, *place*, and *time*. For example, the U.S. Centers for Disease Control and Prevention's (CDC) case definition for an influenza-like illness (ILI) is "Fever (temperature of 100°F [37.8°C] or greater) and a cough and/or sore throat without a known cause other than influenza" (U.S. Centers for Disease Control and Prevention 2014). Patients meeting the case definition of ILI are counted by sex and age category (*person*), characterized by site (*place*), and date of onset (*time*). This conceptually simple process not only characterizes the level, distribution, and spread of ILI in the community but also suggests useful information such as determinants of disease transmission, possible mitigation strategies, and future prevention strategies. Public health surveillance may be performed on all patients, the so-called universal surveillance, or may be performed at designated sites felt to be representative of the population as a whole, the so-called sentinel surveillance. Surveillance may also be described as active, when public health officials contact health-care providers, or passive, when public health officials rely on reports from health-care providers. A wide variety of data sources are used in public health surveillance, including vital statistics, health reports, hospital records, laboratory reports, outpatient visits, registries, and health surveys.

Disease surveillance is commonly recognized for its ability to detect disease outbreaks. Simply put, unless the baseline level of disease is well understood, it is difficult to identify disease levels significantly in excess of what is normal (Thacker and Berkelman 1988). This is an important function, and the early detection of anomalous disease events, particularly the intentional release of pathogens, has received much attention in recent years. Critics point out that disease surveillance, particularly syndromic surveillance, may not catch small outbreaks of disease that remain hidden in the background noise, and also note that diseases with shocking presentations, such as hemorrhagic fevers, are generally identified by astute health-care providers or laboratory technicians (Reingold 2003). Nevertheless, disease surveillance plays a

critical role in the detection and ongoing monitoring of disease outbreaks (Langmuir 1963; Thacker and Berkelman 1988; Thacker 1994; Lombardo and Ross 2007; CIFOR 2009). Importantly, in the case of small- to medium-size outbreaks distributed over a wide geographic area—now common in the case of gastrointestinal outbreaks due to large, centralized food processing plants—coordinated disease surveillance identifies problems that might otherwise go unnoticed in each local jurisdiction (CIFOR 2009). Disease surveillance accomplishes several additional important functions to direct the practice of public health (Thacker and Berkelman 1988). It identifies and quantifies the diseases most burdensome to a given population, allowing for allocation of sometimes scarce resources. Disease surveillance can carefully document how a disease spreads through the population of interest and how it affects individuals over time, and, as a result, can lead to real-time interventions. Importantly, disease surveillance can be used to evaluate public health interventions and identify effective and ineffective public health practices. Finally, disease surveillance can suggest hypotheses, direct research, and detect changes in the practice of clinical (or veterinary) medicine over time. Effective disease surveillance, though not always exciting, is the foundation of successful public health practice.

For centuries, disease surveillance was a paper-based process. In the 1990s, with the emergence of inexpensive, powerful information technology (IT) tools, disease surveillance became an electronic process in wealthy countries (Lombardo and Ross 2007). The incorporation of IT advances led to startling improvements in the timeliness of public health reporting and sophistication of data analysis. These systems initially were stood up to detect a possible intentional biological attack, and as such, their use and acceptance increased exponentially after the events of September 11, 2001 and the anthrax attacks of October 2001. While initially hesitant to adopt these types of systems, public health officials quickly realized their benefit in monitoring the community for the more common conditions such as influenza-like illness, gastrointestinal disease, etc. When systems are used on a daily basis by epidemiologists to monitor their community, they are much more likely to be able to successfully use the system to detect any type of intentional agent release. Such systems have become versatile, commonplace tools in many health departments in the United States, and these electronic disease surveillance tools hold promise to improve health security in resource-limited environments that may benefit from the lessons learned by others to date (Lombardo et al. 2003; Jajosky and Groseclose 2004; The Centers for Disease Control and Prevention 2007; Chretien et al. 2008; Soto et al. 2008). Epidemiologists using electronic disease surveillance not only have the potential to detect anomalous disease activity earlier than traditional laboratory-based surveillance, but they also have the ability to monitor the longitudinal health of their community in the face of a known threat (Lombardo et al. 2003; Jajosky and Groseclose 2004; The Centers for Disease Control and Prevention 2007). Additionally, many electronic disease surveillance systems are able to automatically ingest large amounts of pre-existing electronic data streams for analysis. These data sources, such as insurance claims, prescription data, school absentee data, and commercial sales of over-the-counter medicines, are not traditional health data from medical treatment facilities, yet they often have high public health informational content (Lombardo et al. 2003).

Emerging and re-emerging infectious diseases are among the most serious threats to global public health (Binder et al. 1999; Morens et al. 2004). The World Health Organization (WHO) has identified more than 1100 epidemic events worldwide in the last 10 years alone (The World Health Organization 2007). The emergence of the novel 2009 influenza A (H1N1) virus and the SARS coronavirus in 2002–2003 have demonstrated how rapidly pathogens can spread worldwide (Binder et al. 1999; Morens et al. 2004; Hollingsworth et al. 2007; The World Health Organization 2007). This infectious disease threat, combined with a concern over man-made biological or chemical events, spurred WHO to update their regulations concerning health and the spread of diseases in 2005 (The World Health Organization 2005). These modified International Health Regulations (IHR), a legally binding instrument for all 194 WHO member signatory countries, significantly expanded the scope of reportable conditions and are intended to help prevent and respond to global public health threats. Specifically, the IHR require strengthening of disease detection and response capacities in order to report, within 24 hours of assessment, any public health event of international concern. A clear way forward to satisfy both the letter and spirit of these IHR is to facilitate reporting of events, a well defined benefit of electronic disease surveillance platforms.

In addition to the updated IHRs, there has been growing political interest in the concept of global health security. The WHO and many countries have overtly addressed these "global commons" threats through initiatives such as the Global Health Security Agenda (GHSA) of the United States, whose goal is to accelerate progress in the prevention of, detection of, and response to infectious disease threats over a 5-year period. A key component of the GHSA is public health surveillance. The GHSA specifically targets infectious diseases and includes the topics of novel disease propagation and globalization of trade and travel, in addition to highlighting concerns about increasing antimicrobial drug resistance as well as the threat of disease from the accidental release, theft, or illicit use of a dangerous disease agent. This latter point—accidental release, theft, or illicit use of a disease agent—also draws attention to the growing field of "do-it-yourself (DIY) biology" as well as to research ethics. DIY biology, while often well intentioned and practiced as an after-hours hobby by many trained researchers in academia and corporations, is an unregulated or self-regulated activity. Some in the scientific community fear this DIY work could result in inadvertent or malicious development and release of a biological weapon, heightening the need for increased surveillance capacity.

Also of concern is the ability of scientists to replicate diseases in such a way that modifies their lethality. Although it is truly awe inspiring that science has come so far, charged discussions result when researchers want to share their findings worldwide through publication in peer-reviewed scientific journals, which is the norm for those working in the field. In recent years, there has been debate over the ethics of publishing research that exposes the "recipes" for replicating viruses and changing the virulence of viruses such as avian influenza (H5N1). Many fear that such publications could provide those with nefarious intent with the information needed to develop a "superbug." As scientists continue to make advances in the rapid identification and experimentation of novel pathogens, this debate will likely continue for years at the highest levels of government and academia. In the end, it has proven very difficult to control or contain the spread of such technology, so many public health officials have instead decided to focus on the early detection of a release of such an agent, mainly through enhanced disease surveillance around the globe.

In answer to these challenges, numerous teams of software engineers, analysts, and epidemiologists have been working for more than 15 years to develop advanced electronic disease surveillance technologies, in both the developed setting such as the United States and increasingly in developing settings as well (Dean et al. 1994; Loschen et al. 2007; Burkom et al. 2008; Ashar et al. 2010). Today in the United States, public health professionals in most states have the capability to collect, analyze, and visualize data to assess the health of their communities. Additionally, there are public health "superusers" who are taking electronic disease surveillance to the next level and using the data to investigate many types of public health issues such as chronic disease, injury, and mental health. However, in many places around the world, and particularly in resource-limited environments, public health officials are on the front line of defense against the next epidemic—without the benefit of state-of-the-art electronic disease surveillance capabilities. This book describes the state of the art in technological solutions to disease surveillance.

ORGANIZATION OF THE TEXT

This book will divide the disease surveillance paradigm into two sections, Disease Surveillance Concepts and Disease Surveillance Applications, to aid the reader in their understanding of not only the considerations that must be made when developing and deploying a successful electronic disease surveillance system but also to learn through the provided case studies, what has worked and not worked for various systems in use today. In addition to the continuing maturity of IT tools and the legislation requiring the collection, monitoring, and sharing of these data, there is much work being done in other related domains that warrant discussion. For example, the most valuable systems are far more than just a visualization tool. To provide the most value to public health professionals, advanced analytics must be in place to help public health officials understand nuances of the data. These statistics can vary

from standard epidemiological analyses to complex prediction and early event detection capabilities (Klaucke et al. 1988; Sosin 2003; Buehler et al. 2004).

This book will also provide very useful information in the understanding how to set up and maintain a successful disease surveillance capability for years to come. This is increasingly important in a highly globalized world. People are particularly fearful of a pandemic caused by the global spread of a novel naturally occurring disease such as Middle East respiratory syndrome coronavirus or a pandemic influenza A strain. This fear is understandable given that novel diseases represent the unknown: How quickly and easily does the disease spread from person to person? Who is most susceptible to the disease? What is the likelihood that I or my family will die from the disease if we contract it? These fears are not unfounded, as infectious diseases know no geographic boundaries, and globalization has connected people and parts of the world today more than in any other time in our history. Social and mainstream media can amplify these fears. Many of us have the ability to search the Internet to find more information on a new disease than we can possibly comprehend and to see the ample chatter on social media sites.

In the Concepts section, the authors will discuss the many regulatory, technological, political, and cultural considerations that are involved when establishing a disease surveillance system, as well as the practical considerations of analytics for surveillance and early event detection and effective visualization techniques. In Chapter 2, Katz et al., describe the aforementioned IHR and GHSA and how they have changed the requirements on collection and reporting of public health data. While the WHO is not very detailed in their recommendations and much is left to interpretation at the country level, a core set of capacities has been set forth for countries. This chapter will discuss these core capacities and the timeline countries have in order to implement the core tenets of the IHR.

In Chapter 3, Pavlin et al. discuss the considerations that countries must make when trying to implement an electronic disease surveillance capability. These considerations include the political structure of the public health system in a given country, the information technology and public health capacity of the resident work forces, and the cultural considerations or sensitivities of the population. It is often said that technology is the easiest hurdle to overcome when considering these other very important aspects.

In Chapter 4, Saylors furthers the line of thinking started in Chapter 3 by discussing the lack of standards in clinical case definitions, challenges with respect to long-term system sustainability, and examples of how social and cultural sensitivities can result in further spread of disease, as was the case with Ebola in West Africa in 2014–2015.

Once the reader has a good understanding of the vast challenges that must be overcome in order to implement a successful system, Chapters 5 and 6, by Burkom and Abernethy, respectively, discuss the most effective ways to analyze and visualize the data once the systems are up and running. While sometimes analytic methods and visualization techniques are very person-specific, having the general understanding of how to ensure effectiveness of the selected methods is discussed in these chapters.

Chapters 7 through 11 delve into the application side of disease surveillance in order to give the readers a broad sampling of systems and experiences that have been tried over the years and explain what worked well and what needed further refinement. As public health professionals, we firmly believe that successes, as well as failures, are both worthy of sharing so as to inform others as they approach this space either for the first time or if they are reassessing their current surveillance practices.

In Chapter 7, Brett-Major et al. discuss the reality of the IHR in practice, which complements Chapter 2 that strictly focuses on the policy underlying the IHR. They discuss what is currently in place from the WHO and country perspectives, along with identifying gaps or areas for further improvement.

While disease surveillance is arguably in its infancy when compared with other fields of study within epidemiology and public health, there have been many successes in electronic disease surveillance. In Chapter 8, Perdue et al. discuss possible solutions that have shown promise when considering the sustainability of systems and provide case studies of successful systems in use today in various parts of the world.

Building upon the ideas laid out in the previous chapter, Chapter 9 will discuss the concept of mobile health, or mHealth, and how mobile technologies are expanding the reach of surveillance, particularly in resource limited settings or areas with limited Internet access.

Aside from the technology and the desire for public health professionals to improve surveillance capabilities in their specific work setting, there are legal considerations that must be understood when employing technology solutions and implementing global health policy. In Chapter 10, Hahn discusses some of the legal terminology that is pertinent in the public health and disease surveillance, particularly when introducing technology in a space that utilizes person-based data.

In Chapter 11, case studies are used to describe a variety of systems used for monitoring health during mass gatherings. The contributors to these vignettes have years of experience in developing and conducting electronic disease surveillance in many challenging settings—to include politically, geographically, or financially precarious situations.

Finally, Chapter 12 discusses where the field of electronic disease surveillance can potentially go in the future. For example, cloud computing is frequently discussed as the panacea for health authorities that lack the ability to maintain their own computer equipment, but there are many considerations that must be addressed with respect to data security and privacy before this is readily accepted in a field that utilizes personal health information. Another future area that many people discuss in a variety of domains is predictive analytics. In the field of disease surveillance, this refers to the ability of public health practitioners or scientists to "predict" that an endemic disease will appear in a given geographic location at a particular time thereby allowing health authorities to hone their surveillance accordingly (Buczak et al. 2012). Obviously, having this ability to predict an outbreak allows for the potential to control or mitigate the spread of disease, or ultimately to even prevent the outbreak from starting (Feighner et al. 2009). There are encouraging efforts in this area, but one can imagine that predicting events that are inherently associated with biological systems is much more complex than predicting weather events for instance, which simply rely on physical properties.

CONTROVERSIAL POINTS

As previously mentioned, it is worth noting that electronic disease surveillance, or "syndromic surveillance," while largely accepted by today's public health professionals, represented a cultural shift for many in the workforce for a variety of reasons (Lombardo et al. 2004). For many years, public health performed surveillance activities with pen and paper, and they frequently did not have access to timely data. Any data analysis or research that was conducted retrospectively long after a disease outbreak was well established or known in a given population. The utilization of electronic data, automated data feeds, and automated data processing meant that epidemiologists were no longer waiting to learn about outbreaks, but they were now proactively able to look for possible increases in disease within a given population.

This new capability raised a variety of questions with which epidemiologists struggled. For example, what is the public health authority's obligation to act on an alert picked up by the system? At what frequency should data be reviewed in order to determine if there is an outbreak? What happens once an alert is made? Who gets notified? All of these questions were a natural reaction to a field and workforce undergoing major cultural shifts. For years, health authorities believed that if a detection was made, they were required to follow up on it. It took a number of years for public health officials to become comfortable with the fact that just because a statistical anomaly is detected does not necessarily mean it is epidemiologically significant. As one may imagine, certain times of the year naturally increase the baseline of disease in a community. For example, many parts of the world experience increases in influenza-like illness in the late fall/early winter. When the case counts in the community start increasing, it may indicate there is a rise in disease burden in a given area, but it does not necessarily mean that influenza is running rampant in the community (Henning 2004).

Similarly, once health officials had free access to all these data, the question of how frequently monitoring should occur was among the next questions. Access to "real time" data meant that continuous monitoring for outbreaks was technically feasible, but there were clearly not enough epidemiologists to curate such a system or respond to potential alerts. Over the years and as people gained familiarity with their systems, the general consensus was that receiving data once or twice a day was more realistic in a workforce that was already struggling with personnel reductions. Today, many systems receive data once a day with the ability to increase that data frequency in the event of heightened surveillance needs, such as a mass gathering or some type of emergency situation. Once an alert is made,

the goal is for the system to automatically provide enough information to allow the epidemiologist to quickly make an initial assessment as to whether a potential event is occurring. Information that may help make this determination would be both the level (granularity) of the data as well as the data variables. For example, if the epidemiologist has patient level data, they are able to see line listings of data to determine if there are any common factors among patients within an alert by reviewing the symptoms across the affected population. Similarly, if variables such as time are provided, an initial determination can be made as to whether patients may be connected in any way. Epidemiologists will often not need to take further action after this initial assessment, but the hope is that surveillance systems provide enough specific information to allow a comprehensive outbreak investigation if required.

Surveillance fatigue, or "the boy who cried wolf" syndrome, is something with which every surveillance system must contend. More timely surveillance presents the epidemiologist with the new challenge of understanding the normal fluctuations within their community and balancing this against a statistical alert indicating a potential outbreak of disease. For epidemiologists, this is a balance between understanding this baseline of disease and how it changes over time and when there is need respond to an alert—essentially balancing sensitivity with specificity for outbreak detection. There is limited tolerance, in terms of time, money, and personnel, to investigate alerts that are not "real" events. That said, all alerts represent some type of statistical significance in the change of the baseline health of the community, but the epidemiologist must determine whether the alert is epidemiologically significant.

Overall, the advent of electronic disease surveillance has improved the situational awareness of public health authorities—something they were not accustomed to having given their long reliance on manual data collection and limited routine reporting from the field. Today, while public health professionals will often agree the technologies described herein have had a positive effect on the field of public health as a whole, they also recognize that similar shifts in surveillance practice will continue to occur as data availability and volume increase and analysis and visualization capabilities improve. This will almost certainly require continuous workforce education and refinement of processes within all levels of disease surveillance.

The systematic collection of health information across populations has become easy to accomplish in theory, but the ethics of this process has possibly not kept pace. Questions such as how much data are appropriate to collect, the granularity of the data, how easy is it to associate with individuals, and the accessibility of the data into the future are important to address when establishing a surveillance system. Additionally, there are a variety of cultural and generational norms with respect to the acceptability of surveillance in general that must be considered in each setting.

THE FUTURE

One of the principal responsibilities of a government is to safeguard the health of its population. There are many components of population health, to include vaccination programs, preventive medicine, appropriate access to health care and medicines, and epidemic control. Improving the overall health of a given population has far-reaching effects on the economy and stability of a population, whether it is as small as a village or as large as an entire country. Indeed, improving the health of one population has potential effects on populations worldwide. Even before the GHSA, numerous countries have worked closely with international organizations and across multiple sectors within government to improve global health; but this is certainly a slow and challenging process. Governments around the world, now more than ever, are strongly committed to global health as a means to improve not only health but also global economic and political stability. Members of the public health community worldwide believe that a "public health emergency anywhere is a public health emergency everywhere." Mastering the concepts and practice of disease surveillance with today's technology is required to contribute to this important global effort.

REFERENCES

Ashar, R., S.L. Lewis, D.L. Blazes, and J.P. Chretien. 2010. Applying information and communications technologies to collect health data from remote settings: A systematic assessment of current technologies. *J. Biomed. Inform.* 43: 332–341.

Binder, S., A.M. Levitt, J.J. Sacks, and J.M. Hughes. 1999. Emerging infectious diseases: Public health issues for the 21st century. *Science* 284: 1311–1313.

Buczak, A.L., P.T. Koshute, S.M. Babin, B.H. Feighner, and S.H. Lewis. 2012. A data-driven epidemiological prediction method for dengue outbreaks using local and remote sensing data. *BMC Med. Inform. Decis. Mak.* 12: 124.

Buehler, J.W., R.S. Hopkins, J.M. Overhage, D.M. Sosin, and V. Tong. 2004. Framework for evaluating public health surveillance systems for early detection of outbreaks. *Morb. Mortal. Wkly. Rep.* RR-05: 1–11.

Burkom, H.S., W.A. Loschen, Z.R. Mnatsakanyan, and J.S. Lombardo. 2008. Tradeoffs driving policy and research decisions in biosurveillance. *JHU Appl. Phys. Lab. Tech. Dig.* 27: 299–312.

Chretien, J.P., H.S. Burkom, E.R. Sedyaningsih et al. 2008. Syndromic surveillance: Adapting innovations to developing settings. *PLoS Med.* 5(3): e72. pmed.0050072.

Council to Improve Foodborne Outbreak Response (CIFOR). 2009. Guidelines for foodborne disease outbreak response. Atlanta, GA: Council of State and Territorial Epidemiologists.

Dean, A.G., R.F. Fagan, and B.J. Panter-Connah. 1994. Computerizing public health surveillance systems, Chapter 11. In S.M. Teutsch and R.E. Churchill (eds.), *Principles and Practice of Public Health Surveillance*. New York: Oxford University Press, pp. 200–217.

Feighner, B.H., J.P. Chretien, S.P. Murphy et al. 2009. The pandemic influenza policy model: A planning tool for military public health officials. *Milit. Med.* 174: 557–565.

Henning, K. 2004. Overview of syndromic surveillance: What is syndromic surveillance? *Morb. Mortal. Wkly. Rep.* 53(Suppl.): 5–11.

Hollingsworth, T.D., N.M. Ferguson, and R.M. Anderson. 2007. Frequent travelers and rate of spread of epidemics. *Emerg. Infect. Dis.* 13: 1288–1294.

Jajosky, R.A. and S.L. Groseclose. 2004. Evaluation of reporting timeliness of public health surveillance systems for infectious diseases. *BMC Public Health* 4: 29.

Klaucke, D.N., J.W. Buehler, S.B. Thacker, R.G. Parrish, F.L. Trowbridge, R.L. Berkelman, and the Surveillance Coordination Group. 1988. Guidelines for evaluating surveillance systems. *Morb. Mortal. Wkly. Rep.* 37: 1–18.

Langmuir, A.D. 1963. The surveillance of communicable diseases of national importance, *N. Engl. J. Med.* 268: 182–192.

Lombardo, J., H. Burkom, E. Elbert, S. Magruder, S. Happel-Lewis, W. Loschen, J. Sari, C. Sniegoski, R. Wojcik, and J. Pavlin. 2003. A system overview of the electronic surveillance system for the early notification of community-based epidemics (ESSENCE II). *J. Urban Health: Bull. N. Y. Acad. Med.* 80: i32–i42.

Lombardo, J.S., H. Burkom, and J. Pavlin. 2004. ESSENCE II and the framework for evaluating syndromic surveillance systems. *Morb. Mortal. Wkly. Rep.* 53: 159–165.

Lombardo, J.S. and D. Ross. 2007. Disease surveillance: A public health priority, Chapter 1. In J.S. Lombardo and D.L. Buckeridge (eds.), *Disease Surveillance: A Public Health Informatics Approach.* Hoboken, NJ: John Wiley & Sons, Inc., pp. 1–39.

Loschen, W., J.S. Coberly, C. Sniegoski, R. Holtry, M.L. Sikes, and S. Happel-Lewis 2007. Event communication in a regional disease surveillance system. In *Annual Proceedings of the American Medical Informatics Association 2007*, pp. 483–487. http://www.ncbi.nlm.nih.gov/pmc/articles/PMC2655862/pdf/amia-0483-s2007.pdf.

Morens, D.M., G.K. Folkers, and A.S. Fauci. 2004. The challenge of emerging and re-emerging infectious diseases. *Nature* 430: 242–2492.

Reingold, A. 2003. If syndromic surveillance is the answer, what is the question? *Biosecur. Bioterror.* 81: 177–181.

Sosin, D.M. 2003. Draft framework for evaluating syndromic surveillance systems. *J. Urban Health: Bull. N. Y. Acad. Med.* 80: i8–i13.

Soto, G., R.V. Araujo-Castillo, J. Neyra, M. Fernandez, C. Leturia, C.C. Mundaca, and D.L. Blazes. 2008. Challenges in the implementation of an electronic surveillance system in a resource-limited setting: Alerta, in Peru. *BMC Proc.* 14(2 Suppl. 3): S4.

Thacker, S.B. 1994. Historical development, Chapter 1. In S.M. Teutsch and R.E. Churchill (eds.), *Principles of Public Health Surveillance.* New York: Oxford University Press, pp. 3–17.

Thacker, S.B. and R.L. Berkelman. 1988. Public health surveillance in the United States. *Epidemiol. Rev.* 10: 164–190.

The Centers for Disease Control and Prevention. 2007. Status of state electronic disease surveillance systems—United States, 2007. *Morb. Mortal. Wkly. Rep.* 58: 804–807.

The World Health Organization. 2005. International health regulations. Geneva, Switzerland: WHO.

The World Health Organization. 2007. The World Health Report 2007—A SAFER future: Global public health security in the 21st century. Geneva, Switzerland: WHO.

U.S. Centers for Disease Control and Prevention. 2014. Overview of influenza surveillance in the United States. Accessed February 28, 2014. http://www.cdc.gov/flu/weekly/overview.htm.

2

International health regulations: Policy

REBECCA KATZ, SARAH KORNBLET, ERIN M. SORRELL, CLAIRE STANDLEY, AND JULIE FISCHER

BACKGROUND

Advances in transportation and communications technologies have steadily reduced the time and costs of moving travelers, goods, and information across once-daunting distances. Starting in the nineteenth century, the falling costs of international travel and trade allowed the practical integration of markets across Europe, Asia, and the Americas. Goods and labor began to flow freely between regions, transforming economies worldwide (O'Rourke and Williamson 2000). The factors that lowered barriers to trade also eroded natural barriers to the spread of communicable diseases, contaminants, and other hazards among vulnerable populations. Starting in the early 1800s, successive waves of cholera spread from South Asia along water and railway routes, causing devastating outbreaks in the crowded cities of Europe and the Americas. Each pandemic prompted governments to take steps of varying effectiveness to detect and halt the spread of disease (Evans 1988).

Concerns about the impact of these measures on the movement of travelers and trade goods, coupled with the need to prevent the cross-border spread of infectious disease, catalyzed a series of diplomatic conferences among maritime powers starting in 1851. In 1892, delegates to the seventh of these International Sanitary Conferences agreed to the first International Sanitary Convention, a narrowly focused agreement that addressed quarantine regulations related to cholera along specific westbound maritime routes. By 1938, delegates from an increasing number of participating states, armed with growing awareness of the principles of disease transmission, would negotiate a series of these conventions addressing a short list of priority diseases. Regional organizations in Europe and in the Americas developed to govern disease reporting and information sharing under such agreements, which focused on protecting trade and travel while relying primarily on state mechanisms to prevent the spread of disease at ports and borders (Howard-Jones 1975).

In the mid-twentieth century, the newly created World Health Organization (WHO) became the primary steward for such agreements, which were consolidated into the International Sanitary Regulations, later revised as the International Health Regulations of 1969 (IHR [1969]) (Pizzi 1958). By 1981, revisions had reduced the scope of reportable diseases under IHR (1969) to yellow fever, plague, and cholera—diseases of great historical importance but no longer major public health risks among high-income trading nations. At the same time, globalization and urbanization created risks for the spread of new diseases. Public health leaders worldwide began to report an increasing number of emerging and re-emerging diseases, marked by the transmission of zoonotic diseases along an increasingly complex animal–human interface, often in regions with weak capacities for disease surveillance and response (Jones et al. 2008).

In 1995, the World Health Assembly (WHA), the governing body of the WHO, agreed to revise the IHR with the goal of promoting early detection of and response to epidemics before they became international public health crises. This precipitated nearly a decade of debate on the best approach to an agreement that would allow nations and the global community to anticipate emerging threats, to ensure timely and transparent reporting, and to facilitate evidence-based decision making. The agreement also had to accommodate different national capacities, address concerns over the collection and dissemination of potentially sensitive information, and protect individuals and economies from unmerited actions. In 2003, the spread of severe acute respiratory syndrome (SARS) from China via air travel to more than two dozen countries inspired new action. In 2005, WHA agreed to revise the IHR to "prevent, protect against, control and provide a public health response to the international spread of disease in ways that are commensurate with and restricted to public health risks and which avoid unnecessary interference with international traffic and trade" (WHO 2005a).

IHR ARTICLE BY ARTICLE

The revised IHR include 66 articles and nine annexes, summarized in Figure 2.1. Many of these articles focus on process and form, as is typical of most international agreements. A significant number of articles relate to measures designed to prevent the spread of disease through the international movement of goods and international traffic, primarily the responsibilities of States Parties for infection control and sanitation in ships, aircraft, and ground conveyances and at points of entry (PoE). These measures trace their origins to the IHR (1969) and earlier agreements that sought to harmonize standards for disease control at ports and borders.

Other articles of the IHR (2005) directly address national capacities for disease detection and response. First, every State Party must designate a National IHR Focal Point (NFP) to be responsible for communications to and from the WHO, and dissemination of information on public health events to national stakeholders, on a 24-hour basis. Although a relatively simple measure, this article created a novel network for rapid information sharing on public health events within and across borders. The State Party must also establish a framework to ensure that the NFP has the authority and means to notify the WHO within 24 hours of determining that a domestic event might constitute a potential public health emergency of international concern (PHEIC). Most importantly, articles in the IHR (2005) call upon each State Party to develop the minimum public health capacities required to detect unusual diseases or deaths, assess the risks posed by an outbreak or other event, report pertinent public health information to the most appropriate levels of government and to the WHO when required, and initiate appropriate response measures to control and mitigate the consequences of the event.

In addition to the 66 articles in the IHR, there are nine annexes, each of which provides explicit guidance on how States Parties can achieve an IHR obligation. As with the articles themselves, several of these annexes focus on treatment of travelers and conveyances at designated points of entry (particularly the documenting of ship sanitation), while others clarify the processes by which States Parties implement the detection and reporting of, and response to, public health emergencies.

Articles 1–4: Definitions, purpose, and scope	
Article 1	*Definitions*: The first article focuses entirely on definitions.
Article 2	*Purpose and Scope of the Regulations*: To prevent, protect against, control and provide a public health response to the international spread of disease in ways that are commensurate with and restricted to public health risks, and which avoid unnecessary interference with international traffic and trade.
Article 3	*Principles*: This section sets forth three principles for implementation of the IHR, including that implementation be guided by the Charter of the United Nations and the WHO Constitution, with full respect for human rights and with the goal of protecting all people of the world from spread of disease. Additionally, States have the sovereign right to legislate and to implement policies consistent with the IHR.
Article 4	*Responsible Authorities*: Each State shall designate an NFP for communication to and from the WHO and dissemination of information within the country; in turn, the WHO will designate IHR Contact Points within WHO regional and headquarters organizations.
Articles 5–14: Information and public health response	
Article 5	*Surveillance*: Each State shall develop, strengthen, and maintain the capacity to detect, assess, notify, and report potential PHEICs. The initial capacity-building period is defined as 5 years, with an option for States to request up to two 2-year extensions. The WHO's roles are defined as providing capacity-building assistance to States on request, collecting information regarding public health events, and assessing the potential for diseases to spread internationally.
Article 6	*Notification*: Using the decision instrument in Annex 2, each State will assess public health events and notify the WHO through the NFP within 24 hours of determining that an event constitutes a potential PHEIC. Following initial notification, States shall continue to share pertinent information about the event with the WHO. This article also notes that the WHO will immediately notify the International Atomic Energy Agency (IAEA) if the event is relevant to that organization.
Article 7	*Information Sharing*: If there is evidence of a potential PHEIC within a State's territory, regardless of origin or source, the State shall provide all relevant information to the WHO.
Article 8	*Consultation*: States may ask the WHO for assistance in assessing epidemiologic evidence and consult with the WHO on appropriate health measures, even when the event does not constitute a potential PHEIC.
Article 9	*Other Reports*: The WHO can use reports other than official notifications or consultations to assess whether there is a potential PHEIC occurring. The WHO can use these unofficial reports to seek verification and to consult with States, which are obligated to report any evidence of a potential PHEIC detected outside of their territories to the WHO within 24 hours.
Article 10	*Verification*: The WHO shall inform a State (through the NFP) if a report is received about a potential PHEIC in that State's territories. The State Party must respond to the WHO's inquiry within 24 hours and provide the WHO with available public health information upon request. The WHO shall offer to collaborate with any State to assess potential PHEICs; if the State does not accept the offer of collaboration, the WHO can share information about the event with other States Parties if the Director-General (DG) determines that action is justified.
Article 11	*Provision of Information by the WHO*: The WHO will share relevant information with other International Organizations (IOs) and States Parties as needed to prevent or respond to public health risks but will not make the information generally available unless the event is declared a PHEIC or the WHO determines that the international spread of disease or contamination is either confirmed or inevitable, necessitating immediate action.
Article 12	*Determination of a PHEIC*: The WHO DG determines whether an event is a PHEIC, taking into account information provided by the affected State(s), the Annex 2 decision instrument, the advice of the Emergency Committee (subject-matter experts convened to evaluate potential PHEICs), scientific evidence and principles, and an assessment of the risks to human health, trade, and travel. After making a preliminary determination that a PHEIC is occurring, the DG consults with the affected State; if they do not reach consensus on the determination within 48 hours, the DG proceeds on the basis of advice from the Emergency Committee, as outlined in Article 49. The DG also determines when the PHEIC has ended.

Figure 2.1 IHR articles and annexes. *Note:* Articles and annexes that directly address disease surveillance, reporting, and response mechanisms are highlighted in light purple. Articles directly related to travelers, international traffic and trade, or points of entry are highlighted in dark purple.   *(Continued)*

Article 13	*Public Health Response*: States shall develop, strengthen, and maintain the capacity to respond to public health risks and PHEICs within 5 years (with the option to request up to two 2-year extensions). Should States request assistance in the response to public health risks or events, the WHO shall provide technical guidance and assistance, including the mobilization of international experts, and during a declared PHEIC, can provide further assistance to assess risk and the adequacy of control measures on-site. States Parties are called upon to support WHO-coordinated response activities on request.
Article 14	*Cooperation of the WHO with IOs and Other International Bodies*: The WHO will coordinate with other IOs or international bodies to implement the IHR, particularly when an event is primarily within the competence of other IOs.
Articles 15–18: Recommendations	
Article 15	*Temporary Recommendations*: Once an event has been determined a PHEIC, the DG shall issue temporary recommendations on measures that States Parties can take to reduce the international spread of disease and avoid unnecessary interference with travel and trade. These recommendations expire after 3 months, but they may be modified or extended for additional 3-month periods.
Article 16	*Standing Recommendations*: The WHO may make standing recommendations for appropriate health measures for specific public health risks to prevent or reduce the international spread of disease.
Article 17	*Criteria for Recommendations*: When issuing, modifying, or terminating temporary or standing recommendations, the DG shall consider advice of the Emergency Committee, views of States Parties, scientific principles and evidence, non-restrictive health measures, international standards, and activities taken by other relevant international bodies.
Article 18	*Recommendations with Respect to Persons, Baggage, Cargo, Containers, Conveyances, Goods, and Postal Parcels*: This article outlines the type of advice the WHO may recommend, including reviews of travel history, quarantine, isolation, refusing entry of persons or goods, and implementation of exit screening.
Articles 19–22: Points of entry (PoE)	
Article 19	*General Obligations*: States will develop capacities to detect, assess, report, and respond to potential PHEICs at designated PoE, identify competent authorities at each designated PoE, and provide information on specific public health risks at PoE to the WHO.
Article 20	*Airports and Ports*: States shall designate airports and ports that will be responsible for developing capacities per Annex 1 and list all ports authorized to offer Ship Sanitation Control Certificates. The WHO may arrange to certify that an airport or port has met these obligations, and the WHO will publish certification guidelines and lists of certified airports and ports.
Article 21	*Ground Crossings*: States may designate ground crossings as PoE, taking into account the public health risks and volume of international traffic.
Article 22	*Role of Competent Authorities*: The competent authority at each PoE shall monitor conveyances and property (such as baggage, cargo, containers, or goods) departing and arriving from affected areas; ensure that facilities used by travelers are sanitary; supervise deratting, disinfection, or decontamination of conveyances and property; advise conveyance operators of intent to apply control measures; supervise safe disposal of any contaminated substances from conveyances; monitor and control discharge by ships that might contaminate waterways; supervise services concerning travelers and property, including medical examinations and inspections; develop contingency plans for public health events; and communicate with the NFP.
Articles 23–34: Public health measures for movement of people and goods	
Article 23	*Health Measures on Arrival and Departure*: States may require information from travelers for public health purposes upon arrival or departure, including itinerary, contact information, and applicable health records, and may require a noninvasive medical examination (limited to the least intrusive exam required to meet the public health objectives). Medical exams, vaccinations, or other health measure require informed consent and must be done per international safety guidelines. Baggage and other goods may be inspected.

Figure 2.1 (*Continued*) IHR articles and annexes. *Note:* Articles and annexes that directly address disease surveillance, reporting, and response mechanisms are highlighted in light purple. Articles directly related to travelers, international traffic and trade, or points of entry are highlighted in dark purple. (*Continued*)

Article 24	*Conveyance Operators*: Conveyance operators must comply with WHO recommended health measures adopted by the State, inform travelers of these health measures, and keep conveyances free from infection or contamination.
Article 25	*Ships and Aircraft in Transit*: No health measures shall be applied to ships passing through a State Party's territories (including ships from unaffected areas that stop only to take on fuel and supplies, or any ship that does not stop at all) or to aircraft in transit at an airport, although the movement of passengers and materials may be restricted.
Article 26	*Civilian Lorries, Trains, and Coaches in Transit*: Unless authorized by international agreements, no health measures shall be applied to trucks, trains, or buses from unaffected areas that are only passing through a territory.
Article 27	*Affected Conveyances*: If evidence of a public health risk (such as clinical signs or symptoms or sources of infection or contamination) is found on board a conveyance, the competent authority may take appropriate control measures. If the competent authority is not able to carry out control measures, the authority can allow the affected conveyance to depart after notifying competent authorities at the next known PoE (and, for ships, documenting the required measures).
Article 28	*Ships and Aircrafts at PoE*: A ship or aircraft will not be prevented from calling on a point of entry for public health reasons, but in the case that a PoE is not equipped to carry out the IHR requirements, the ship or aircraft may be ordered to proceed at its own risk to the nearest suitable PoE. The movement of travelers and cargo from ships and aircraft (including taking on water, food, fuel, and supplies) should not be prevented for public health reasons, unless measures are needed to prevent the spread of disease or contamination first. Officers in command of ships or aircraft must notify port/airport authorities of any infections or other health risks as soon as possible before arrival. Suspect ships and aircrafts that land or berth elsewhere than their expected ports/airports shall inform the nearest competent authority without delay so that appropriate health measures may be applied. Any emergency measures taken by the officer in command of a ship or pilot to protect the health and safety of travelers shall be communicated to the competent authority.
Article 29	*Civilian Lorries, Trains, and Coaches at PoE*: The WHO shall develop guiding principles for the application of health measure to trucks, trains, and buses at PoE and ground crossings.
Article 30	*Travelers Under Public Health Observation*: A traveler placed under public health observation at arrival may continue on if the traveler does not pose an imminent public health risk.
Article 31	*Health Measures Relating to Entry of Travelers*: States Parties may subject travelers to medical examinations, vaccinations, or other prophylaxis to determine whether a public health risk exists as a condition for residence, or as a condition for entry. The traveler can refuse to consent but may be denied entry. If there is evidence of an imminent public health risk, the State Party may advise or compel the traveler to undergo a medical exam, vaccination, or measures such as quarantine, isolation, or observation (in accordance with national laws).
Article 32	*Treatment of Travelers*: Travelers shall be treated with respect for dignity, human rights, and freedoms, taking into account gender, sociocultural, ethnic, or religious concerns. Travelers who are quarantined, isolated, or subject to other public health measures must be provided with adequate food, water, accommodations, medical treatment, and means of communication.
Article 33	*Goods in Transit*: Goods, other than live animals, in transit shall not be subject to health measures or detained for public health purposes.
Article 34	*Container and Container Loading Areas*: States Parties shall ensure that container shippers use containers that are free from infection or contamination, that container loading areas are kept free from infection or contamination, and that competent authorities conduct inspections.
Articles 35–41: Health documents and charges for travelers	
Article 35	*General Rule*: No health documents (other than those provided under the IHR or WHO recommendations) shall be required in international traffic, except for travelers seeking temporary or permanent residence. Travelers may be required to complete contact forms or questionnaires for public health purposes.

Figure 2.1 (*Continued*) IHR articles and annexes. *Note:* Articles and annexes that directly address disease surveillance, reporting, and response mechanisms are highlighted in light purple. Articles directly related to travelers, international traffic and trade, or points of entry are highlighted in dark purple.   (*Continued*)

Article 36	*Certificates of Vaccination or Other Prophylaxis*: A traveler who has a certificate of vaccination or other prophylaxis shall not be denied entry as a consequence of the disease on the certificate.
Article 37	*Maritime Declaration of Health*: The master of a ship has to declare the health status of those on board before the vessel's arrival in port.
Article 38	*Health Part of the Aircraft General Declaration*: The pilot should supply any information on the health of those on board, when appropriate, to the competent authority.
Article 39	*Ship Sanitation Certificates*: Ship Sanitation Control Certificates, which note that a ship is free of contamination or infection, are valid for 6 months.
Article 40	*Charges for Health Measures Regarding Travelers*: With the exception of travelers seeking temporary or permanent residence, the State Party cannot charge travelers for measures to protect public health (rather than for the benefit of the traveler), including isolation and quarantine, vaccinations that are not a published requirement, or medical exam required for entry. If the State Party does level charges for health measures, they must be uniformly applied, must not exceed the costs of service, and must be published.
Article 41	*Charges for Baggage, Cargo, Containers, Conveyances, Goods, or Postal Parcels*: When there are charges for health measures, there can only be one tariff that does not exceed the costs of service and applies to all equally.
Articles 42–46: General provisions for health measures	
Article 42	*Implementation of Health Measures*: Health measures under the IHR should be implemented without delay, transparently, and nondiscriminatorily.
Article 43	*Additional Health Measures*: IHR does not prevent States from adopting health measures for specific public health risks or emergencies that achieve the same or greater health protection than WHO recommendations, in accordance with national and international laws. These measures shall not be more restrictive of international trade or more invasive/intrusive to persons than reasonably available alternatives, and should be based on scientific principles, evidence, or specific guidance from the WHO. If a State Party's actions interfere with international travel and trade, national authorities must notify the WHO of the measures and the rationale for implementing them within 48 hours. The WHO will share this information with other States Parties and may request that the State reconsider the action. This article also applies to mass gatherings.
Article 44	*Collaboration and Assistance*: States shall collaborate with each other and, to the extent possible, provide support for detection and response, technical assistance, financial assistance, and logistical support to help build and maintain core capacities. The WHO will collaborate upon request to evaluate and assess public health capacities, facilitate technical assistance, and mobilize financial resources. This assistance may be provided through multiple channels.
Article 45	*Treatment of Personal Data*: Health information collected or received by a State shall be kept confidential and processed per national laws. Personal information may be disclosed to assess and manage a public health risk, although it must be treated fairly and lawfully.
Article 46	*Transport and Handling of Biological Substances, Reagents, and Materials for Diagnostic Purposes*: States Parties shall facilitate the transport, processing, and disposal of biological substances, reagents, and other materials for diagnostic purposes, subject to national laws and international guidelines.
Articles 47–53: IHR roster of experts, emergency committee, and review committee	
Article 47	*IHR Roster of Experts Composition*: The DG shall establish a roster of experts in all fields relevant to the IHR. The DG shall also appoint one member at the request of each State Party and relevant IO.
Article 48	*Emergency Committee Terms of Reference and Composition*: The DG shall establish an Emergency Committee to provide views on whether an event constitutes a PHEIC, and, if so, to propose temporary recommendations. The DG selects experts for the Emergency Committee from the IHR Roster of Experts, including at least one expert nominated from the State experiencing the event, and from other WHO advisory panels.

Figure 2.1 (*Continued*) IHR articles and annexes. *Note:* Articles and annexes that directly address disease surveillance, reporting, and response mechanisms are highlighted in light purple. Articles directly related to travelers, international traffic and trade, or points of entry are highlighted in dark purple. (*Continued*)

Article 49	*Emergency Committee Procedure*: The DG convenes the Emergency Committee (including via teleconference, videoconference, or other electronic communication) to consider potential PHEICs and invites the State Party in whose territory the event originated to make presentations to the Committee. After each meeting, the Emergency Committee summarizes and forwards its findings and recommendations to the DG. Based on this advice, the DG makes the final determination on whether an event constitutes a PHEIC and communicates the temporary recommendations and the views of the Emergency Committee to the States Parties and subsequently to the public.
Article 50	*Review Committee Terms of Reference and Composition*: The Review Committee provides the DG with technical advice on the IHR themselves and on standing recommendations. Members are appointed from the IHR Expert Roster or other WHO technical advisory panels and shall be representative of gender, geography, development, and scientific opinions.
Article 51	*Review Committee Conduct of Business*: Decisions of the Review Committee shall be taken by majority.
Article 52	*Review Committee Reports*: For each session, the Review Committee shall draw up a report to submit to the DG. Dissenting professional reviews can be expressed.
Article 53	*Review Committee Procedures for Standing Recommendations*: Proposals for standing recommendations/modifications/termination may be submitted to the Review Committee through the DG. The DG can appoint technical experts to advise the committee.
Articles 54–66: Final provisions	
Article 54	*Reporting and Review*: States Parties and the DG shall report on implementation of IHR to the WHA, which will periodically review the functionality of the IHR. The WHO will periodically conduct studies to review the functionality of Annex 2.
Article 55	*Amendments*: Amendments to the IHR may be proposed by any State Party or the DG and submitted to the WHA for consideration.
Article 56	*Settlement of Disputes*: States Parties should first attempt to settle disputes regarding IHR application through negotiation. If that fails, the issues can be referred to the DG. States Parties may agree to accept the DG's arbitration as compulsory; alternatively, they may resort to dispute settlement mechanisms under other international agreements or organizations to which they may be parties. Disputes between the WHO and a State Party shall be submitted to the WHA.
Article 57	*Relationship with Other International Agreements*: IHR should be compatible with other international agreements, and IHR shall not affect the rights and obligations derived from other agreements. Nothing in the IHR shall prevent States Parties from concluding special treaties or arrangements to facilitate application of the IHR.
Article 58	*International Sanitary Agreements and Regulations*: IHR replaces the previous International Sanitary Agreements and Regulations. It does not replace the Pan American Sanitary Code, except for relevant IHR articles.
Article 59	*Entry into Force*: Period for Rejection or Reservations: The period for rejection of reservations shall be 18 months. The IHR enter into force 24 months after adoption, unless a State has rejected the IHR or an amendment, the State has made a reservation, or a State becomes party to the IHR after the date of notification.
Article 60	*New Member States of the WHO*: Any State that becomes a member of the WHO after 2005 has 12 months to communicate any reservations or rejections.
Article 61	*Rejection*: If a State notifies the DG of a rejection to the IHR or an amendment, the IHR will not enter into force for that State. In this case, the previous international health agreements (listed in Article 58) remain in force for that State.

Figure 2.1 (*Continued*) IHR articles and annexes. *Note:* Articles and annexes that directly address disease surveillance, reporting, and response mechanisms are highlighted in light purple. Articles directly related to travelers, international traffic and trade, or points of entry are highlighted in dark purple.   (*Continued*)

Article 62	*Reservations*: States Parties may notify the DG of reservations to the IHR, either before or after the regulations enter into force. The DG shall notify the other States Parties of the objections; if one-third of the other States Parties object to the reservation within 6 months, the DG shall notify the State to consider withdrawing the reservation. If one-third of States do not object, the reservation stands. If the State does not withdraw its reservation despite objections from one-third of States Parties, the DG can refer the matter to the Review Committee at the State's request. The DG submits the reservation and any views of the Review Committee to WHA, which determines whether the reservation will be accepted or not by majority vote.	
Article 63	*Withdrawal of Rejection and Reservation*: A rejection or a reservation may be withdrawn at any time through notification of the DG.	
Article 64	*States Not Members of the WHO*: A State that is a member of previous international sanitary regulations, but not a member of the WHO, may become a party to the IHR through notification to the DG.	
Article 65	*Notification by the DG*: The DG shall notify all States and other parties to any international sanitary regulation of the adoption of the IHR, as well as any amendments.	
Article 66	*Authentic Texts*: The IHR will be equally authentic in Arabic, Chinese, English, French, Russian, and Spanish.	
Annexes		
Annex 1	*Part A. Core Capacity Requirements for Surveillance and Response*: Part A of Annex 1 defines the minimum core capacities required of States Parties at the local/community level (to detect unusual disease or deaths, report essential information to the appropriate level, and implement preliminary control measures); the intermediate level (to support control measures, confirm and assess events, and report essential information to the national level); and the national level (to assess reports or urgent events within 48 hours, notify the WHO of potential PHEICs, determine control measures, provide technical and logistical support to local investigations, share information and coordinate actions across levels and sectors, and establish a national public health emergency response plan and multisectoral rapid response teams). Annex 1 calls on States to meet these requirements through existing structures and resources, developing plans of action to strengthen them as necessary after a 2-year assessment period.	*Part B. Core Capacity Requirements for Designated Airports and Ground Crossings*: Part B delineates the core capacities required at designated points of entry at all times (to provide appropriate medical services and transport for ill travelers, train personnel to inspect conveyances, and ensure the safety and sanitation of PoE facilities) and during events that might constitute a PHEIC (establish a public health emergency contingency plan, evaluate and care for affected travelers and animals, isolate or quarantine affected travelers as necessary, apply entry and exit controls to travelers, treat goods and conveyances as necessary to prevent or remove public health risks, and equip and train personnel for the safe transport of travelers who might carry infection or contamination).
Annex 2	*Decision Instrument for the Assessment and Notification of Events That May Constitute a PHEIC*: This instrument provides an algorithm for States to determine when an event constitutes a potential PHEIC that should be notified to the WHO.	
Annex 3	*Model Ship Sanitation Control Exemption Certificate/Ship Sanitation Control Certificate*: This Annex provides examples of certificates that States Parties can adapt and use to document ship inspections at designated PoE.	
Annex 4	*Technical Requirements Pertaining to Conveyances and Conveyance Operators*: This Annex provides detailed information about the role of conveyance operators and control measures to be applied to conveyances at designated PoE.	
Annex 5	*Specific Measures for Vector-Borne Diseases*: This Annex details how to treat conveyances and other measures to reduce the threat of vector-borne diseases at designated PoE.	

Figure 2.1 (*Continued*) IHR articles and annexes. *Note:* Articles and annexes that directly address disease surveillance, reporting, and response mechanisms are highlighted in light purple. Articles directly related to travelers, international traffic and trade, or points of entry are highlighted in dark purple. (*Continued*)

Annex 6	*Vaccination, Prophylaxis, and Related Certificates*: This annex specifies that only WHO-approved vaccines or prophylaxis should be administered under the IHR, and when they are given, travelers will be provided a certificate (a model of which is provided in the annex).
Annex 7	*Requirements Concerning Vaccination or Prophylaxis for Specific Diseases*: This annex provides the specific recommendations and requirements associated with vaccination and documentation of vaccination against yellow fever.
Annex 8	*Model of Maritime Declaration of Health*: This is an example of a form that can be adapted and used by States Parties for documentation by masters of ships for submission to competent authorities at designated PoE.
Annex 9	*Health Part of the Aircraft General Declaration*: This document is part of the Aircraft General Declaration promulgated by the International Civil Aviation Organization (ICAO) for use in declaring health conditions for persons on board a flight with illness other than airsickness or accidents.

Figure 2.1 (*Continued*) IHR articles and annexes. *Note:* Articles and annexes that directly address disease surveillance, reporting, and response mechanisms are highlighted in light purple. Articles directly related to travelers, international traffic and trade, or points of entry are highlighted in dark purple.

Annex 1: Part A. Core capacity requirements for surveillance and response

Annex 1 of the IHR provides the clearest guidance in the regulations for the infrastructure States must develop, strengthen, and maintain at all levels of government. Annex 1 calls on each State to conduct an assessment of existing national infrastructure and resources to meet minimum requirements for surveillance, reporting, notification, verification, response, and collaborating activities within 2 years of the treaty entering into force. Based on this initial assessment, States are to develop and implement plans of action to ensure that core capacities are developed and maintained.

Annex 1 calls for the development of different capacities at different levels of government. At the local level, States must be able to detect unexpected disease or deaths, report essential information to the appropriate level (intermediate or national) based on national systems, and implement initial control measures. At the intermediate level (e.g., a state, province, territory, county, or other identified administrative entity between the local and national level), the public health system must be able to confirm reports from the local level, support control measures, assess the urgency of events, and report relevant information up to the national level. Finally, at the national level, States must be able to assess reports from the local and intermediate levels within 48 hours, and when appropriate, notify the WHO through the NFP. The national level is also responsible for supporting the public health response on a 24-hour basis, through determination of control measures, laboratory analysis, logistical assistance, and epidemiologic support. The national level ensures communications among all appropriate government ministries and manages dissemination of relevant information from the national level and from the WHO to clinics, hospitals, points of entry, laboratories, and other pertinent entities. The national level must also develop and maintain a public health emergency response plan that includes the ability to deploy multidisciplinary rapid response teams within 48 hours of an event.

Annex 1: Part B. Core capacity requirements for designated airports, ports, and ground crossings

Part B of Annex 1 outlines the core capacities required at points of entry at all times. Points of entry shall provide access to medical services to ill travelers, provide equipment and personnel to transport ill travelers when necessary, have trained personnel available to inspect conveyances, and ensure a safe environment for travelers. States should also provide trained personnel to control vectors and reservoirs near points of entry. Points of entry shall also have an emergency response plan, with a coordinator and contact points. As part of a response, States shall have the capacity to care for ill travelers or animals, have arrangements in place for isolation and treatment at appropriate facilities, have private space for interviews with affected travelers, have quarantine capability away from the point of entry, and be able to disinsect, derat, disinfect, and decontaminate any goods. States must be able to apply entry or exit controls. The State is also responsible for applying entry and exit controls for travelers and being able to transport using the appropriate equipment and personnel any infected traveler.

Annex 2: Decision instrument for the assessment and notification of events that may constitute a PHEIC

Annex 2 of the IHR replaces what was once—in previous international sanitary agreements—a fixed list of notifiable diseases with a decision algorithm designed to anticipate emerging infections and other unusual or unexpected events. This algorithm has a list of four "always notifiable" diseases: smallpox, wild-type polio, new subtypes

of human influenza, and SARS. If a single case of any of these diseases is detected, the State must notify the WHO through the NFP. The algorithm also lists a series of diseases that can cause serious public health events; any case of these diseases necessitates that the State utilize this instrument to determine whether the event is a potential PHEIC. These diseases include cholera, pneumonic plague, yellow fever, viral hemorrhagic fevers, West Nile fever, or other diseases of national or regional concern, such as dengue or dengue hemorrhagic fever. For these diseases and for all other public health events, the State should assess whether the event is serious, whether it is unusual or unexpected, whether there is a significant risk of international spread, and whether there is a significant risk of international travel or trade restrictions. This assessment will lead to the determination of whether the NFP should notify the WHO under the IHR (Figure 2.2).

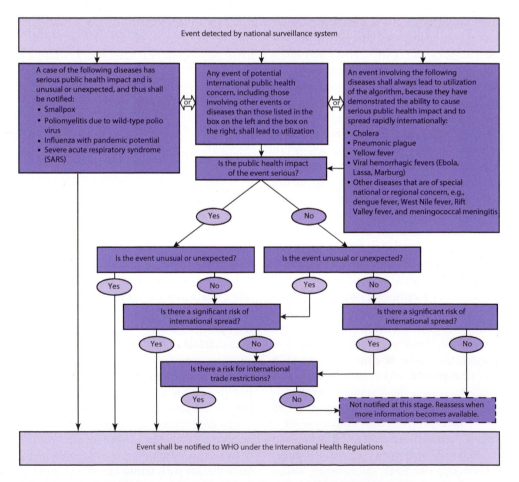

Figure 2.2 Annex 2 decision instrument for determination of a potential PHEIC.

Each State develops its own processes for making national assessments under Annex 2 and then reporting potential PHEICs to the WHO. In the United States, reports of unusual or unexpected events come from clinicians or laboratories to the local health departments. Local health departments then report the information to the state-level health department, which voluntarily sends information forward to the federal level. At the federal level, the public health event is assessed with the assistance of relevant agencies. Human health communicable disease events are assessed by the U.S. Centers for Disease Control and Prevention, whereas zoonotic disease events may be assessed by U.S. Department of Agriculture. Once an assessment is made at the relevant agency, the finding is sent to the U.S. Department of Health and Human Services Operations Center, which is the official NFP for the United States. The United States then makes several simultaneous notifications. The NFP notifies the relevant WHO authorities in the Pan American Health Organization (PAHO)—the WHO Regional Office for the Americas—and the WHO Regional Office for the Western Pacific (WPRO), since the United States spans both regional organizations (see Figure 2.5). The NFP simultaneously informs other federal agencies through their Emergency Operations Centers, the localities from which the event originates, and both Canada and Mexico through trilateral agreements. Once the report is received by the WHO regional offices, it is forwarded to WHO headquarters, which then makes an assessment. The reports to the WHO are done through an electronic notification system that only relevant authorities can access. As at the national level, the WHO will bring in the relevant expertise of other IOs when appropriate. The assessment is then forwarded to the DG, who will call together an Emergency Committee, which will make a recommendation back to the DG on whether the event constitutes a PHEIC and what travel and trade recommendations they advise. Once an event is declared a PHEIC, the WHO is then in charge of coordinating communication and governance of the event.

Other guidance

Since the IHR entered into force in 2007, the WHO has released an extensive collection of guidance documents, procedures, monitoring tools, and training materials to support States as they build, strengthen, and maintain capacity and work to implement the regulations. These guidance documents range from tutorials on how to use the Annex 2 decision instrument (WHO 2014d) to case definitions for the "always notifiables" (WHO 2014a). In response to requests for guidance on legal issues related to IHR implantation, the WHO created a *Toolkit for Implementation in National Legislation*. The document includes a section on general questions and answers, legislative references, and a tool on how to conduct internal assessments of laws and regulations (WHO 2009a). There is also a toolkit to assist countries in establishing the function of NFP (WHO 2009b).

The WHO has provided links to specific guidance related to building laboratory capacity (WHO 2014c) and extensive guidance related to points of entry. The guidance on points of entry includes handbooks for inspection of ships and issuance of ship sanitation certificates (WHO 2011) and guidelines for public health contingency planning at points of entry (WHO 2012b) and how to test the efficacy of insecticides in planes (WHO 2012a). There are also sample passenger locator cards, certificates, and activity reports.

Most relevant to developing national capacities for surveillance and response is the WHO guidance called the IHR Core Capacity Monitoring Framework, initially published in 2010 and then updated yearly. The Monitoring Framework, and an accompanying Monitoring Tool, provide a set of country-level indicators for IHR implementation that link to eight core capacities (National Legislation, Policy, and Financing; Coordination and NFP Communications; Surveillance; Response; Preparedness; Risk Communications; Human Resources; Laboratory), as well as points of entry and four specific hazards (zoonotic diseases, food safety, chemical, and radiological and nuclear events). For Surveillance, the WHO determined that each State should have indicator-based surveillance that includes an early warning function for the detection of public health events and an event-based surveillance system. Response indicators include surveillance for antimicrobial resistance and systems for infection prevention and control.

For each of the 13 core capacities, the WHO identified attributes within each country-level indicator and then a series of 256 actions. These attributes are sorted into capability levels: foundational capacities are categorized as <1; inputs and

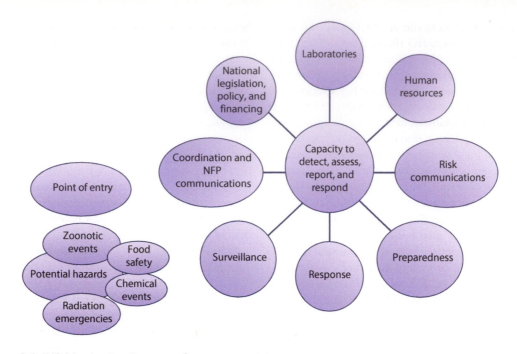

Figure 2.3 IHR Monitoring Framework: core capacities.

processes as Level 1; outputs and outcomes as Level 2; and "additional" attributes that reflect advanced capabilities as Level 3 (WHO 2013). Defining these baseline capacities and capabilities assists countries in implementing the IHR (2005) but offers flexibility to countries in defining how activities fit into their own systems and priorities (Figure 2.3).

Issues not covered by IHR

While IHR addresses many aspects of detection, reporting, and response to a public health emergency, the IHR do not address preventive or curative health services comprehensively. For example, the IHR do not call for countries to engage in preventative actions unrelated to an existing emergency, such as vaccinating against childhood diseases, ensuring preventative health-care checkups for the population, or guaranteeing access to clinical care. The IHR do not address chronic disease, so although the public health community may describe obesity or other conditions as public health emergencies, these types of conditions are not applicable to the IHR. And while Article 46 of the IHR calls for the transport and processing of reagents and other materials for diagnostic

purposes, the IHR does not obligate States to share biological samples with other States Parties.

IHR IN USE: DECLARED PHEICs

Recent and ongoing infectious disease outbreaks around the world, such as pandemic (H1N1) 2009 influenza and the novel Middle East respiratory syndrome coronavirus (MERS-CoV), are examples of how countries are using the IHR and confronting these challenges while building their capacities to detect, assess, report, and respond to such events. The 2009 H1N1 pandemic was the first-ever declared PHEIC under the IHR. The second declared PHEIC was wild-type polio in May 2014, representing a very different use of the IHR. The Ebola virus disease outbreak in West Africa was declared a PHEIC in August 2014. MERS-CoV has been circulating since 2012, and while it has been debated on multiple occasions, it has not been declared a PHEIC under the IHR (as of January 2015).

H1N1 influenza pandemic of 2009

The 2009 H1N1 influenza A virus pandemic was the first declared PHEIC by the DG under the IHR. The United States and Mexico both reported cases of novel influenza to the WHO, per the text of the Regulations. The WHO then assessed the reports, consulted back with the United States and Mexico, convened an Emergency Committee to provide travel and trade recommendations, and on April 25, 2009, the DG declared a PHEIC (Katz 2009). The IHR were followed to the letter with regard to declaring, reporting, and ongoing communication for global governance of the pandemic. The timely alert of the H1N1 outbreak to the WHO allowed other countries to put their pandemic plans into action and prepare at the community level, allowing for faster reaction. Most agree the overall response under the revised IHR was efficient, especially in comparison with responses during previous global outbreaks (Katz and Fischer 2010). The creation of NFPs enabled real-time communication and facilitated information sharing and notification.

There were, however, countries that ignored the WHO and Emergency Committee evidence-based recommendations and took their own national actions to control disease, including some actions that have less evidentiary support (Katz and Fischer 2010). And while the WHO was criticized for how and when it declared H1N1 an official pandemic (June 11, 2009)—leading to a revision of the pandemic planning documents to take into account severity along with global spread—the IHR worked as intended.

Countries such as Mexico have used the lessons learned during the 2009 H1N1 influenza pandemic to strengthen national capacities and thus enhance IHR implementation efforts. Despite the relatively early detection of cases, close coordination with PAHO, and quick information sharing with other North American countries, Mexico's laudable surveillance efforts were still not sufficient to instigate successful containment and did not prevent the spread of cases (Leung and Nicoll 2010). Mexico benefited from having an existing pandemic influenza preparedness plan, developed using WHO guidelines. This plan was successfully adapted to handle the emergence of H1N1 in 2009, and in particular facilitated multisectoral coordination and enhanced surveillance. However, the biology of pandemic (H1N1) 2009 influenza virus as a less pathogenic but more readily transmitted infection challenged Mexico's diagnostic capabilities and revealed that there was a significant lack of capacity at the state level that could handle viral identification and diagnosis. Since this time, Mexico has invested significantly in its peripheral health facilities and now has 28 laboratories at the state level that can perform molecular diagnosis for influenza (Bell et al. 2009).

Polio—The second declared PHEIC

On May 5, 2014, based on the recommendation of the IHR Emergency Committee, the DG declared the second PHEIC in response to the renewed spread of polio. The global community had been moving toward polio eradication, with renewed efforts and a flood of resources lowering global prevalence to all-time lows in 2013 (WHO 2014e). In early 2014, however, the number of cases had increased, and the location and status of affected States increased the risk of international spread of the disease. The WHO identified Pakistan, Cameroon, and Syria as the States posing the greatest risk of exporting the disease. These States are experiencing internal conflict and are surrounded by fragile States, leading to weak health systems and fruitful conditions for spreading polio. Domestic conflict in Syria caused vaccination coverage to drop from 95% in 2010 to just 45% in 2013, and in Pakistan, vaccination workers have been targeted by militants, who have killed approximately 25 health workers to date (BBC News 2013; Shah Sherazi and Watkins 2014).

The WHO and the IHR Emergency Committee decided that the increased rates of infection and the geographic location of these new cases constituted a PHEIC, and the WHO called upon a discrete list of countries—Afghanistan, Equatorial Guinea, Ethiopia, Iraq, Israel, Somalia, and Nigeria—to conduct vaccination campaigns and document vaccination coverage for travelers. States currently exporting polio—Pakistan, Cameroon, and Syria— were called upon to ensure that all residents and visitors receive vaccinations and all those engaging in international travel be vaccinated and demonstrate proof. In this instance, the WHO decided to use the power of the IHR to try to contain a resurgence of a known disease and ensure affected nations take all necessary action to eliminate cases.

Ebola—The third declared PHEIC

In December 2013, a 2-year-old boy in Guinea became sick and died; he would later be described as the index case of the largest Ebola virus disease outbreak in history (Baize et al. 2014). The disease spread for more than 2 months in the rural forest region of Guinea, misdiagnosed first as cholera and then as Lassa fever, until samples sent to laboratories in Europe tested positive for Ebola virus in March 2014. Guinea immediately reported the cases to the WHO, and by the end of March 2014, Liberia had also reported laboratory-confirmed cases to the WHO. In response, WHO issued a public alert as well as a subsequent emergency flash appeal for financial resources to assist in the response. In April, Médecins Sans Frontières (MSF)—the nongovernmental organization on the front lines of treating Ebola cases—described the outbreak as "unprecedented" because of the broad geographical distribution of cases, including in Guinea's capital Conakry, as well as the rapid increase in case numbers. In June, MSF declared the outbreak to be "out of control" (MSF 2014). Ebola continued to spread throughout the region, with case counts exploding in Sierra Leone after its initial confirmed case in May and a cluster of cases reported in Nigeria, which were fortunately controlled relatively quickly through massive contact tracing efforts. Despite the exponential case counts and clear evidence of international spread, including by air in the case of Nigeria, the WHO did not declare the outbreak a PHEIC until August 8, by which point the virus had spread widely throughout Guinea, Liberia, and Sierra Leone. Later in 2014, Ebola virus spread to additional countries, including Mali—two separate introductions, both of which required intensive contract tracing efforts to stop transmission; the United States—two cases imported from West Africa and two health-care workers infected through caring for the first patient; Spain—one imported case and a health-care worker secondarily infected; the United Kingdom—one imported case; and several other European nations that took care of individuals who were evacuated from West Africa (WHO 2015).

The Ebola virus disease outbreak presented all the hallmarks of a true public health emergency of international concern, yet the international response was sluggish. When the WHO finally made the PHEIC declaration, the Emergency Committee issued evidence-based travel and trade recommendations, but fear, public opinion, and political pressure led some nations to take aggressive actions outside of the recommendations, including border closures and flight restrictions that may have further hampered the response effort. The PHEIC declaration also did not trigger the level of resources necessary to contain the outbreak, although individual nations, foundations, and philanthropists came forward with assistance. Several weeks after the PHEIC declaration, WHO released a "roadmap for response," which outlined the steps needed to curb the outbreak as well as a request for the financial, technical, and logistical resources required to implement the roadmap (WHO 2014b). The global community began to make significant financial contributions. Despite these investments, the outbreak continued to grow such that in September 2014, the United Nations Secretary-General took responsibility for the response, noting that the Ebola outbreak had moved beyond just a public health response, and required a coordinated multiagency effort. The WHO still managed the health aspects through IHR mechanisms, but overall responsibility was transferred to the United Nations Mission for Ebola Emergency Response (UNMEER), headquartered in Accra, Ghana.

The West Africa Ebola virus outbreak demonstrated the efficacy of the IHR, but only to a point. Guinea and the WHO shared information effectively and efficiently in the days leading up to the initial formal notification, and Guinea promptly reported the outbreak through formal channels as soon as laboratory confirmation was made. WHO also chose, per the IHR, to share publically relevant information regarding the outbreak. However, despite the failure of early efforts to stem transmission, clear evidence of international spread, and the subsequent rapid escalation of cases, WHO did not declare a PHEIC until 5 months after the initial report from Guinea. Perhaps, if the PHEIC had been declared earlier, the global community might have taken comprehensive mitigating actions more promptly. Similarly, the initial delay in detecting and diagnosing the disease, capacities mandated by the IHR, likely contributed to the spread of the disease. Had these West African nations more fully implemented the IHR, they would have been better equipped to detect, report, and respond in a timely fashion.

Anticipating new challenges: The current status of MERS-CoV surveillance

As the 2009 H1N1 influenza virus pandemic demonstrates, even where preparedness plans are in place and executed well, challenges can arise with respect to adequate surveillance systems. The MERS-CoV emerged in the Middle East in 2012 and has since spread throughout the region, with occasional cases in other regions of the world. Most of the reported cases of human-to-human transmission of MERS-CoV have involved nosocomial transmission and family clusters, with limited evidence of widespread community-acquired cases. However, the number of cases is still rising, as is the list of countries in which cases are being confirmed. The IHR Emergency Committee has met several times to discuss whether MERS-CoV constitutes a PHEIC, but as of January 2015, they have not recommended that a declaration be made. While MERS-CoV has yet to be declared a PHEIC, the global community is using the IHR framework to monitor the situation, provide guidance, and continue to assess the situation. The situation highlights the challenges in remaining diligent in conducting active surveillance and response activities around MERS-CoV, while continuing to increase global capacity and willingness to detect, report, and respond to emerging public health threats.

TIMELINE AND CURRENT STATUS

Per Article 5, States Parties were given 5 years from entry into force to establish national core capacities, with the opportunity to apply for a 2-year extension in June 2012, and in exceptional cases, a second 2-year extension in June 2014. It is not clear at this time what will happen in 2016—whether the WHO will continue to require monitoring of capacity-building efforts or whether the IHR will converge with other international efforts to build global capacity to address public health emergencies (Figure 2.4).

In 2012, only 40 of the then-196 States Parties reported that they had achieved the core capacities for implementation by their own self-assessments. An additional 118 countries requested and received 2-year extensions and submitted action plans for building the necessary capacities for implementation. The remaining 38 States failed to submit a national plan for achieving compliance with the IHR (Inglesby and Fischer 2014). When nations reported again in 2014, the numbers had not greatly improved. After two more years, only 65 States Parties reported they had fully implemented the IHR. Eighty-one requested another 2-year extension, and 48 failed to report (WHO 2005b).

The inability of so many nations to develop and implement capacities to detect, assess, report, and respond to public health emergencies successfully illustrates the challenge of meeting the IHR's ambitious scope. For many countries, IHR

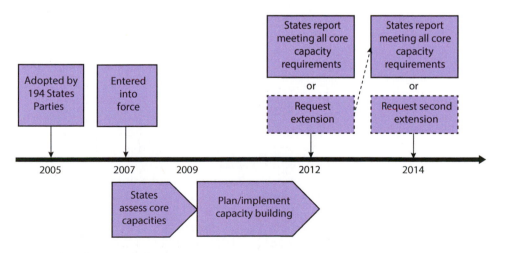

Figure 2.4 Timeline for IHR implementation.

requires the development of surveillance and diagnostic platforms upon very minimal foundations. Detecting and controlling disease at points of entry demands resources and a framework for communication and coordination across borders that are simply not available in many nations and regions. Anticipating these challenges, WHA included Article 44 in the IHR (2005), calling upon countries to work together to ensure that all states have adequate health capacity.

In February 2014, the U.S. government, in partnership with 27 other nations, the WHO, the World Organization for Animal Health, and the United Nations Food and Agriculture Organization, launched the Global Health Security Agenda (GHSA). GHSA is, in part, designed to accelerate progress toward building the capacities described in the IHR, moving toward a world that is protected from infectious disease threats and is better able to prevent, detect, and respond to public health emergencies (U.S. HHS 2014). In September 2014, President Obama hosted the now 44 members of the GHSA, along with WHO, World Organization for Animal Health (OIE), and Food and Agriculture Organization of the United Nations (FAO), to reaffirm commitments to the GHSA and to devote resources toward 11 different action packages that were designed to align with many of the core capacities mandated under the IHR. Hopefully this effort, and others like it, will guide nations toward capacity building, eventually enabling all nations of the world to detect, assess, report, and respond to a public health emergency (Figure 2.5).

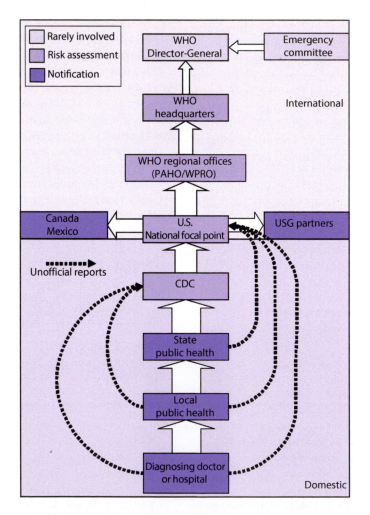

Figure 2.5 U.S. process of reporting a potential PHEIC.

REFERENCES

Baize, S., D. Pannetier, L. Oestereich et al. 2014. Emergence of Zaire Ebola virus disease in Guinea. *N. Engl. J. Med.* 371: 1418–1425.

BBC News. 2013. Polio outbreak fears in war-ravaged Syria. October 21. http://www.bbc.com/news/health-24607136.

Bell, D.M., I.B. Weisfuse, M. Hernandez-Avila, C. del Rio, X. Bustamante, and G. Rodier. 2009. Pandemic influenza as 21st century urban public health crisis. *Emerg. Infect. Dis.* 15: 1963–1969.

Evans, R.J. 1988. Epidemics and revolutions: Cholera in nineteenth-century Europe. *Past Present* 120: 123–146.

Howard-Jones, N. 1975. *The Scientific Background of the International Sanitary Conferences 1851–1938.* Geneva, Switzerland: World Health Organization. Accessed June 2014. http://whqlibdoc.who.int/publications/1975/14549_eng.pdf.

Inglesby, T. and J.E. Fischer. 2014. Moving ahead on the global health security agenda. *Biosecur. Bioterror.: Biodef. Strat. Pract. Sci.* 12: 63.

Jones, K.E., N.G. Patel, M.A. Levy, A. Storeygard, D. Balk, J.L. Gittleman, and P. Daszak. 2008. Global trends in emerging infectious diseases. *Nature* 451: 990–994.

Katz, R. 2009. Use of revised international health regulations during influenza A (H1N1) epidemic, 2009. *Emerg. Infect. Dis.* 15(8): 1165–1170.

Katz, R. and J. Fischer. 2010. The revised International Health Regulations: A framework for global pandemic response. *Global Health Governance*, Vol. 3. Accessed June 2014. http://ghgj.org/Katz%20and%20Fischer_The%20Revised%20International%20Health%20Regulations.htm.

Leung, G.M. and A. Nicoll. 2010. Reflections on pandemic (H1N1) 2009 and the international response. *PLoS Med.* 7: e1000346.

Médecins Sans Frontières. 2014. *Ebola in West Africa: 'The Epidemic Is Out of Control.'* June 23. http://www.msf.ca/en/article/ebola-west-africa-epidemic-out-control.

O'Rourke, K.H. and J.G. Williamson. 2000. When did globalization begin? NBER working paper no. 7632. Cambridge, MA: National Bureau of Economic Research.

Pizzi, M. 1958. International Sanitary Regulations, World Health Organization, Amended 1956. 129 pp. Ill. Geneva, Switzerland, World Health Organization, 1957. *Am. J. Trop. Med. Hyg.* 7(4): 470.

Shah Sherazi, Z. and T. Watkins. 2014. Attack targets polio workers in Pakistan, Kills 11. *CNN News*, March 1. Accessed July 2014. http://www.cnn.com/2014/03/01/world/asia/pakistan-attack/.

U.S. HHS (U.S. Department of Health and Human Services). 2014. Global health security agenda: Toward a world safe & secure from infectious disease threats. Accessed June 2014. http://www.globalhealth.gov/global-health-topics/global-health-security/GHS%20Agenda.pdf.

WHO (World Health Organization). 2005a. *Fifty-Eighth World Health Assembly: WHA58.3 Revision of the International Health Regulations.* Geneva, Switzerland: World Health Organization. Accessed June 2014. http://www.who.int/csr/ihr/WHA58-en.pdf.

WHO. 2005b. International Health Regulations (2005) monitoring framework. Accessed March 2015. http://www.who.int/gho/ihr/en/.

WHO. 2009a. International Health Regulations (2005): Toolkit for implementation in National Legislation. Geneva, Switzerland: World Health Organization. Accessed June 2014. http://www.who.int/entity/ihr/publications/WHO_HSE_IHR_2009.4.4/en/index.html.

WHO. 2009b. Toolkit for implementation in National Legislation: The National Focal Point (NFP). Geneva, Switzerland: World Health Organization. Accessed June 2014. http://www.who.int/ihr/NFP_Toolkit.pdf.

WHO. 2011. *Handbook for Inspection of Ships and Issuance of Ship Sanitation Certificates.* Geneva, Switzerland: World Health Organization. Accessed June 2014. http://www.who.int/entity/ihr/publications/handbook_ships_inspection/en/index.html.

WHO. 2012a. *Guidelines for Testing the Efficacy of Insecticide Products Used in Aircraft.* Geneva, Switzerland: World Health Organization. Accessed June 2014. http://www.who.int/entity/ihr/publications/aircraft_insecticides/en/index.html.

WHO. 2012b. *International Health Regulations (2005): A Guide for Public Health Emergency Contingency Planning at Designated*

Points of Entry. Geneva, Switzerland: World Health Organization. Accessed June 2014. http://www.who.int/entity/ihr/publications/9789290615668/en/index.html.

WHO. 2013. IHR core capacity monitoring framework: Checklist and indicators for monitoring progress in the development of IHR core capacities in states parties. Geneva, Switzerland: World Health Organization. Accessed April 2014. http://www.who.int/ihr/checklist/en/.

WHO. 2014a. Case definitions for the four diseases requiring notification in all circumstances under the International Health Regulations (2005). Accessed June 2014. http://www.who.int/ihr/survellance_response/case_definitions/en/.

WHO. 2014b. Ebola response roadmap. Accessed March 2015. http://www.who.int/csr/resources/publications/ebola/response-roadmap/en/.

WHO. 2014c. Laboratory. Accessed June. http://www.who.int/entity/ihr/laboratory/en/index.html.

WHO. 2014d. Tutorials on the use of annex 2 of the International Health Regulations, 2005. Accessed June. http://www.who.int/entity/ihr/annex_2_tutorial/en/index.html.

WHO. 2014e. WHO Statement on the Meeting of the International Health Regulations Emergency Committee Concerning the International Spread of Wild Poliovirus, May 5. Accessed June 2014. http://www.who.int/mediacentre/news/statements/2014/polio-20140505/en/.

WHO. 2015. Ebola Situation Report—4 February 2015. Accessed March 2015. http://apps.who.int/ebola/en/ebola-situation-report/situation-reports/ebola-situation-report-4-february-2015.

3

Public health surveillance system considerations

CARMEN C. MUNDACA-SHAH, JOHN MARK VELASCO, AND JULIE A. PAVLIN

INTRODUCTION

Public health surveillance is vital to understanding the impact of diseases, targeting resources, detecting and mitigating outbreaks of disease and evaluating prevention programs. In public health, competition for scarce resources can be high in both developed and developing settings, and thus surveillance is of vital importance to determine priorities for intervention (Morse 2007). In addition, many emerging diseases in recent years have started in areas of the world with fewer public health capacities, either nascent or degraded (Jones et al. 2008). These areas have often experienced large growths in population and also have a history of antibiotic use that results in faster resistance rates. Historically, countries may also have reluctance to report disease outbreaks due to impacts on tourism and trade (Morse 2007).

USE OF ELECTRONIC AUTOMATED SURVEILLANCE TOOLS

With the perceived threat of bioterrorism in the 1990s, many organizations researched ways to improve the detection of unexpected or unusual disease outbreaks. These early efforts were eventually termed syndromic surveillance. The definition of syndromic surveillance varies but is generally described as a health surveillance system that emphasizes (1) data availability in real time or near real time, (2) reliance on non-specific clinical signs or other proxies of health status vs. confirmed diagnoses, (3) data collected for purposes other than disease surveillance and are available automatically without additional work on behalf of health-care providers, and (4) the availability of algorithms to automatically alert public health officials of aberrations in the data that may indicate a disease outbreak of public health significance (Katz et al. 2011).

While rapid recognition of infectious disease outbreaks drove early research efforts and is still an important goal (Pavlin et al. 2003), health departments are finding the most use for situational awareness, confirming or ruling out an event, assisting with case finding and epidemiologic investigations, and in analyzing trends (Uscher-Pines et al. 2009). Syndromic surveillance systems are also used to find and notify health officials of reportable diseases and to share expected disease signs and symptoms with clinicians. Even when the data are not timely enough, does not have sufficient coverage in the population, or the algorithms are not sensitive enough to detect an unexpected or emerging public health threat, most health departments find the systems a useful adjunct to traditional public health surveillance, especially in providing early warning to a start of an expected event (e.g., influenza) or situational awareness to monitor the impact of a known threat or document that there is no significant public health threat (Triple-S 2013).

The proliferation of electronic health data ran parallel with the development of syndromic surveillance. The advent of "big data" and the availability of a myriad number of databases that could potentially be mined to determine the health status of a population has changed the landscape from too little information, to potentially too much. Beyond availability and cost, developers of systems need to consider other criteria to include timeliness, reliability, completeness, quality, flexibility, investigability, and overall usefulness in meeting the goals of the particular surveillance system (Mandl et al. 2004).

Data sources that are commonly used in syndromic surveillance systems include a range from medical encounter data to nondirect health behaviors that may change when a person becomes ill. The closer the data source is to a medical encounter, the more reliable it is as an indicator. Commonly used data sources include those associated with a medical visit such as the patient chief complaint when presenting to an emergency room,

diagnostic codes or other early clinical diagnoses which are often nonspecific without laboratory test results (e.g., acute respiratory infection, gastroenteritis), ambulance dispatch activity and reasons for calls, the number of admissions to a hospital or intensive care unit, laboratory and radiology tests ordered, and prescriptions written. Near medical encounters are calls to nurse advice lines, querying health websites for specific information and over-the-counter sales of medications. Furthest from an actual health visit, but with high volume and potentially very timely are queries on Internet search engines, absenteeism from work or school, posts on social media such as Twitter and even participatory epidemiology where members of the general public are invited to share their health status on a routine basis (Chunara et al. 2015).

Once appropriate data sources have been selected, it must be determined how to extract and transmit the data. Often, the data can be incorporated into an existing reporting schedule, but sometimes a data collection system will need to be developed. After it is determined if and how the data can be transmitted, a way to view the data must be developed. Data need to be aggregated and viewed in a way that facilitates public health analysis and response. Syndromes in syndromic surveillance are defined as a group of symptoms or signs that can serve as a proxy of disease in a population. With health encounters, actual diagnoses of disease such as influenza based on rapid tests or clinical diagnoses can be included along with less accurate diagnoses such as fever or diarrhea. There will be a trade-off between sensitivity and specificity when determining which indicators to include, with data furthest from the health-care encounter being more susceptible to lack of specificity. Some examples of syndromes commonly used include influenza, other respiratory illnesses, gastrointestinal illnesses, heat and cold injuries, disease after natural disasters (volcanic ash, dust storms, etc.) or those specific to bioterrorism threats (e.g., botulism-like symptoms). Data can also be aggregated by geographic level, by the health facility location, or if available, by the home or work address of the individual person. Data can also be displayed with a temporal aggregation, with most early detection systems looking at daily impact. However, weekly or even monthly views may be appropriate for following up seasonal epidemics or determining impact after occurrence, and more frequent aggregation (hourly) may provide early evidence of an outbreak with a short incubation and steep epidemic curve. If available, data can also be aggregated by demographic information such as age.

Typical syndromic surveillance systems are usually based on a software platform and are flexible in accepting and transforming various data sources. Examples of syndromic surveillance systems in the United States are the Electronic Surveillance System for the Early Notification of Community-based Epidemics (ESSENCE) (Lombardo et al. 2003; Holtry et al. 2010) and the Suite for Automated Global Electronic bioSurveillance (SAGES), which uses the ESSENCE framework (information on SAGES at http://www.jhuapl.edu/sages/), EpiCenter (information at https://www.hmsinc.com/service/epicenter.html), the North Carolina Disease Event Tracking and Epidemiologic Collection Tool (NC DETECT) (information at http://www.ncdetect.org/) and the National Syndromic Surveillance Program run by the U.S. Centers for Disease Control and Prevention (information at http://www.cdc.gov/nssp/overview.html). In Europe, the Syndromic Surveillance Survey Assessment towards Guidelines for Europe (Triple S-AGE) includes 24 organizations from 13 countries and reviews and analyzes syndromic surveillance activities across member states (Triple-S Project 2011). Guidelines for designing and implementing syndromic surveillance and an extensive review of European projects can be found at http://www.syndromicsurveillance.eu.

The use of syndromic surveillance systems worldwide has been increasing commensurate with the availability of health and health-related data sources. Along with the expansion of systems has come a revised understanding of how best to use them to augment traditional surveillance and a better understanding of how to balance the need for sensitivities in different systems at different times. When the World Health Organization (WHO) revised the International Health Regulations in 2005 (IHR 2005) to improve the timeliness and scope of health hazard surveillance, syndromic surveillance was not included as a way to meet the IHR (2005) requirements (WHO 2001b). Since this assessment was completed in 2001, the utility of various systems has been proven, and the Triple S-AGE has made compelling arguments that syndromic surveillance programs at the subnational level with enough population representation can assist in detecting and assessing public health emergencies in a timely manner and should be included in support of the IHR (2005) (Ziemann et al. 2015). With the capability of obtaining data sources in resource-limited settings also improving, the use of electronic automated programs such as syndromic surveillance can assist any country in complying with the IHR (2005) and improving their awareness and response to new and old diseases of public health impact.

CONSIDERATIONS FOR DEVELOPING SETTINGS

Since the 2002 SARS outbreak, many changes have been encouraged and enacted on a global basis for disease surveillance (Hitchcock et al. 2007; Chan et al. 2010). The WHO not only reports disease information in near real time to national and international stakeholders and the public for better worldwide visibility (WHO 2014), they also have implemented the International Health Regulations (2005) (IHR 2005), which require prompt notification by all 194 States Parties for events that may constitute a public health emergency of international concern (PHEIC) (Morse 2012). A PHEIC is defined as "an extraordinary event which is determined to constitute a public health risk to other States through the international spread of disease and to potentially require a coordinated international response" (WHO 2008). Of note, these include any illness or medical condition that can present harm to humans from any origin or source (WHO). In addition to reporting requirements, since 2002 the ability to detect and identify new pathogens through advanced sequencing techniques has become rapidly more available, even in traditionally resource limited settings (Lipkin 2013). This capability has allowed more rapid responses to new diseases to prevent spread and also to develop new treatments and vaccines.

However, in many places around the world, infrastructure to collect and transmit health data is either lacking or falling into disrepair as funds become less available for public health problems. There are still locations where surveillance programs are fragmented and cannot provide a comprehensive picture of disease trends for the country and region. Many disease surveillance systems are specific for a particular disease, which results

Table 3.1 Traditional reasons for disease surveillance and potential enhancements through automated, electronic systems

Disease surveillance purpose	How potentially enhanced by electronic surveillance
Detect outbreaks and monitor disease trends	Use of methods to expand surveillance coverage with inexpensive tools such as SMS may provide a more comprehensive and timely way to detect and track outbreaks
Determine current public health status (situational awareness)	May improve timeliness of information access and dissemination and depending on local capabilities, may increase reach to areas previously not captured
Determine public health priorities	May provide a more comprehensive picture of public health needs in a community, especially if expanded to include chronic diseases and injuries
Guide planning and implementation of programs to prevent and control disease or injury	Better understanding of where interventions are most needed and may also provide methods for those responsible for implementation to communicate on acceptability and effectiveness
Evaluate prevention measures	May provide less biased information from routine typically non-disease surveillance data sources compared to manual reporting
Support epidemiologic research	Databases may be more complete and allow comparison between different surveillance markers

in missing emerging outbreaks in other diseases. Many systems are also reactive rather than proactive in looking for potential new problems and mitigating them before they become serious public health issues (Morse 2007).

Understanding local needs and the ability to sustain health surveillance systems is instrumental in developing an effective, useful system in any location. It is also crucial to remember the multiple reasons to create disease surveillance systems, which go far beyond outbreak detection, and which can possibly be improved with electronic systems even, and perhaps especially, in resource-limited settings as described in Table 3.1.

BUILDING SUSTAINABLE DISEASE SURVEILLANCE SYSTEMS IN RESOURCE-LIMITED SETTINGS

The public health community in resource-limited countries has embraced an increased access to technological tools with the hope that this technology will strengthen their disease surveillance capabilities. However, one of the greatest challenges in the developing world has been to implement or upgrade systems without creating parallel ones and without increasing the workload for surveillance

staff (Chretien and Lewis 2008). Therefore, focusing on sustainability of new or upgraded systems is a key issue in these settings.

The planning phase

When planning the implementation or upgrade of a disease surveillance system, certain elements should be assessed before a decision is made to start this process. In order to build the path for a sustainable system, it is essential to secure support from high level authorities at the organization or institution where the system will be implemented (WHO 2003a, 2005; Domeika et al. 2009). Once surveillance has been identified as a clear need, the authorities should translate their commitment to this process with five actions: (a) the development of a strategic vision and plan (WHO 2005; PHRPlus 2006); (b) the generation of legislative action that supports the activities and processes associated with the system (Domeika et al. 2009; Wamala et al. 2010); (c) the dedication of financial and other resources necessary to not only initiate but also sustain the system (Soto et al. 2008; Domeika et al. 2009; Kebede et al. 2011); (d) the provision of technical assistance to provide oversight to this process (Franco et al. 2006; Robertson et al. 2010;

Lukwago et al. 2012); and (e) the establishment of coordination mechanisms between organizations and within the different levels of the system (WHO 2003b; Gueye et al. 2006).

STRATEGIC VISION AND PLAN

The system should reflect the priorities of the organization where it will be implemented. Without such a vision, donors or other external organizations involved could drive the system toward their own interests instead of following the organization's needs (PHRPlus 2006). The plan of action should map out a sustainability strategy for the disease surveillance system that aims to integrate the system into the organization or institution where it will be implemented. This plan should provide the system with an adequate organizational structure by outlining clear roles and responsibilities for every level of the system (WHO 2003b, 2005; Franco et al. 2006), including a monitoring and evaluation framework and an articulated workforce development plan.

LEGISLATIVE ACTION

Enacting legislation and developing a national directive is among the initial steps in the context of implementing a national electronic disease surveillance system (WHO 2003b, 2005; Kebede et al. 2011). Legislation and a national directive allow health workers and other staff to take responsibility for performing the identified surveillance tasks. It also signifies that surveillance staff can be held accountable for their actions or inactivity once they had been provided with the tools and training to use the disease surveillance system. On the other hand, national or regional surveillance team leaders can reference the legislation or national directive to reward personnel who exhibited exemplary work performance which can serve as a potential motivator for continued employee excellence.

As important as it is to have legislation and a national directive, it is equally important to include clear and precise guidelines within the directive. The directive should specify the system's components, all the steps of the disease surveillance processes, and the resources required to accomplish the surveillance tasks. Surveillance activities should be designed according to what was described in the directive. If it is not written in the directive, support for necessary surveillance activities may be difficult to marshal. In addition,

flexibility and responsiveness to changes in disease surveillance systems and in the directive or legislation that guided them can facilitate the implementation process. A change in the public health situation in a country, for instance, may necessitate a change in the country's disease surveillance system that should be reflected in the directive. Finally, the existence of legislation related to disease surveillance virtually guarantees continuity in the organization's commitment. Regardless of changes in high level administrative positions, existing legislation or a directive means that established disease surveillance priorities would continue to be maintained and supported. The dissemination of these documents to all the surveillances sites is important to ensure that the authorities at the surveillance sites provide support to the surveillance staff for the fulfillment of the surveillance tasks. In situations where a system is being implemented or pilot tested in one region, city, or even hospital system, the same principles apply. Even though national legislation will not be enacted, the political or administrative oversight needs to provide official directives.

FINANCIAL SUPPORT

The third key element that should be obtained in support of a system, given institutional or organizational commitment, is financial support (Robertson et al. 2010). Ideally, such resources would come from the organization where the system is to be implemented (WHO 2003b; PHRplus 2006). However, due to the limited resources for disease surveillance in developing countries, it is not uncommon for such systems to be implemented with the financial support of an external donor (Jefferson et al. 2008; Domeika et al. 2009; Huaman et al. 2009; Kant and Krishnan 2010; Robertson et al. 2010; Kebede et al. 2011; Ear 2012; Lukwago et al. 2012; Rajatonirina et al. 2012). The certainty of the funding source for the system and the duration of the sponsorship should be clearly stated (Sow et al. 2010). It is advisable to convene a meeting of interested donors to discuss surveillance needs, planned activities, and resource requirements. Such a donor meeting would be beneficial in determining the levels of commitment intended by each potential donor.

Implementers must ensure adequate financial support for the system in order to build the capacity needed for surveillance and empower the surveillance community in the country, thus avoiding the problem of creating dependency on donors in the long term (WHO 2005). One of the major concerns about the external funding of surveillance systems is that such funding is typically of limited duration. Therefore, the use of resources that the organization already has in place should be encouraged (Soto et al. 2008; Domeika et al. 2009).

One issue to address when external organizations support the implementation process of a disease surveillance system is the system staff perception of the ownership of the system. If members of the surveillance team believe that what is asked of them originates from an external organization, individuals might feel less compelled to complete the assigned tasks. It is important that the organization deliver to staff a clear message of system ownership, making sure the surveillance staff understands that rather than being externally owned, the system belongs to the organization (Ear 2012).

TECHNICAL SUPPORT

In addition to financial support of the system, another consideration at this level is the need for technical assistance. The institution should assign skilled staff from the institution or develop an agreement with an organization that can provide the expertise required. Ministries of Health (MOH) have extensive experience in disease surveillance but are open to receiving technical support from other organizations such as the WHO, or the U.S. Centers for Disease Control and Prevention (CDC) (WHO 2003b; Sow et al. 2010; Wamala et al. 2010; Lukwago et al. 2012). The aim for an organization providing technical support should be to build capacity within the recipient organization in order to develop a team that ultimately would be able to lead the implementation process (Robertson et al. 2010). Technical support should continue to the point that the organization is able to administer the process independently. The implementation process might fail if the organization takes over the surveillance process prematurely.

COORDINATION

System coordination has to be clearly defined and established at the highest administrative levels. Most MOHs have several organizations that use different surveillance systems to provide epidemiological surveillance data, including laboratory and clinical public health data. Although each surveillance system collects information from the same patients, many of them do not share these data. One of the key elements in the sustainability of disease surveillance is the coordination of and eventual integration of these disparate systems in order to meet the need for timely and more complete surveillance data (WHO 2001a, 2003b; Domeika et al. 2009; Kant and Krishnan 2010).

It is also critical that institutions develop partnerships with other institutions in order to enhance their surveillance capabilities (Curioso et al. 2005; Domeika et al. 2009; Wamala et al. 2010; Kebede et al. 2011). In particular, it is imperative to establish a collaborative relationship with any other surveillance initiatives in the same area, to be able to provide mutual support (Kant and Krishnan 2010). Finally, it is quite important to develop a relationship of trust between members of the external funding organization and in-country personnel that facilitates positive working relationships and considers cultural aspects when establishing this process.

Building surveillance teams

A national team is generally created to oversee the implementation process of a disease surveillance system. In order to provide closer support to the surveillance sites in a timelier manner, the national team should rely, when available, on regional and district teams for this purpose. At the national, regional, and district levels, the characteristics of these teams and the functions performed are essential for the generation of quality and timely data at the local surveillance sites.

SETTING UP NATIONAL AND LOCAL TEAMS

The essential activities of training, monitoring, supervising, and providing feedback can only be accomplished if the surveillance teams are skilled, highly committed, and available. This group of people has to be interested, actively involved in surveillance, convinced of its usefulness, and experienced in surveillance itself or working in the organization in which the system will be implemented.

When recruiting personnel for these teams, motivation should be an important attribute. Inside the team, is recommended that at least one person has a clear vision of the system and is able to effectively interact across various levels in hierarchical organizations. The national team is the link between all of the surveillance sites and the highest level authority in the organization or institution.

The experience of the national implementing team with the surveillance system and the implementation process contributes to a more efficient and effective implementation. The same surveillance system, for example, was implemented in the Peruvian Navy, Army, and Air Force at different times but in the order indicated. It was observed that the implementation process was faster and easier once the team had gained more experience, identified more effective strategies, and structured the training.

Surveillance staff values the surveillance skills and knowledge of the surveillance instrument that the national surveillance team will be using. A disease surveillance system requires effective user support, training, and technical expertise to maintain the tool. Technical support assigned to the national surveillance team should have expertise in the specific software program used to develop the tool.

As the implementation process evolves, it is important to maintain an advanced level of training for surveillance supervisors. Lack of analytical skills is common even at the national level team in resource-limited settings. These skills are necessary to be able to translate data into action. However, addressing this issue is especially challenging. The cost of continuing surveillance education, the long hours of work experienced by supervisors, and the small salary of supervisors as government employees serve as barriers to meeting the continuing education needs of these key individuals.

The national surveillance team should create a local, on-site surveillance team instead of assigning this task to one person. It is unrealistic to expect that one person could be dedicated exclusively to surveillance. Therefore, having multiple people engaged in surveillance efforts eases the overall impact of the task and enables personnel to comply more effectively with surveillance expectations. One person can be assigned responsibility for disease surveillance, but everyone at the site needs to collaborate in the event that help is required. It is important to identify and recruit for this team those health workers who are more interested in the system and who would be able to disseminate messages about its importance.

TRAINING

Training is recognized as one of the most important activities when implementing a disease surveillance system (Curioso et al. 2005; WHO 2005; Sow et al. 2010). It is needed for the successful implementation of a surveillance program and as a way to address challenges such as staff turnover, workload, and limited surveillance skills. The key outcome of disease surveillance is to have access to reliable and timely information in order to make decisions. Therefore, human resources need to be motivated and trained in order to be able to effectively and efficiently collect and transmit this information.

Opportunities should be created to train as many personnel as possible considering the limited resources available (Rajatonirina et al. 2012). Training that ultimately reaches all surveillance levels—district, regional, and central—are most likely to yield successful implementation of a system. Implementing a new tool or broader surveillance systems typically requires an initial training at the central level of the institution or organization. Once training of the central level team is completed, training is instituted at the regional level. Staff at the central and regional levels are then able to join forces to train district-level end users. If an external group provides initial training, this group should make themselves available for clarification or support during the initial phase of system implementation.

Trainers have to consider their audience when developing surveillance training courses. Healthcare workers and other professionals differ in their expectations of and need for information. When communicating with high-level authorities, for instance, the designers of a training experience should pay attention to institutional context and the level of public health background of this population. Instructional designers need to tailor training content and terminology to ensure a clear understanding of disease surveillance by nonpublic health professionals. Adapting the training is sometimes necessary to meet the needs of senior personnel who typically have less experience with technology than younger trainees.

Several strategies are used to deliver surveillance training: (a) large-scale training at one central location, (b) combining training by surveillance supervisors with scheduled on-site supervisory visits to surveillance units, and (c) training using an online environment. Surveillance staff training may be conducted at a central or regional location, which means surveillance staff members from all areas of the country are invited to participate in these training courses. An advantage of this format of training is that experiences shared during the training help supervisors and surveillance staff to develop closer relationships, which is essential for future communication about the system. Relationship building may also increase staff motivation to comply with disease reporting guidelines. In addition, scheduling the presence of a high-level authority at a training course emphasizes to attendees the importance of disease surveillance. Training may also be undertaken as part of periodic supervisory visits to surveillance sites.

Online training might prove a beneficial option, particularly as a means of addressing resource constraints and allowing more flexibility for participants to attend trainings. E-mail and telephone communications should also be used to reinforce the training that personnel receive, to clarify staff doubts, send documentation and information, as well as establish permanent contact with surveillance staff being supervised.

In delivering training designed to meet the needs of surveillance staff, implementers should consider two aspects. Training has to be maintained continuously and performed in a comprehensive way. A system cannot survive without continuous training especially considering high staff turnover. Training should not only be offered on an on-going basis but also be conducted as frequently as possible (Wuhib et al. 2002; PHRPlus 2006; Siswoyo et al. 2008; Kant and Krishnan 2010). A region in Peru with the most successful disease surveillance network included monthly training sessions for the surveillance staff at the district level that focused on various surveillance-related topics. Frequent on-going staff training was considered one of the most important contributing factors to their exceptionally good performance in disease surveillance. It is advisable that implementers develop an annual plan for training in epidemiology and disease surveillance for their organization, and ultimately incorporate this training into health workers curricula.

The format and content of the training course is essential to the success of a system. A recommendation for the initial phase is to have training courses no longer than 2 days duration. Longer courses may overwhelm health-care workers and make it difficult for them to retain the concepts needed to start reporting. The objective of this methodology is to give the end users information that could be immediately used when they return to their sites. Surveillance staff should be able to start this new task immediately after they receive training.

The content addressed in training should, at minimum, include the following: (a) the purpose and importance of disease surveillance, (b) the role of health-care workers in surveillance, (c) the data collection and disease reporting process, (d) data analysis and interpretation, and (e) the detection of an appropriate response(s) to disease outbreaks or events. Training should include content on concepts related to surveillance and functions that disease surveillance systems serve, the legislation that mandates and guides surveillance, and information about the most prevalent and relevant diseases in their community, region, country, and internationally. Trainers should explain how the disease surveillance information will be used for making public health decisions. The reporting process has to be clearly explained, with time assigned for trainees to practice using the data collection tool and reporting system. It is recommended that training provides surveillance staff skills to understand and interpret the data. Surveillance staff need training that enables them to identify disease outbreaks and other events and appropriately respond to them. Having this information empowers staff and reinforces the importance of their disease surveillance task.

The train-the-trainer approach is simple and replicable and has proved useful for disease surveillance by enabling those who have been trained to train personnel at their sites. Trainees then became trainers, thus contributing to a more rapid spread of knowledge about electronic disease surveillance (Soto et al. 2008; Rajatonirina et al. 2012). For instance, one organization in Peru instituted the effective strategy of having every person who was trained replicate this training for the rest of their site's team. A train-the-trainer strategy allows more frequent and widely disseminated training to be available.

MONITORING AND EVALUATION

While training is key to providing the required skills and surveillance staff motivation, system monitoring is a core activity in the maintenance of an effective electronic disease surveillance system

(WHO 2005; Soto et al. 2008). At least one trained person should be assigned to monitor the system, including assessing data quality and ensuring reporting accuracy and timeliness (Soto et al. 2008). The designated system monitor is responsible for communicating with surveillance sites, clarifying issues and addressing questions from staff at the site, and engaging in supervisory visits. National surveillance team members hold primary responsibility for system monitoring.

Monitoring is important to identify surveillance areas or functions that are not working effectively. This is accomplished through the measurement of indicators (WHO 2003b). When indicator data are not forthcoming, training and supervision visits should be conducted in an effort to respond to what is identified as a problem. It has been observed that contacting surveillance staff when data reporting was overdue or missing increased timeliness of reporting from 64.6% to 84% (Huaman et al. 2009). Evaluation of the system is important in an effort to ultimately assess the effect of implemented health promotion and disease prevention measures (PHRPlus 2006; Weber 2007; Soto et al. 2008).

FEEDBACK

Bidirectional feedback is one more function of the national surveillance team that was deemed essential (Wuhib et al. 2002; WHO 2005; Weber 2007; Sow et al. 2010). The national surveillance team should establish channels that the end users utilize to communicate the problems they had with the system or the tool and any suggestions for change. On the other end, surveillance staff receives feedback on the information they collect and send. Activities such as the creation of bulletins and reports are very useful (WHO 2003b; Lukwago et al. 2012). The frequency of these reports should consider the national team's capacity and take advantage of electronic tools to export that information when needed (Soto et al. 2008). These reports may be sent both by e-mail and by printed format. Even when it takes considerable time for a printed report to reach recipients, surveillance staff value having a document to show their supervisors and coworkers the work they are doing. The surveillance staff deemed it essential to see the information collected in a way that is useful to them; data usefulness is helpful in motivating surveillance site personnel. Providing end users feedback on their performance can also be quite rewarding (WHO 2003b). Strategies such as creating a ranking of sites according to their overall performance and timely reporting and congratulations on this ranking has improved staff morale.

SUPERVISION

Supervisory visits should accompany monitoring and evaluation activities whenever possible (WHO 2003b; Franco et al. 2006; Sow et al. 2010). Supervisory visits depend on the budget and the resources available. The implementers' plan should include supervisory visits based on the needs of the system, while also considering their geographic accessibility to the units. When providing on-site supervision, the quality of reporting increases and the act of supervision motivates the surveillance staff in several ways (John et al. 1998; Huaman et al. 2009). The simple fact of visiting the surveillance staff in these sites helps to build a relationship with them. Listening and learning about their local problems, difficulties, and challenges are also an important part of these visits. The supervisory team should provide information of what is expected from the sites before supervising them. During the visit, the team compares the data reported, which appeared on the electronic system, with the one registered in the site records book. If any problems are identified, the team retrains the surveillance staff to clarify any misunderstandings (WHO 2003b). In addition, the team would meet with all the personnel at the site to let them know about the system and request their commitment to the task.

This visit is also an opportunity for the national team to learn about the site, the resources in place, the process in place, and the surveillance staff's morale. This understanding is important to the team to determine what is feasible to ask from the surveillance staff and not to put in place unfair accountability measures. After the visit, a report is prepared with recommendations for improvement if needed. The team should be careful to emphasize the objective of the visit as a way to improve their tasks and the final report as constructive and not punishment.

SUPPORT

The perception of support teams available to surveillance staff is quite important. Disease surveillance systems that function effectively are characterized by constant communication and the presence of a surveillance team that surveillance staff know they can call when problems arise (Gueye et al. 2006; Weber 2007). Team availability and responsiveness to the concerns of staff at any level contributes to the development of trusting relationships that ultimately facilitate a more effective surveillance system.

In summary, the national and regional teams should be composed of highly motivated and skilled personnel (Sow et al. 2010). The critical functions of training, monitoring, supervision, and feedback address critical points of providing skills and increasing motivation of reporting staff to conduct the surveillance task, ensuring high performance at the surveillance sites. At the same time, the national team has the critical function of informing the institutional administrative level of the diseases and events under surveillance. By presenting analysis of data collected in a useful way to the high authorities of an organization or institution, evidence can be translated into measures that would benefit the population under surveillance (Wuhib et al. 2002).

Generating timely and quality data at the surveillance site

While the support of high level authorities is critical to start the surveillance implementation process, without human resources at the surveillance site that are skilled and motivated and the provision of a local enabling environment, a system will not be able to function properly (Rajatonirina et al. 2012).

SURVEILLANCE AWARENESS

Implementers of disease surveillance systems sometimes have to work to change the views of surveillance staff, particularly those who see their task as merely routine or inconsequential (WHO 2005). They should aim to increase staff's awareness of the purpose and importance of surveillance and specifically the significance of the surveillance roles and tasks. Some surveillance staff needs to be educated about disease surveillance in order to understand the importance of their surveillance tasks and the critical role they and the data they collect ultimately play in disease prevention (Soto et al. 2008).

While awareness of surveillance staff is critical for engagement on the reporting tasks, all health-care workers in the surveillance sites should be educated about the disease surveillance system, the importance of surveillance, and their role in the documentation of disease (WHO 2003b). Physicians at disease surveillance sites, for instance, need to know how to accurately record the symptomatology and diagnosis of patients they interview and treat.

Dissemination of information about the existence and products of a disease surveillance system is a key component to create this awareness of the importance of the system (Weber 2007). It not only informs personnel about a system integral to the organization but also gives them the opportunity to become involved, share her or his perspectives, and ultimately support surveillance personnel in the tasks they had to perform. When the highest ranked person at the site knows about the system and the need to comply with it, the chance that the task would be accomplished by the organization is heightened.

INCENTIVES

As described earlier in this chapter, training, monitoring, and feedback can be staff motivators. Moreover, working in an environment where the resources required to fulfill surveillance tasks are present also increases motivation among the surveillance staff. Even when resources available are limited at a site, site directors who recognize the importance of surveillance may facilitate access to support.

Implementers should also consider the positive impact of non-financial incentives on the morale of surveillance staff. An assessment of surveillance staff is essential to identify incentives of value to them. For instance, a national "Epidemiology Day" was designated in the Peruvian Army to increase awareness of disease surveillance and to honor those who demonstrated excellent performance. This effort was very well received among the surveillance staff in the Peruvian military as the recognition came from their highest leadership.

ACCOUNTABILITY

In the case of delays in surveillance report submissions, organizations might address accountability by means of written formal documentation of the incident. Implementers should be cautious when enforcing compliance to the system as it might hurt the surveillance staff morale. It is advisable to have a more flexible approach to such problems.

Direct contact with surveillance staff should be the initial effort to assess the reason for the delay and, if reasonable, to provide a deadline extension. It is important that staff compliance to reporting deadlines is not based on avoidance of sanctions (Wuhib et al. 2002).

FEASIBILITY

The effectiveness of a surveillance system depends on making surveillance a feasible task in terms of the processes and tools employed. Ensuring feasibility involves simplicity, flexibility, and standardization of both processes and tools, each of which will be discussed in the following section.

Surveillance processes need to be as simple as possible to enable surveillance staff to meet expectations and avoid disruption of their other assigned activities (Wuhib et al. 2002; Sow et al. 2010). Surveillance systems tend to fail in the presence of two problems: (a) the system or its component processes are too complex or (b) administrators or others held unrealistic expectations for collection of a great quantity of information that ultimately proved to be impossible for staff to manage.

Implementers should assess which aspects of a disease surveillance system can be simplified in an effort to contribute to the potential success of the system (Robertson et al. 2010). As part of this effort, strategies such as prioritizing the list of events to survey (WHO 2003b; Weber 2007), simplifying data collection instruments, reducing report frequency, and simplifying training efforts could potentially contribute to the success of an electronic disease surveillance system.

When determining report frequency and type of surveillance data (e.g., individual versus grouped) to be collected, consideration should be given to several issues: the need for the data, how data will be used, the resources available, the data collection process to be employed, the complexity of data collection forms, the kind and complexity of data analysis, and the frequency of report submissions. In addition to facilitating data collection, simple, user-friendly surveillance tools are also noted to facilitate data reporting. For instance, it is advisable to develop a simple tool that users could quickly load on to every computer, even those with slow Internet connections common in most areas outside the capital of developing countries. Surveillance staff at the local level should be able to use the system without extensive information technology knowledge. At the same time, the staff should have the sufficient tools to conduct a complex analysis of data if needed.

It is important to standardize the processes to collect and report data at every surveillance site and, when possible, adapt the processes to the tool used to report the data (WHO 2003b; Franco et al. 2006). Processes should be standardized in every location where patients initiate contact with a health-care facility such as emergency rooms, ambulatory offices, and hospital admissions. However, one of the problems commonly observed is data consistency: not every site records the same data. Having a reminder card with the patient data or events that are required to be collected has proven useful. Accordingly, data collection guidelines should clearly specify the parameters of data to be collected and reported.

Flexibility as a means of adaptability serves as a key attribute of successful electronic disease surveillance systems. Flexibility is important not only when developing the disease surveillance tool but also throughout the entire process of implementation. For instance, surveillance actors with an inflexible vision of the system could jeopardize the implementation process. A disease surveillance system should be adaptable to different epidemiological scenarios and international recommendations, and allow for the modification of laws or regulations to take into account differing needs for information.

Due to limited resources at surveillance sites, reporting deadlines should be adjusted to reflect what is feasible for surveillance staff considering limited staff, efforts to attend to competing tasks, slow Internet connectivity, availability of records used to complete the report, and the availability of a means of communication used to send the report. Differences among surveillance sites regarding differing levels of resources, including communication resources and expectations for field work, should be considered when holding these sites accountable to the same reporting standards.

Flexibility in delivery of surveillance reports, such as computers with Internet connectivity, landline telephones, mobile phones (Singh et al. 2011), and even radio communication (WHO 2003b), allows members at higher levels of the surveillance system to reach surveillance staff in towns or other areas where Internet access is unavailable (Siswoyo et al. 2008; Soto et al. 2008; Lukwago et al. 2012; Rajatonirina et al. 2012).

Implementers need to establish a mechanism to obtain user requests for surveillance tool modifications that facilitate the reporting process. These requests should be assessed and prioritized by the technical assistance team. Having a team of engineers or technical experts as part of a surveillance team to assess and respond to requests for changes may not only improve the flexibility of the tool but also improve the timeliness with which the team responds to such requests.

In summary, in order to generate timely and quality data, the reporting staff needs to be skilled and motivated (Robertson et al. 2010); have access to adequate resources to collect and transmit the data collected and be assigned a feasible task. Feasibility requires having simple, flexible, and standardized procedures in place, including the surveillance tool used by the system.

SUMMARY

Success in implementing electronic disease surveillance systems is related to several factors at different stakeholder levels: the institutional administrative level, the national and regional disease surveillance team level, and the surveillance site level. A list of factors associated with successful implementation is highlighted in Table 3.2.

Existing and additional systems should work synergistically and span the full spectrum of public health problems specific to that country.

Table 3.2 Factors associated with successful implementation of electronic disease surveillance systems in resource-limited countries

Political will	• At every level of the system • Clear articulation of needs • Legislation provided to act • Local champion at the regional/local level
Strategic vision and plan	• Map out sustainability • Include monitoring, evaluation, and workforce development plan
Adequate financial support	• Build capacity and empower surveillance community • Avoid creating dependency on donors
Trained and available workforce	• Can be challenge for developing countries • Provides skill to produce high quality data • Need to ensure analysis of data collected is possible
Performance improvement plan	• Nurture culture to keep surveillance staff motivated • Use non-financial incentives • Provide regular feedback to end users
Flexibility and adaptability	• Personnel and software need to adapt to changing environment • System must be able to incorporate different and new data sources
System is intuitive to end users	• Average surveillance staff should be able to use the system • Simple and complex analyses can be performed
Useful at all levels	• From local users to the national level • Feedback is important
Data transparency	• Develop data use agreements • Ensure data sharing is legal and ethical
Start small	• System should be tested and proven before it is expanded in large scale

Source: Mundaca, C., A best practices model for implementing successful electronic disease surveillance systems: Insights from Peru and around the globe, PhD dissertation, Uniformed Services University of the Health Sciences, Washington, DC, 2013.

Interventions or new systems should not be implemented at the cost of sacrificing other health priorities, and there should be a balance between country-specific needs, donor-driven requirements, and international interests. Intrinsic challenges related to human resources should be considered, political commitment and support should be evaluated, and if there is a need, resources should be focused first in strengthening the existing health systems prior to introducing changes. Measures such as these may be more beneficial and sustainable in the long run for regulators, funders, and recipient nations in improving global public health disease surveillance.

DISCLAIMER

The views expressed are those of the authors and do not necessarily reflect the official views of the Uniformed Services University of the Health Sciences, the Henry M. Jackson Foundation for the Advancement of Military Medicine, Inc., or the Department of Defense.

REFERENCES

Chan, E.H., T.F. Brewer, L.C. Madoff et al. 2010. Global capacity for emerging infectious disease detection. *Proc. Natl. Acad. Sci. U.S.A.* 107: 21701–21706.

Chretien, J.P. and S.H. Lewis. 2008. Electronic public health surveillance in developing settings: Meeting summary. *BMC Proc.* 2 (Suppl. 3): S1.

Chunara, R., E. Goldstein, O. Patterson-Lomba, and J.S. Brownstein. 2015. Estimating influenza attack rates in the United States using a participatory cohort. *Sci. Rep.* 5: 9540.

Curioso, W.H., B.T. Karras, P.E. Campos, C. Buendia, K.K. Holmes, and A.M. Kimball. 2005. Design and implementation of Cell-PREVEN: A real-time surveillance system for adverse events using cell phones in Peru. *AMIA Annu Symp Proc.* 2005: 176–180.

Domeika, M., G. Kligys, O. Ivanauskiene et al. 2009. Implementation of a national electronic reporting system in Lithuania. *Euro Surveill.* 14: 1–6.

Ear, S. 2012. Emerging infectious disease surveillance in Southeast Asia: Cambodia, Indonesia, and the U.S. Naval Area Medical Research Unit 2. *Asian Secur.* 8: 164–187.

Franco, L., J. Setzer, and K. Banke. 2006. Improving performance of IDSR at district and facility levels: Experiences in Tanzania and Ghana in making IDSR operational. Bethesda, MD: The Partners for Health Reform*plus* Project, Abt Associates, Inc. Accessed September 1, 2015. http://www.urc-chs.com/uploads/resourcefiles/idsrsynthesisreport.pdf.

Gueye, D., K. Banke, and P. Mmbuji. 2006. Follow-up monitoring and evaluation of integrated disease surveillance and response in Tanzania. Bethesda, MD: The Partners for Health Reform*plus* Project, Abt Associates, Inc. Accessed March 17, 2014. http://pdf.usaid.gov/pdf_docs/PNADG241.pdf.

Hitchcock, P., A. Chamberlain, M. Van Wagoner, T.V. Inglesby, and T. O'Toole. 2007. Challenges to global surveillance and response to infectious disease outbreaks of international importance. *Biosecur. Bioterror.* 5: 206–227.

Holtry, R.S., L.M. Hung, and S.H. Lewis. 2010. Utility of the ESSENCE surveillance system in monitoring the H1N1 outbreak. *Online J. Public Health Inform.* 2: e3028.

Huaman, M.A., R.V. Araujo-Castillo, G. Soto et al. 2009. Impact of two interventions on timeliness and data quality of an electronic disease surveillance system in a resource limited setting (Peru): A prospective evaluation. *BMC Med. Inform. Decis. Mak.* 9: 16.

Jefferson, H., B. Dupuy, H. Chaudet et al. 2008. Evaluation of a syndromic surveillance for the early detection of outbreaks among military personnel in a tropical country. *J. Public Health* 30: 375–383.

John, T.J., R. Samuel, V. Balraj, and R. John. 1998. Disease surveillance at district level: A model for developing countries. *Lancet* 352: 58–61.

Jones, K.E., N.G. Patel, M.A. Levy et al. 2008. Global trends in emerging infectious diseases. *Nature* 451: 990–994.

Kant, L. and S.K. Krishnan. 2010. Information and communication technology in disease surveillance, India: A case study. *BMC Public Health* 10(Suppl. 1): S11.

Katz, R., L. May, J. Baker, and E. Test. 2011. Redefining syndromic surveillance. *J. Epidemiol. Glob. Health* 1: 21–31.

Kebede, S., J.B. Gatabazi, P. Rugimbanya et al. 2011. Strengthening systems for communicable disease surveillance: Creating a laboratory network in Rwanda. *Health Res. Policy Syst.* 9: 27.

Lipkin, W.I. 2013. The changing face of pathogen discovery and surveillance. *Nat. Rev. Microbiol.* 11: 133–141.

Lombardo, J., H. Burkom, E. Elbert et al. 2003. A systems overview of the Electronic Surveillance System for the Early Notification of Community-based Epidemics (ESSENCE II). *J. Urban Health* 80(2 Suppl. 1): i32–i42.

Lukwago, L., M. Nanyunja, N. Ndayimirije et al. 2012. The implementation of Integrated Disease Surveillance and Response in Uganda: A review of progress and challenges between 2001 and 2007. *Health Policy Plan.* 28: 30–40.

Mandl, K.D., J.M. Overhage, M.M. Wagner et al. 2004. Implementing syndromic surveillance: A practical guide informed by the early experience. *J. Am. Med. Inform. Assoc.* 11: 141–150.

Morse, S.S. 2007. Global infectious disease surveillance and health intelligence. *Health Affairs* 26: 1069–1077.

Morse S.S. 2012. Public health surveillance and infectious disease detection. *Biosecur. Bioterror.* 10: 6–16.

Mundaca, C. 2013. A best practices model for implementing successful electronic disease surveillance systems: Insights from Peru and around the globe. PhD dissertation, Uniformed Services University of the Health Sciences, Washington, DC.

Pavlin, J.A., F. Mostashari, M.G. Kortepeter et al. 2003. Innovative surveillance methods for rapid detection of disease outbreaks and bioterrorism: Results of an interagency workshop on health indicator surveillance. *Am. J. Public Health* 93: 1230–1235.

PHRplus. 2006. Georgia immunization MIS and disease surveillance reforms: Achievements, lessons learned and future directions. Working paper, Bethesda, MD: Partners for Health Reform*plus*, Abt Associates, Inc. Accessed September 1, 2015. http://www.curatiofoundation.org/uploads/other/0/149.pdf.

Rajatonirina, S., J.-M. Heraud, L. Randrianasolo et al. 2012. Short message service sentinel surveillance of influenza-like illness in Madagascar, 2008–2012. *Bull. World Health Organ.* 90: 385–389.

Robertson, C., K. Sawford, S.L. Daniel, T.A. Nelson, and C. Stephen. 2010. Mobile phone-based infectious disease surveillance system, Sri Lanka. *Emerg. Infect. Dis.* 16: 1524–1531.

Singh, V., R. Madhusudan, and J. Mohan. 2011. An evaluation of mobile phone technology use for Integrated Disease Surveillance Project (IDSP) in Andhra Pradesh, India. Paper presented at the *Annual Meeting of the International Society of Disease Surveillance*, Atlanta, GA.

Siswoyo, H., M. Permana, R.P. Larasati, J. Farid, A. Suryadi, and E.R. Sedyaninqsih. 2008. EWORS: Using a syndromic-based surveillance tool for disease outbreak detection in Indonesia. *BMC Proc.* 2(Suppl. 3): S3.

Soto, G., R.V. Araujo-Castillo, J. Neyra et al. 2008. Challenges in the implementation of an electronic surveillance system in a resource-limited setting: Alerta, in Peru. *BMC Proc.* 2(Suppl. 3): S4.

Sow, I., W. Alemu, M. Nanyunja, S. Duale, H.N. Perry, and P. Gaturuku. 2010. Trained district health personnel and the performance of integrated disease surveillance in the WHO African region. *East Afr. J. Public Health* 7: 16–19.

Triple-S. 2011. Assessment of syndromic surveillance in Europe. *Lancet* 378: 1833–1834.

Triple-S. 2013. Guidelines for designing and implementing a syndromic surveillance system. Accessed May 21, 2015. http://www.syndromic surveillance.eu/Triple-S_guidelines.pdf.

Uscher-Pines, L., C.L. Farrell, S.M. Babin et al. 2009. Framework for the development of response protocols for public health syndromic surveillance systems: Case studies of 8 U.S. states. *Disaster Med. Public Health Prep.* 3(2 Suppl.): S29–S36.

Wamala, J.F., C. Okot, I. Makumbi et al. 2010. Assessment of core capacities for the International Health Regulations (IHR [2005])—Uganda, 2009. *BMC Public Health* 10(Suppl. 1): S9.

Weber, I.B. 2007. Evaluation of the notifiable disease surveillance system in Gauteng Province, South Africa. MMed dissertation, University of Pretoria, Pretoria, South Africa. Accessed March 17, 2014. http://upetd.up.ac.za/thesis/available/etd-07302008-141155/.

World Health Organization (WHO). 2001a. Integrated disease surveillance in the African region: Regional strategy for communicable diseases 1999–2003. Accessed March 17, 2014. http://whqlibdoc.who.int/afro/2001/AFR_RC_48_8.pdf.

World Health Organization (WHO). 2001b. Revision of the International Health Regulations. Progress report, February 2001. *Wkly. Epidemiol. Rec.* 76: 61–63.

World Health Organization (WHO). 2003a. Documentation of integrated disease surveillance and response implementation in the African and Eastern Mediterranean regions. Accessed March 17, 2014. http://whqlibdoc.who.int/hq/2003/WHO_CDS_CSR_LYO_2003_5_eng.pdf.

World Health Organization (WHO). 2003b. Implementing integrated disease surveillance and response. *Wkly. Epidemiol. Rec.* 78(27): 229–240.

World Health Organization (WHO). 2005. Global consultation on strengthening national capacities for surveillance and control of communicable diseases. World Health Organization.

Accessed March 17, 2014. http://whqlibdoc.who.int/hq/2005/WHO_CDS_CSR_LYO_2005_18_eng.pdf.

World Health Organization (WHO). 2014. International Health Regulations implementation: Global outbreak alert and response operations. Accessed March 14, 2014. http://www.who.int/ihr/about/02_Global_Outbreak.pdf.

World Health Organization (WHO). Notification and other reporting requirements under the IHR (2005). Accessed March 14, 2014. http://www.who.int/ihr/publications/ihr_brief_no_2_en.pdf.

Wuhib, T., T.L. Chorba, V. Davidiants, W.R. Mac Kenzie, and S.J. McNabb. 2002. Assessment of the infectious diseases surveillance system of the Republic of Armenia: An example of surveillance in the Republics of the former Soviet Union. *BMC Public Health* 2: 3.

Ziemann A., N. Rosenkotter, L. G-C. Riesgo et al. 2015. Meeting the International Health Regulations (2005) surveillance core capacity requirements at the subnational level in Europe: the added value of syndromic surveillance. *BMC Public Health* 15: 107.

4

Surveillance challenges in resource-limited settings

KAREN SAYLORS

Disease surveillance in emerging infectious disease hotspot regions of the world is essential to early disease detection and pandemic disease prevention.

BACKGROUND

Surveillance for emerging infectious diseases in human and animal populations is a global health imperative and represents an enormous challenge to government authorities, particularly in resource-limited settings (King et al. 2006; Keusch et al. 2009). Despite widespread agreement on the need for coordinated surveillance activities that unite public health and animal health objectives, there are few examples of surveillance programs that utilize expertise from both sectors and attempt to simultaneously monitor both clinical disease and animal disease outbreaks. Public agencies dedicated to human and animal health have different stakeholders, and disease control objectives for protecting human health and the livelihood of animal producers are often in conflict, resulting in competition rather than cooperation (Jones et al. 2008).

Despite challenges in coordination between animal and human health agencies, there is international recognition of the need for consistent surveillance that is globally linked, whereby disease outbreaks are immediately reported and responded to, both to contain their spread and to communicate about circulating transmissible agents at a global scale.

The purpose of a public health surveillance system is to ensure that problems of public health importance are monitored and managed efficiently and effectively and to be able to respond quickly to public health threats (e.g., outbreaks of emerging infectious diseases and bioterrorism). Consistent with the Centers for Disease Control's Guidelines (2001), a surveillance system must address: (a) the integration of surveillance and health information systems, (b) the establishment of data standards, (c) the electronic exchange of health data, (d) changes in the objectives of public health surveillance to facilitate the response of public health to emerging health threats (e.g., new diseases), and (e) a communications infrastructure built on principles of public health informatics, including agreements on data access, sharing, and confidentiality. Such ongoing, systematic monitoring of health-related data is intended to be used to develop a toolbox of potential public health responses to be used in responsive action to outbreak events or in high prevalence/incidence situations to reduce morbidity and mortality and to generally improve population health. In order to assure outbreak response readiness, a surveillance system must constantly measure the burden of disease, including understanding changes in health factors, identification and knowledge of high-risk populations and emerging health trends or concerns, and be able to detect changes in health practices or incidence early in the process. In resource-rich settings, a surveillance system necessarily engages commitments to the allocation of resources to eventual outbreaks or public health crises, but in resource-limited settings, public policy around disease surveillance may be in place, but necessary financial commitments may not be available or may not be designated for public health response in the case of an epidemic.

Each country's public health network must define what constitutes a public health risk in the local landscape to determine what diseases need regular monitoring. Health-related events that affect many persons or that require large expenditures of resources are most often considered of public health importance. However, health-related events that affect few persons might also be important, especially if the events cluster in time and place (e.g., a limited outbreak of a severe disease). There are various standardized measures that help with the prioritization of diseases, such as indicators of frequency (total number of cases and/or deaths, incidence/prevalence rates, or quality-adjusted life years [QALYs] or disability-adjusted life years [DALYs]), severity indicators, evaluation of health disparity or access to care related to a specific disease, or cost of treatment of a specific disease. However, in many cases of resource-limited settings, such evaluation measures are not in place or consistently tracked, so the World Health Organization (WHO) has mandated certain diseases of significant risk to public health be reportable through the International Health Regulations 2005 requirements. Generally, a country's ministry of health works with the WHO to define approximately 20–25 reportable diseases that will be tracked through the local surveillance system. One challenge is that such surveillance approaches are usually passive, relying on usually irregular weekly reporting of clinical cases, most of which are suspected reportable disease findings and not lab-confirmed diagnoses. In cases of a disease that is considered virulent enough for active monitoring (e.g., Ebola), if someone has died or the illness severity is such that a person has sought medical care and the symptoms sound the alarm based on standard clinical definitions, suspected cases may be followed up on by a clinical or epidemiology team in order to control the spread of infection. This type of active surveillance response varies from country to country, depending on resource availability and the stage and sophistication of the surveillance system in place, the quality and extent of laboratory facilities in the country, and the funds available for follow-up of the disease incident.

THE NEED FOR STANDARDIZED CLINICAL CASE DEFINITIONS

One challenge of being able to conduct consistent surveillance is variance in case reporting due to a lack of standardized case definitions of certain reportable or neglected tropical diseases. In addition to the challenge of sometimes inconsistent provincial- or district-level disease reporting, there is often enormous variance in clinical case definition, exacerbated by a lack of lab infrastructure in many resource-limited settings, resulting in an absence of lab confirmation. One example of the challenge of case definitions is the case of buruli ulcer (BU), a chronic, indolent necrotizing disease of the skin and underlying tissues caused by *Mycobacterium ulcerans*, which belongs to the same family of organisms that causes tuberculosis and leprosy. In 2002, Médecins Sans Frontières (MSF) opened a BU treatment program in Cameroon in collaboration with the Ministry of Health's national disease control program. In March 2007, MSF conducted a cross-sectional study in one health district in the most endemic region of Cameroon to (1) estimate the prevalence of BU in the target population of the project, (2) estimate the proportion of BU cases visiting the MSF project at least once (coverage), and (3) estimate the proportion of patients visiting another service provider such as a traditional healer or peripheral health center at least once (health-seeking behavior). We also aimed to describe the spatial distribution of the prevalence as well as that of health seeking behavior to help target the most affected areas and to address access problems for certain communities (Porten et al. 2009).

Determining BU prevalence is challenging, and difficulties include undiagnosed cases due to fears of stigmatization, little knowledge of the disease among both the population and health workers, and variability in clinical presentation of the disease. Furthermore, BU occurs primarily in remote rural areas where the population has limited access to health care. Although BU is a notifiable disease in Cameroon, such reporting rarely happens at the health district level. In the course of the Akonolinga cross-sectional study, health delegates worked with local health clinics and traditional healers and went door-to-door to identify suspected BU cases. In working with health professionals across the district, people with many other types of ulcers and skin diseases were identified, making it clear that standardized clinical case definitions for BU were not well known, even in an area of disease endemicity. In the context of the BU study, the lesion was inspected, measured, and categorized according to clinical criteria using the clinical case definitions by the study team, which was made up of one doctor/nurse experienced in BU, one medical assistant, and one interviewer who performed the consultations and interviews at the central screening location.

LIMITED LAB CAPACITY IN LOW-RESOURCE AREAS

Another challenge faced by this public hospital (and many others like it) was the fact that there was no laboratory confirmation process for determining the exact identity of the disease agent. Suspected BU samples were sent weekly to the Centre Pasteur de Cameroun, the reference lab in the capital city 2 hours away, in order to identify and confirm BU cases. A lack of lab infrastructure is common in most clinical settings in low-resource countries,

and as a result, many surveillance systems are based only on suspected and not confirmed case reporting. In cases where samples are sent to a reference lab, whether in the same city, another city, or even another country, confirmed laboratory diagnoses do not always get captured accurately or in a timely manner within the surveillance database.

Due to the widely recognized challenge of limited lab capacity in low-resource settings, several U.S. Department of Defense (DoD) organizations have engaged in lab capacity building within foreign military settings, with the goal of enhancing disease surveillance capacity. Through a combination of Armed Forces Health Surveillance Center (AFHSC), Global Emerging Infectious Disease Surveillance (GEIS) funding and the DoD HIV/AIDS Prevention Program (DHAPP), the Cameroon military has been able to renovate the capital city's military hospital bacteriology lab, and using Foreign Military Financing available through the U.S. embassy, equipment and supplies have been purchased to furnish the renovated lab. This lab now supports sexually transmitted infectious disease surveillance efforts, including HIV testing and treatment monitoring and an antibiotic-resistant gonorrhea study. In addition, through support from AFHSC-GEIS, the Military Health Research Centre (CRESAR) laboratory facility at the Yaoundé army base was renovated in 2008–2009, to include both human and animal sample processing laboratories. The renovation allowed for necessary facility improvements, specifically a 2000 L water backup tank, a 250 kVA automatic-switch generator, and a liquid nitrogen plant. Also available are −80°C freezers, an automatic temperature-monitoring system, and certified biosafety cabinets. These system improvements have allowed for field surveillance, sample storage, and lab analyses of both human and zoonotic influenza, efforts that have been ongoing since 2009. Standardizing surveillance reporting is in place for sentinel sites across Cameroon, allowing for the monitoring of seasonality effects and viral subtyping, in a global effort to prevent the emergence of pandemic strains of influenza.

Not having clinical services and laboratory diagnostic capacities co-located means greater reliance on human medical expertise and consistent clinical case definitions. Having a human-skills-reliant system necessitates regular training of medical service professionals and regular review of standardized case definitions that are clear and simple, that are based on criteria (clinical, biological, epidemiological), and that may include well-defined classification (possible, probable, confirmed) and TPP (time–place–person) information. When setting up a new surveillance system, education and discussion around clinical case definitions must be integrated into the training and engagement phase of system users to assure that case reporting is not all over the map.

ONGOING INFECTIOUS DISEASE MONITORING

Although public health infrastructures, specifically ministries of health, in resource-limited settings may attempt to establish exhaustive surveillance efforts, such as cancer registries and notifiable disease reporting, such systems are not actually exhaustive, usually because of resource limitations. Public health surveillance in such settings is often event based and reactive in response to a concerning health event, rather than based on automated technologies that monitor health-related information in a daily or weekly manner. An exhaustive surveillance effort requires standardized data collection that is rarely observed or possible in low-resource settings. Additionally, information dissemination about health events to health authorities is not always efficient or consistent, and with breaks in the communication chain, the surveillance system stalls (Velasco et al. 2014). However, with changing technological and social media paradigms, and with the availability of open-source software, basic surveillance systems that could function in resource-limited settings are becoming more viable.

INFORMATION TECHNOLOGY CHALLENGES

In low-resource settings, especially in central Africa, one of the main challenges of surveillance is the lack of information technology (IT) infrastructure. Often, the ministerial hierarchy in power in much of central Africa does not invest in a centralized IT platform that could support a surveillance system. Government public health agencies tend to avoid the fiscal investment: paying the necessary upfront hardware and software costs and the required long-term maintenance and support costs, whether because of a lack of funding or because surveillance is not considered a high

priority. When international investors show interest in offering surveillance architecture options to ministry leaders, the consistent problems are maintenance, system oversight, and, at the end of the funding cycle, sustainability.

PILOTING AN OPEN-SOURCE ELECTRONIC SURVEILLANCE SYSTEM IN CAMEROON

From 2012 to 2014, Metabiota (formerly Global Viral Forecasting Incorporated) and its central Africa nongovernmental organization counterpart, Global Viral (GV), worked with AFHSC-GEIS and the Johns Hopkins University Applied Physics Laboratory to conduct a pilot study of the Suite for Automated Global Electronic bioSurveillance (SAGES) project, in collaboration with the Cameroonian Ministry of Defense and Ministry of Health, to explore possible uses of the SAGES tools for creating an electronic disease surveillance system in Cameroon. Metabiota and GV worked with identified partners at the Ministry of Defense, Ministry of Justice, and Ministry of Health to conduct a needs assessment, to collect information on possible system architectures for disease surveillance, to provide technical assistance for disease surveillance, and to advocate for the integration of this task force in country. The task assigned Metabiota and GV as the technical implementing partner was to conduct IT, public health, and clinical capacity assessment for Cameroon military health facilities in the countries, and these assessments were to be used to establish an advocacy plan for integrating SAGES into military surveillance efforts.

After advocating for and securing Ministry of Defense military health buy-in, the technical team focused on the reinforcement of the military health surveillance network, with the goal of providing technical assistance to facilitate infectious disease surveillance using SAGES in Cameroon. This new technology was intended to build the capacity of military health professionals and establish better tools for surveillance data acquisition, thereby facilitating data sharing among network partners. The project was intended to provide Military-Civilian-Military aid to the Cameroonian military in order to bring their public health reporting system into closer alignment with the International Health Regulations, 2005 (IHR 2005) requirements, as mandated by the WHO. The Cameroon

Ministry of Health has outlined 23 reportable diseases that are to be tracked through this electronic surveillance system.

During the course of the SAGES project, there have been numerous challenges with implementing the electronic biosurveillance system in Cameroon. One ongoing issue has been the need for our civilian technical team to provide regular IT support to military data entry personnel, to interface with the software developers to install remotely provided updates and system patches, and to troubleshoot. These technically complex tasks would have been impossible for the military team to accomplish on its own, which would have stalled the project and prevented regular disease surveillance from occurring. This type of feedback is critical to the development team. As a result, newer versions of the SAGES software simplify some of the application-specific IT tasks, allowing them to be performed by non-IT personnel. However, the ability to provide routine system patches to the hardware on which the application is installed will remain an issue without the appropriate IT workforce. Another challenge within the military team was the regular turnover of staff assigned to the hospital-based disease tracking and data entry at the four implementation sites: Yaoundé, Bertoua, Ebolowa, and Douala. This resulted in a regular need for retraining and reconfiguring work teams, which led to inconsistent data capture.

Another challenge with maintaining an electronic biosurveillance system within the military health system was the commitment required from the military hierarchy for active supervision of the data collection/entry team in order for the system to be successful. This military buy-in is required at multiple levels—from the Direction of Military Health as a superstructure as well as from military leadership at each military hospital or clinic site—in order for daily data capture to be conducted and proactively monitored for problems.

An ongoing challenge has been end-user engagement: encouraging the clinical directors and the military hierarchy to use the system, to be responsive to the system's alerts and proactively investigate the nature of the signaled outbreak in order to understand whether there is an actual public health risk or some reporting erraticism. As Metabiota approaches the end of its technical assistance pilot phase, the sustainability test will be whether the military hierarchy assumes ownership of the project and continues to use the biosurveillance system.

The mechanical aspects of the handover will be assured, as the server and equipment will be transferred to the Direction of Military Health, but whether engagement with daily or weekly notifiable disease tracking will be maintained, and greater still, whether the IT dimension of engaged support will be consistently continued, remains to be seen.

An additional challenge is that in resource-limited settings, there are often few IT technicians because although some individuals may have gone to school or held technical internships in developed countries, there is often a problem of "brain drain" whereby highly trained intellectuals often immigrate to more developed countries where jobs are more plentiful and pay is higher than at home, so the "best and brightest" often end up leaving their home countries for job opportunities.

Another issue that often arises is that when a system infrastructure is put in place and hardware is distributed, individuals in power sometimes decide that the server, laptops, or cell phones designated for surveillance data collection and analysis would be better used for personal or administrative purposes, effectively disassembling the surveillance infrastructure.

A FRAMEWORK FOR A SUCCESSFUL INFORMATION TECHNOLOGY APPROACH

Despite the challenge of having a comprehensive, functional IT platform that spans regional, provincial, or national levels, resource-constrained settings are in great need of surveillance coverage. By adhering to a simple system architecture and sticking with realistic data reporting, a basic surveillance system can be created and maintained. The key is simplicity, assuring the system utilizes inexpensive and accessible technology such as electronic media (e-mails, websites, and cell phones [texts] or fax, if available) and is

- Reliable and fast
- Low frequency (requiring only daily, weekly, or monthly input)
- Secure
- Regular, punctual, and exhaustive

The success of such a system requires that technologically savvy early adopters advocate for it and that the leadership in power buy into and support the concept, cost of implementation, and human resources mandatory for its long-term continuation.

SUSTAINABILITY

Surveillance systems require extensive and regular funding to maintain consistent data, and often such systems are difficult to sustain in resource-limited settings. In the central African Congo Basin, which is considered an infectious disease hotspot because of the regular emergence of a large number of pathogenic agents there—notably known hemorrhagic fevers and fevers of unknown origin—there is a pressing need to assure that both animal and human disease outbreaks are monitored and controlled to avoid spread to larger populations.

SENTINEL SURVEILLANCE SYSTEMS

As described previously, sentinel surveillance systems are used when high-quality data are needed about a particular disease but cannot be obtained through a passive reporting system. Whereas passive systems usually received data from a large number of health facilities, a sentinel system involves only a limited number of carefully selected reporting sites (WHO 2014), usually with the aim of being representative of the larger population or in areas where there is high prevalence or incidence of a specific disease. Sentinel surveillance often focuses on high-frequency diseases (e.g., seasonal flu), occupationally exposed individuals, and high-risk key populations (e.g., sex workers, military) in order to signal trends and monitor the burden of disease in these communities, which often serve as precursors to disease trends in the general population.

ZOONOTIC DISEASE MONITORING

Since 2010, USAID has supported a consortium of research organizations in the concurrent monitoring of human outbreaks and animal die-offs through the Emerging Pandemic Threats (EPT) PREDICT program. Systematic surveillance of high-risk animal-to-animal and animal-to-human priority pathogens of known epidemic and unknown pandemic potential has been ongoing in "geographic hotspot regions" (Jones et al. 2008) in an effort to shift the emerging infectious disease prevention and surveillance paradigm. In a retrospective analysis of outbreaks of new diseases over the past 50 years, zoonotic pathogens

have been found to be most concentrated in lower-latitude regions of tropical Africa, Asia, and Latin America, with intense concentrations in the Congo Basin, the Gangetic and Indus River plains of India, eastern China and southeast Asia, the Niger Delta in West Africa, and the Rift Valley region of East Africa. PREDICT conducts sentinel surveillance in these regions in the hope that in better characterizing dangerous pathogens, actively monitoring animal reservoirs, better understanding amplification mechanisms for viruses that may jump the animal–human barrier, and efficiently targeting behavioral change interventions aimed at human behaviors that amplify disease transmission, this targeted global sentinel surveillance effort may minimize zoonotic disease spillover, amplification, and spread.

An example of successful regional coordination efforts recently occurred in relation to a monkeypox* outbreak among chimpanzees in a primate reserve in eastern Cameroon. For many years, monkeypox has been a reportable and actively monitored human disease in the Democratic Republic of Congo, although the animal vector has not been clearly identified. This disease has been loosely associated with animal die-offs, but the surveillance focus in the Democratic Republic of Congo has been primarily on humans. In July 2014, there were suspect cases of pox-virus infection among chimpanzees at a rescue center in Cameroon. The Ministry of Health, Ministry of Forest and Fauna (Wildlife), and Ministry of Fisheries, Livestock and Animal Production (MINIPIA) worked with GV/PREDICT to collect diagnostic samples, which were transferred to the CRESAR-Ministry of Defense lab to test for pox-viruses, as chimps had shown symptoms consistent with orthopox-virus. Real-time Polymerase Chain Reaction (PCR) assays specific for monkeypox were received from the National Institutes of Health/National Institute of Allergy and Infectious Diseases and tested in the GV PREDICT lab, and analyses indicated the presence of the Congo Basin strain of monkeypox virus. The rapid response to this outbreak was remarkable and demonstrates the importance of multisectorial collaboration and open communication among partners, as well as strong field surveillance and laboratory diagnostics, for a successful surveillance system to function in resource-limited settings.

* Administrative communication from GV PREDICT to Cameroon Ministry of Health, July 2014.

SOCIO-CULTURAL CHALLENGES OF DISEASE SURVEILLANCE

Often the disease surveillance and outbreak response systems that international agencies put in place come into direct conflict with a local population's social or cultural beliefs, norms, and perceptions of illness. With pandemic diseases like HIV, where transmission routes are multiple and may not be clearly understood, there is often misinformation and accusations that Western governments or international nonprofits are infecting people with HIV when they come for HIV prevention and surveillance efforts. Conspiracy theories are often circulated in local populations about donated condoms being infected with HIV, and this is cited as a reason for individuals not protecting themselves during sex. This phenomenon is often associated with surveillance efforts: when foreigners come into resource-limited settings, there is suspicion of and hesitation toward outsiders, especially if they are introducing novel ideas or technology that may be new or even contradictory to a local population's cultural or religious worldview.

When organizations like the WHO or MSF come into a country in response to an outbreak, they must be extremely sensitive to the local perceptions of their arrival, especially when they are outfitted in personal protective devices (PPDs). During the 1994–1995 Ebola outbreak in remote villages in Gabon's Ogooué-Ivindo Province (Georges et al. 1999), local people were terrified when a WHO responder came into the village already wearing their PPD. Although the WHO employee was following protocol to avoid contagion, locals thought that an alien from outer space had descended to bring infection to their village (qualitative interviews conducted by author, 2012). This impression persisted for some time, and as a result, preventative messages to curb the spread of Ebola in the village, where burial practices were spreading the disease among family members, were not listened to. Ebola is most contagious in a human body when the body has just died, and many family members were infected by hugging and washing the corpses of relatives. After this experience, WHO adjusted their protocol for bringing PPD to the village, allowing the outbreak response team to meet the local population before suiting up.

International outbreak response organizations must communicate clearly with local populations to explain what they are doing and why. Without such early and frank communication, there is often misperception and a distorted idea of what such agencies are doing in the country. In the case of the 2014–2015 Ebola outbreak in West Africa, there is a local perception that international nonprofit organizations are bringing the disease to intentionally infect the local population. Especially in Guinea, where in the early months of the outbreak there were more than twice as many deaths as in neighboring Sierra Leone and Liberia, aid group staff from Doctors without Borders and the Red Cross were threatened with knives, stones, and machetes, with the local population saying, "Wherever those people have passed, the communities have been hit by illness" (Nossiter 2014). Such a response is based on the fear and panic that people feel in an outbreak situation, but it has roots in a wariness of outsiders, a strong belief in traditional religion, and a reliance on traditional healers rather than Western medicine. One village chief said, "We are absolutely afraid, and that is why we are avoiding contact with everybody, the whole world. We do not accept their [aid organizations] presence at all. They are the transporters of the virus in these communities" (Nossiter 2014). The fact that medical teams wear head-to-toe suits and masks, burning them after use, exacerbates fear levels even further. Clear communication about the purpose of PPDs and an explanation of aid organizations' strategies are fundamental in attempting to alleviate the fear and misinformation associated with outbreak response.

After more than a year of Ebola raging through West Africa, and with more than 11,134 deaths since February 2014, fear, mistrust, and mob mentality have driven people to flee the Ministry of Health holding centers into dense communities in Liberia, Sierra Leone, and Guinea, creating a difficult public health situation. The Ebola crisis in particular is "overwhelming inadequate public health systems already battling common deadly diseases such as malaria," according to the AFP (Dosso and Fowler 2014). Fear and distrust of outside doctors are prevalent in the West Africa region, and in Liberia, rumors of cannibalism and people being drained of their blood in Ebola clinics is leading to violence. Health workers say that "the testimony of survivors is crucial to proving the myths wrong" (Dosso and Fowler 2014) because it reinforces the importance of engaging the local community to understand and negotiate the nuances of socio-cultural and traditional/religious beliefs in surveillance and outbreak situations.

Surveillance and outbreak response efforts require clear and early communication with the local village chiefs, administrative prefects, and rural communities, to describe the approach and to enroll their assistance with passing on behavioral change messages. It is only by engaging local populations to help them understand the importance of the surveillance effort or outbreak response approach and involving them in the work that those populations will adjust their behaviors to better protect themselves from disease exposure or transmission risks.

HIV POINT PREVALENCE STUDIES ACROSS CENTRAL AFRICA

Through DHAPP funding, Metabiota and GV have conducted HIV/syphilis surveillance and research in the central African region since 2000, focusing on HIV testing, sample collection, and lab testing, in pursuit of generating improved military and public health data in central Africa and within the global HIV research community. Metabiota has been influential in the development of HIV research and prevention programs that have provided information on the genetic diversity of HIV, prevalence statistics, and the behavioral risks associated with the spread of the disease in key populations in central Africa. In particular, we have conducted regular surveillance of HIV and syphilis in the military in eight central African countries (Cameroon, Central African Republic, Chad, Democratic Republic of Congo, Equatorial Guinea, Gabon, Republic of Congo, and São Tomé and Príncipe) every 3–4 years, providing point prevalence data for all eight countries.

In terms of awareness raising and engagement, between 2002 and 2010, Metabiota conducted advocacy campaigns in the region that were initially focused on sensitizing military high commands to the importance of HIV prevention and the necessity of supporting health programs for servicemen and women. In a region where military health is one of the least funded branches of the armed forces and often there is limited interaction between ministry of health and ministry of defense officials regarding jurisdiction of health care, the sensitization was imperative for regional surveillance of HIV. Through strategic campaigning and

partnership throughout central Africa, Metabiota's advocacy eventually led to authorization to provide technical assistance to central African militaries for the implementation of HIV prevention and surveillance activities, the development of military HIV prevention programs, and the gathering of baseline information on the disease's circulation in the region. Through this program, we have provided more than 17,000 military men and women with voluntary HIV counseling and testing services, and a cumulative number of 140,000 military men and women have received health education messages. Moreover, in a region where health statistics are difficult to obtain, the prevalence rates provided through these studies in all eight countries have established a baseline of HIV prevalence rates in military and most-at-risk populations (MARPs), such as sex workers and men who have sex with men (MSM), significantly aiding civilian public health interventions. The importance of formative research and strong collaboration is paramount in working with sentinel high-risk key populations. Conducting regular surveillance with these key populations allows for monitoring of different emerging infectious disease trends and behavioral risk factors at the country and regional levels.

PUBLIC HEALTH IMPLICATIONS OF SURVEILLANCE IN UNDER-RESOURCED SETTINGS

Based on Alexander Langmuir's (1963) definition, public health surveillance is the ongoing, systematic collection, analysis, interpretation, and dissemination of data regarding a health-related event for use in public health action to reduce morbidity and mortality and to improve health (CDC, 2001). Specific to dissemination, public health surveillance data must be presented to relevant target groups to facilitate their use in real-life contexts and for appropriate outbreak containment efforts (Goodman et al. 2000). Key target groups include public health practitioners; health-care providers; professional, volunteer, and international health organizations; and policy makers. One major challenge with often-disjointed surveillance efforts in resource-limited settings is the tendency to over- or under-report to satisfy mandated quotas, as often happens with vaccination campaigns in rural areas, and the impetus to hide or compensate for coverage or performance gaps is detrimental to the larger goal of a comprehensive and standardized surveillance effort. In informal systems where data are often collected with pen and paper records, and data documentation is often a postscript effort after clinical care has been provided, there are regular breakdowns in the communication chain, making timely data dissemination or public health response quite difficult.

CHALLENGES WITH REAL-TIME EPIDEMIOLOGICAL ANALYSIS AND FEEDBACK

Ideally, in the case of a reportable disease incident, each health service level (facility, district, province, etc.) should rapidly analyze the data received and initiate action within the framework of pre-set standard procedures, but reporting up the chain should not be delayed (WHO 2008). The central surveillance team should prepare summary epidemiological reports of overall findings and recommendations for action and immediately present them to the national authorities; disseminate them quickly to local authorities and organizations involved in public health activities; and once an action plan is decided upon with local health authorities, provide feedback to the reporting units. In an organized, well defined system, such an ideal analysis and dissemination plan could occur, but in overtaxed public health systems in resource-limited settings, even though the will and effort to monitor and control public health crises are usually present, limited funds and human resources often make high-level operational implementation unrealizable.

THE CHALLENGE OF ENGAGING STAKEHOLDERS

In order for surveillance networks to work, stakeholders must be engaged and take advocacy roles from the beginning of the effort. Stakeholders are people or organizations who use data for the promotion of healthy lifestyles and the prevention and control of disease, injury, or adverse exposure. In a sophisticated and evolved surveillance system, engaged public health stakeholders might be interested in defining questions to be addressed by the surveillance system evaluation to test efficacy or data quality. However, in real-life situations in resource-constrained settings, data findings are generally used by public health practitioners: health-care providers; data collectors and users; representatives of affected communities; governments at the local, state, and federal levels; and professional and private nonprofit organizations. Stakeholders can provide input and political advocacy to ensure that the public health surveillance system addresses appropriate questions and assesses pertinent attributes and that its findings will be acceptable and implementable. The challenge of engaging stakeholders is identifying individuals or organizations that have the financial and administrative capacity for advocating for the prolonged maintenance of a surveillance system, as well as the political will to do so.

An essential part of the equation for the success of a surveillance network is regular and strategic communication with public health stakeholders. Communication must be systematic and regular, such as a weekly report on health status of population. Surveillance communication must also be adapted for a variety of target audiences, including policy decisions makers, public media, and public health actors in hospitals and clinics, as well as for other professionals in outbreak response situations. Public health surveillance messaging is most powerful when it is communicated briefly and succinctly to public health practitioners who can disseminate it appropriately and in the proper context, based on the urgency of the public health situation.

CONCLUSION

Granted, setting up and maintaining surveillance networks and systems in low-resource settings has its challenges, especially with so many immediate and deadly public health concerns burdening the public health clinics and hospitals that field medical crises and whose medical personnel often detect outbreaks first. In many developing regions of the world, economic hindrances force public health and international aid agencies to prioritize surveillance and disease outbreaks as they can, with endemic, debilitating diseases, like malaria, tuberculosis, or cholera, often taking precedence. With the chronic problem of "brain drain" in Africa and many developing countries, where promising young scientists, doctors, or systems administrators seek brighter futures elsewhere, workforce issues remain a constant challenge in developing world settings. Despite these challenges and those discussed earlier, there is a growing understanding and appreciation of the advantages of proactive tracking of reportable diseases, especially as our world becomes increasingly interconnected by air travel and regional road systems that are constantly built up and reinforced by extractive industry interested in moving lumber, coal, and other natural resources toward the West. One of the repercussions of our global advancement toward more interconnected systems, with international markets and trade, nearly universal Internet and cell phone coverage, easier migration, and global transport, is the very real issue of diseases migrating with us, introducing illness that might have once been endemic to a small region to a much more global scale. As we live in this interconnected reality, we must proactively develop a global disease surveillance network where we communicate among ourselves about emerging disease risks and trends, tracking alerts and concerns at an international level. As we have seen with the 2014 Ebola crisis, the problems faced in resource-limited settings quickly become all of our concern in this global public health system where all of our health is interconnected. It is important to recognize that the trend in public health in resource-limited settings is encouraging. "One lesson learned from recent successes against AIDS, malaria and TB is that victory comes only when the whole infrastructure of health, including the active involvement of local people, is promoted. In epidemics, even more than in individual cases of disease, prevention is far, far better than cure" (Unseating the First Horseman 2014). So, as a global community of public health professions, we continue efforts to vigilantly monitor and prevent the emergence of the next public health crisis.

REFERENCES

Centers for Disease Control. 2001. Guidelines for evaluating public health surveillance systems. *Morb. Mortal. Wkly. Rep.* 50(RR13): 1–35.

Dosso, Z. and J. Fowler. August 20, 2014. Liberia imposes curfew as Ebola crisis grows. Agence France-Presse.

Georges, A.-J., E.M. Leroy, A.A. Renaut et al. 1999. Ebola hemorrhagic fever outbreaks in Gabon, 1994–1997: Epidemiologic and health control issues. *J. Infect. Dis.* 179(Suppl. 1): S65–S75.

Global Epidemiological Surveillance Standards for Influenza. 2013. World Health Organization. WHO Press, Geneva, Switzerland.

Goodman, R.A., P.L. Remington, and R.J. Howard. 2000. Communicating information for action within the public health system. In S. Teutsch and R.E. Churchill (eds.), *Principles and Practices of Public Health Surveillance.* Oxford University Press, p. 168.

Jones, K.E., N.G. Patel, M.A. Levy, A. Storeygard, D. Balk, J.L. Gittleman, and P. Daszak. 2008. Global trends in emerging infectious diseases. *Nature* 451(7181): 990–993.

Keusch, G.T., M. Pappaioanou, M.C. Gonzalez, K.A. Scott, and P. Tsai (eds.). 2009. *Sustaining Global Surveillance and Response to Emerging Zoonotic Diseases.* Washington, DC: The National Academies Press.

Key Elements for Planning a Health Information/ Surveillance System. 2008. Managing WHO humanitarian response in the field—Annexes, June 27, pp. 92–94. http://www.who.int/hac/techguidance/tools/annexes.pdf.

King, D.A., C. Peckham, J.L. Waage, J. Brownlie, and M.E. Woolhouse. 2006. Epidemiology. Infectious diseases: Preparing for the future. *Science* 313(5792): 1392–1393.

Langmuir, A.D. 1963. The surveillance of communicable diseases of national importance. *N. Engl. J. Med.* 268: 182–192.

New York Times, The (NYT). (2014b). Those Who Serve Ebola Victims Soldier On. Adam Nossiter and Ben C. Solomonaug. Aug 23, 2014. Accessed October 6, 2014. http://www.nytimes.com/2014/08/24/world/africa/sierra-leone-if-they-survive-in-ebola-ward-they-work-on.html?_r=0.

Porten, K., K. Saylors, E. Comte et al. 2009. Prevalence of Buruli ulcer in Akonolinga Health District, Cameroon: Results of a cross sectional survey. *PLoS Neglect. Trop. Dis.* 3(6): e466.

Unseating the first horseman: The price of global health is eternal vigilance. The Economist, August 16, 2014. http://www.economist.com/news/leaders/21612155-price-global-health-eternal-vigilance-unseating-first-horseman.

Velasco, E., T. Agheneza, K. Denecke, G. Kirchner, and T. Eckmanns. 2014. Social media and internet-based data in global systems for public health surveillance: A systematic review. *Milbank Quart.* 92(1): 7–33.

World Health Organization. 2008. *International Health Regulations (2005)*, pp.74. ISBN: 9789241580410.

5

The role and functional components of statistical alerting methods for biosurveillance

HOWARD S. BURKOM

ANALYSIS CONTEXT

This chapter discusses analytical tools for prospective disease surveillance. We first establish the practical context of these tools and present them not as isolated mathematical methods, but as part of a multi-step process beginning with a monitored population whose true, instantaneous disease levels cannot be known. Figure 5.1 illustrates this process schematically. The health department or other monitoring institution routinely collects data streams believed to be useful for detecting and tracking outbreaks and other health events of interest. The data streams are aggregated and filtered in an attempt to highlight these events (Burkom et al. 2004). Prospective surveillance systems are intended to summarize information from these data streams for rapid comprehension by human monitoring staffs with limited time for analysis and investigation.

For these systems, the role of analytical methods is to summarize for quick understanding by a limited human staff the current, relevant health concerns of this population. Concerns that are relevant depend on the monitoring institution and recent pathogenic threats. Early electronic surveillance systems were mainly concerned with human outbreaks of infectious disease with emphasis on bioterrorism detection, based primarily on Emergency Department patient record data (Lombardo et al. 2003; Mandl et al. 2004). As of 2015, current systems are increasingly designed with an all-hazards approach including surveillance for chronic disease risk factors (Berkelman and Buehler 1990), toxic exposures (Law et al. 2014), and livestock outbreaks (Vial and Berezowski 2015). However, useful analytics require information relevant to threats of interest.

Among the features of Figure 5.1, this chapter deals with (a) the filtering of the data streams to

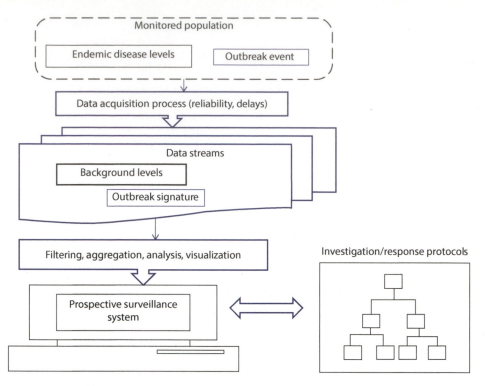

Figure 5.1 Schematic of biosurveillance context.

capture as much of a presumed outbreak signature and as little of the background and systematic noise as possible and (b) analytic methods to recognize and characterize an outbreak signal sooner and more clearly than possible without the analytics. The discussion below omits research areas focusing on the top of the figure, such as population-based disease transmission models or agent-based models tracking the behavior of individuals (Burke et al. 2006; Jiang and Cooper 2010; Dawson et al. 2015). While these areas have potential for public health planning and decision support for institutions, sections below focus on the process-driven environment of the health monitor routinely working with data. Also not covered are data acquisition and cleaning processes, visualization techniques, and investigation/response protocols. However, without reliable acquisition processes producing quality input data, outputs of subsequent analytic methods have little value; and without user-friendly visualization and adequate response protocols, these outputs have little purpose. In some instances, analysis methods can adjust for known data behavior issues such as systematic late reporting and reporting bias, and techniques are summarized below. An evaluation of utility of a disease surveillance system should consider all features of Figure 5.1.

To provide the proper perspective on using alerting algorithms for surveillance system users, the Suite for Automated Global Electronic bioSurveillance (SAGES) system (Lewis et al. 2011) provides the following online guidance:

General considerations for use and interpretation of statistical alerting methods include the following:

1. These methods are not intended to positively identify outbreaks without supporting evidence. Their purpose is to direct the attention of a limited monitoring staff with increasingly complex data streams to data features that merit further investigation. They have also been useful for corroboration of clinical suspicions, rumor control, tracking of known or suspected outbreaks, monitoring of special events and health effects of severe weather, and other locally important aspects of situational awareness. Successful users value these methods mainly for the latter purposes and do not base public

health responses solely on algorithm alerts.

2. All of these algorithms are one-sided tests that monitor only for unusually high counts, not low ones. Low counts could result from an emergency situation because data reporting could be interrupted, but there are many common reasons for low counts (such as unscheduled closings or system problems), so the algorithms do not test for abnormally low counts.

3. In addition to data- and disease-specific considerations below, algorithm selection was also driven by system considerations. Users need to monitor many types of data rapidly. External covariates such as climate data or clinic schedules are not available for prompt analysis. Many methods in the literature, armed with substantial retrospective data of a certain type, depend on analysis of substantial history. Day-to-day users, often with only a small fraction of time available for monitoring, will not wait several minutes for each query. In the absence of data history and data-specific analysis time for each stream, these methods have been adapted from the literature and engineered to system requirements.

4. If the time series monitored by algorithms represent many combinations of clinical groupings, age groups, and geographic regions, excessive alerting may occur simply because of multiple testing. For this reason, default alert lists should be limited to results from those time series of concern to the user, either by system design or by active specification by the user. A general method of reducing the default alert list is to restrict algorithms to all-age time series groupings. Depending on the scope of the user's responsibility, the alert list may also be restricted according to both epidemiological interest and the resources available for investigation. For example, a monitor of a national-level system with algorithms applied to many facilities may be interested only in alerts with at least 5–10 cases. In circumstances of heightened concern, these restrictions can be relaxed, or the user can use advanced querying methods to apply algorithms to age groups and/or sub-syndromes.

This guidance was tailored to everyday use of SAGES systems to clarify the role of the analytical methods. Similar guidance is important for appropriate interpretation of algorithmic results in other surveillance systems to achieve practical investigation and reporting procedures.

DATA AGGREGATION AND FILTERING

Necessary for a prospective analytical method to yield useful guidance are consistent data streams appropriate to both the outcome of interest and the capability to investigate and respond. Highlighting the importance of this section, Lescano et al. (2008) noted that in the sometimes neglected "initial implementation stage, epidemiologists should study the completeness and timeliness of the reporting, and describe thoroughly the population surveyed and the epidemiology of the health events recorded" and emphasized that "where too many symptom combinations or other potential outcomes exist and can be surveyed, data analyses can target a few carefully selected outcomes to monitor routinely in order to minimize false positive alerts and avoid an unnecessary burden on public health professionals." Effort must be budgeted and expended to be sure data streams are appropriate and consistent, including both recent data and any historical data to be used for baseline or model-training purposes.

Among the operations required to prepare a data stream for prospective analysis, this chapter omits the nontrivial, often cumbersome tasks of record deduplication and verification of expected data field completeness and formatting (Burkom 2007). Also beyond the chapter scope is removal of bias because input data streams were designed or coded for billing or other purposes, not for surveillance (Ziemann et al. 2012; Triple S-AGE 2015). Relative to detection and tracking of increases in disease incidence or transient outbreaks—the data-independent true population status in Figure 5.1—others sources of bias are changes in diagnosis coding, available treatment, and access to care. For example, vaccination for hepatitis A was recommended for all U.S. children after May 2006, and there was a sharp, sustained drop in reportable cases (CDC Division of Viral Hepatitis 2015). Thus, the pre-2006 reportable levels for baseline values overestimated subsequent prospective levels and were not useful for detection of subsequent outbreaks. Such bias sources can rarely be accounted for in biostatistical models. More systematic bias sources such as cyclical trends and routine clinic schedules are modeled in various ways, as addressed in the next section. We focus here on how time series used as algorithm inputs are derived from cleaned data records. The ability to detect and analyze changes in the data background caused by outbreak-attributable patient records is influenced by data aggregation decisions.

Effect of spatial data aggregation

To begin with spatial aggregation, there is a thematic trade-off in the data window size, as illustrated by Figure 5.2, repeated from Burkom et al. (2008a). Increasing the window better reveals typical patterns and cycles that can be modeled and possibly more outbreak cases, but the added data may also worsen the masking of the outbreak signal. The left half of Figure 5.2 plots counts of daily respiratory-related clinical visits for 3+ years of data on three levels: the entire state, a large treatment facility (with a median daily respiratory visit count exceeding 100), and a small facility (median daily visit count approximately 10). The right side of the figure shows the same data restricted to a single influenza season to distinguish series behavior on a smaller time scale. At the statewide level, visible cyclic features in the time series are amenable to regression modeling, but these features weaken as the spatial scale decreases. Reducing the scale will better distinguish a localized event, but a broader scale is needed to detect an event distributed over a wider population with limited effects in any locality (Parker 1989). Reis et al. have advocated simultaneous surveillance on multiple spatial scales (Reis et al. 2003, 2007), and this umbrella approach must be weighed against Lescano's recommendation to make pragmatic aggregation choices driven by local analysis and investigation capacity (Lescano et al. 2008).

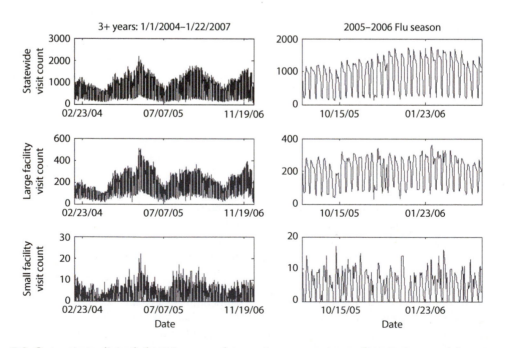

Figure 5.2 Outpatient clinic daily visit counts for respiratory syndrome for varying spatial aggregation and temporal scale.

Effect of temporal aggregation

Before 1990, most surveillance-motivated studies focused on annual or monthly data (Cates et al. 1978; Parker 1989). Since then, growing concerns over the global threat of bioterrorism combined with rapid progress in informatics have pushed health monitoring institutions toward weekly, daily, and increasingly toward real-time monitoring (Mandl et al. 2004).

Increasing the frequency of data monitoring poses analytic challenges. For example, the data underlying the plots in Figure 5.3 come from the accidental anthrax release at Sverdlovsk in 1979. The solid curve shows the number of newly symptomatic cases on each day after the release, with symptoms appearing in the first case on day 4. The dotted and dashed curve shows the numbers of cases at 3-day and 7-day intervals, respectively. Suppose that these values were attributable counts added to a time series of background cases without knowledge of the release. In a stable background, the 7-day aggregation shows the clearest signal with the large peak of 27 cases in the second week. Researchers have modeled epidemic curves with lognormal distributions, but only the series of 3-day counts from these authentic data provides a good lognormal fit.

The daily aggregation shows the weakest signal, with no more than 5 additional cases on any day. Multiple analytic strategies have been applied to achieve detection performance at daily and more frequent intervals. In the progression from weekly to daily monitoring, studies have shown that daily monitoring can afford a mean detection advantage of several days (Xing et al. 2011), but public health planners should consider the value of this lead time according to their objectives and capabilities. Beyond analytic considerations, essential practical questions are: Are accurate data reliably available at the desired frequency? Can the analysis be conducted and presented fast enough? Especially, what is the public health value—can more timely alerts provide an advantage in terms of investigation, response, and situational awareness? As the time interval for analysis decreases, these questions become more demanding of public health protocols and capacities.

General aggregation considerations

One approach to detecting events at multiple, indeed variable, scales in both space and time is the use of scan statistics (Kulldorff et al. 2005), discussed in the next section, and its effective use

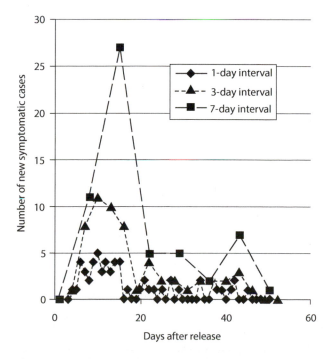

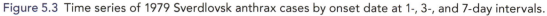

Figure 5.3 Time series of 1979 Sverdlovsk anthrax cases by onset date at 1-, 3-, and 7-day intervals.

depends on availability of relevant location information in the data records, on estimates of baseline spatial data distributions, and on the capacity to investigate significant clusters (Xing et al. 2009).

The filtering and aggregation decision that requires most epidemiological and medical domain expertise is classifying medical encounters and other care-seeking behaviors by category of patient complaint, a classification effort that has generalized the usage of the term *syndrome* from a characteristic cluster of symptoms to a method of grouping records to produce data streams useful for monitoring a population for signals related to outcomes of interest. Early syndromic surveillance systems focused on diagnosis codes assigned during emergency department visits. For example, medical experts debated the set of codes that should be pooled and counted to monitor for acute gastrointestinal illness, a *GI syndrome*. Key issues were how many syndromes to monitor and which codes should belong to each. An early classification system may be found at (CDC Office of Public Health Preparedness and Response 2015). Inspection of this system shows three levels of specificity for most of these syndromes, indicating the differing opinions of the participating medical epidemiologists and the sensitivity/specificity trade-off described above. Validation of these groupings requires a sufficient number of authentic events with well labeled data, a difficult challenge. For methodologies based on confirmed diagnoses, see the influenza-like illness study performed by Marsden-Haug et al. (2007) and the broad, regression-based study by van den Wijngaard et al. (2008).

Some health-monitoring institutions did not use syndromes derived from diagnosis codes, partly because the codes are not available soon enough after medical encounters for processing. Among many local health departments, syndromes are formed according to free text in chief complaint fields, often the only other complaint-based classifier that is promptly available from all reporting facilities. A variety of methods, ranging from weighted keyword groups (Sniegoski 2004) to machine-learning algorithms (Dara et al. 2008), have been used to form syndromes from free text. See Conway et al. (2013) for a review of these methods.

The generalization of the syndrome concept to classification and monitoring of groups of records has been extended to sources of evidence beyond human medical encounters as population health monitoring efforts seek to broaden situational awareness capability. One of the first such extensions was to purchase records of over-the-counter (OTC) sales remedies. Among early studies, Okhusa et al. aggregated sales of all types of common cold remedies to track influenza-like illness (ILI) "because use of such medications has long been accepted in Japanese society as the first and most common treatment for" ILI (Okhusa et al. 2005). Edge et al. used sales of anti-emetics and anti-nauseants to track gastrointestinal illness (Edge et al. 2004). Hogan et al. used sales of pediatric electrolytes to monitor for pediatric GI outbreaks (Hogan et al. 2003) and found evidence of earlier signals than in their clinical data. Subsequent research used more complex analytical methods to seek optimal product groups, the syndrome analogue. Magruder et al. used a two-stage process, first forming many small product groups based on qualitative observations, and then using a hierarchical clustering process to obtain 16 super groups for prospective monitoring (Magruder et al. 2004). Wallstrom et al. developed an unsupervised clustering algorithm using a Bayesian Monte Carlo Markov chain model for categorizing OTC products (Wallstrom and Hogan 2007).

Another data source for which syndromic classification has recently expanded is that of veterinary laboratory data (Dorea et al. 2014). Hoinville et al. reported on an inaugural 2011 global conference dedicated to standardization of terms and concepts to promote veterinary surveillance (Hyder et al. 2011) and as of 2015, the global community is mobilizing rapidly. This effort is motivated by worldwide concerns over zoonotic transmission of emerging diseases and the potential for bioterrorist attacks on livestock. As for human data categorization, intensive syndrome formation research efforts have already begun. Warns-Petit et al. (2010) applied a three-step procedure to classifying wildlife necropsy data, including hierarchical clustering similar to that of Magruder's procedure for OTC, but after initial data reduction using principal components analysis. Dorea et al. (2013b) compared three approaches for veterinary laboratory test orders categorization using truth data formed with the help of three clinical and biological specialists. The approaches were rule-based, Naïve Bayes, Decision Tree classifiers, and their study found that the rule-based method outperformed the machine-learning ones.

The final subtopic treated here on aggregation and filtering of data sources for surveillance is the application to various forms of social media. The use of social media channels to monitor population health is rapidly growing in multiple directions, not only because of the rapid rise and emerging public health potential of these methods, but also because data sets are less constrained by privacy and proprietary barriers than clinical data sets. Eysenbach introduced the term *infodemiology* as "the science of distribution and determinants of information in an electronic medium, specifically the Internet, or in a population, with the ultimate aim to inform public health and public policy." He included in this broad definition web queries, tweets, health-related Internet sites, and other online evidence sources (Eysenbach 2006), and this expansive concept stimulated work on filtering strategies for many such sources. For example, among many published efforts investigating the utility of web searches, Hulth et al. applied a partial least-squares regression method to find web queries that displayed the same pattern as clinical syndromic indicators during epidemics (Hulth et al. 2009). Twitter data have been the subject of considerable research. For example, Collier et al. classified tweet using support vector machines and Naïve Bayes classifiers based on unigrams, bigrams and, regular expressions (Collier et al. 2011). Sophisticated natural language processing techniques have been applied to long text streams from websites involving public health reports (Collier 2012). For example, Chanlekha et al. developed a linguistics-based spatiotemporal zoning scheme to classify web documents, and validation using inter-rater agreement from a group of human annotators was promising (Chanlekha and Collier 2010). Far more research on the optimal use of natural language processing for classifying online documents and web searches will likely be available by the time this article is published. As this research corpus grows, the ultimate application and value to public health of these social media evidence sources are still being determined.

A final observation about the aggregation and filtering of data for prospective disease surveillance involves adaptability. Health monitors have called for this flexibility in the case definitions, syndrome groups, product categories, query sets, and other derived classifications for rapid adaptation to perceived new threats (German et al. 2001). Thus, algorithms used for monitoring these classifications must be robust to these adaptations.

STATISTICAL ALERTING METHODS BY OBJECTIVE

Having discussed the role of analytical methods and the filtering and aggregation decisions crucial to effective monitoring, this section presents basic concepts and some recent trends in statistical alerting methods. While the previous section outlined the use of machine learning and other advanced analytical techniques for data classification; this section focuses on analytical methods for prospective alerting given appropriate and available data streams. Several review papers attempting to cover these methods are available (Farrington and Andrews 2003; Sonesson and Bock 2003; Buckeridge et al. 2005; Shmueli and Burkom 2010). A recent, comprehensive effort is the review by Unkel et al. (2012) that classifies applications as regression techniques, time series methodology, statistical process control, methods incorporating spatial information, and multivariate. Those authors recognize the interrelated nature of these method types and note that "this classification is chosen only to help our presentation of material and is not based on any rigorous taxonomy." The current section lists primary objectives for alerting methods and then addresses the component issues of calculating expectations, deriving test statistics, and setting thresholds for each objective. No comprehensive catalog of applications is intended, and the examples selected are not purported to be the best available.

The discussion below is presented with examples from univariate alerting methods, the most commonly applied alerting algorithms in global surveillance systems because of data availability.

Primary objectives

A student's online searches for alerting methods in biosurveillance will uncover a variety of unrelated material and perspectives, and this paragraph gives the context of the current section.

We first distinguish (a) alerting based on recognition of individual cases or on known scenarios of epidemiological importance vs. (b) alerting based on unexplained statistical aberrations in chosen data streams.

CASE-BASED ALERTING

For example, the U.S. National Poison Data System contains queries for volume-based alerts seeking statistical aberrations, and for case-based alerts of any individuals with specified combinations of symptoms. The accurate selection of trigger records may require substantial data analysis, but once the criteria for individual-based alerts are established, algorithms are not required. Case-based alerting is in the domain of the previous section, while the concern in the following paragraphs is "volume-based" alerting requiring recognition of anomalous observed numbers or proportions of data records.

SCENARIO-BASED ALERTING

Bioterrorism concerns have stimulated interest in scenarios involving infection of monitored populations with weaponized diseases, and these concerns have driven efforts to detect deliberately caused outbreaks as soon as possible to save lives and mitigate morbidity. Researchers have attempted to combine models of disease transmission and progression, population movement, and atmospheric dynamics to develop rapid scenario detection capability. The approach of these alerting methods is to monitor for combinations of circumstances in the included data sets that give a high probability of the disease scenario of concern. In such attempts, the modeler must find computational compromises that are efficient but sufficiently representative of the real-life disease process in the monitored population. For example, Hogan et al. modeled an outdoor aerosol release of anthrax, a plausible bioterrorist scenario (Hogan et al. 2007). Their model employed emergency department visit data including diagnosis codes with meteorological data to estimate "a posterior distribution over the location, quantity, and date and time conditioned on a release having occurred." These efforts involve the large corpus of research with agent-based models instantiating and tracking individuals in a monitored population. For example, Shen and Cooper built Bayesian networks of large populations to monitor competing hypotheses of multiple diseases (Shen and Cooper 2009). As an example of the compromises required to execute complex, agent-based models, they used equivalence classes to capture transmission-relevant properties of modeled individuals. More recent efforts have introduced particle filter methods of physics to remove the need to instantiate multiple individuals and relax simplifying assumptions about disease progression (Dawson et al. 2015)

In addition to surveillance for effects of rare, weaponized pathogens, a common scenario that has received wide research attention is the seasonal influenza epidemic. This scenario is important for several reasons: seasonal influenza is responsible for high global mortality and morbidity every year, multiple strains with changing antigenic presentation present a perennial pandemic threat, and the patient presentation of most weaponized diseases begins with influenza-like-illness symptoms. Furthermore, some historical data sets do exist and have been used for analysis and model development. A community of prominent researchers has modeled ILI visit count data as a Markov process with epidemic and endemic states. Le Strat and Carrat published a Hidden Markov Model (HMM) with a likelihood function for distinguishing the two states and to allow classification of the current time as endemic or epidemic (Le Strat and Carrat 1999). They did not directly propose a prospective alerting algorithm but provided results using authentic data and supporting the assertion that HMM's "provide the most natural way of making inferences about such phenomena, by assigning different probability distributions to the [endemic and epidemic] dynamics." Thus, the alerting approach is to promptly recognize a high probability of being in the epidemic state. Most HMM applications assume Gaussian or other distributions for multiple states, infer the parameters of the discrete distributions from the data, and then calculate the probability of being in either state. However, simple underlying distributions do not capture the seasonal behavior of ILI data, and Le Strat and Carrat discussed computational challenges of capturing systematic data behavior in the HMM formulation. Subsequent modelers have taken up this challenge. Martinez-Beneito et al. used historical time series of ILI rates and applied autoregressive modeling to detrended series obtained by differencing (Martinez-Beneito et al. 2008). They then modeled the current process as white noise or autoregressive. They obtained a prospective algorithm with Bayesian inference for prompt epidemic alerting. Conesa et al. advanced this approach by taking into account incidence rate magnitudes and by treating these rates as stochastic quantities (Conesa et al. 2015). These increasingly representative and complex efforts require substantial processing for the Bayesian inference and the authors describe efficiencies in their application of Monte Carlo Markov Chain modeling.

Representing another prominent approach in prospectively distinguishing epidemic states from ILI data, Frisen et al. questioned the utility of fully parametric methods because of substantial year-to-year differences in the onset date, shape, and peak level of the influenza epidemic curve (Frisen et al. 2009). They presented a semi-parametric approach based on maximum likelihood estimation of the beginning of flu season, implemented and available in the downloadable R program *OutbreakP*.

GENERAL ABERRATION DETECTION

The above discussion involves monitoring for specific cases or for known rare or common scenarios whose details can shape detection approaches. We consider methods for general alerting in which the goal is to detect statistical anomalies that may or may not signify public health events of concern.

COMPONENTS OF ABERRATION DETECTION METHODS

Preconditioning tactics

Assuming that the filtering and aggregation processes of the previous section have produced time series that plausibly contain signals of interest, univariate and multivariate statistical hypothesis tests may still produce excessive false alarms for many reasons. Researchers have applied preconditioning strategies to reduce excess alerting. Some hypothesis tests assume input time series with Gaussian distributions, and developers have applied square root or other normalizing transformations to obtain expected background distributions (Hafen et al. 2009). The differencing stratagem of Martinez-Beneito reported above may be helpful for detrending. Some data quality issues may be treated analytically. One common problem is that of late reporting of data, so that the most recent, hence the most critical, time series entries are underestimated. Noufaily et al. applied a proportional hazards model that revealed temporal influences on relatively short delays (Noufaily et al. 2015). Another common problem is that a monitored time series may comprise data streams from multiple care facilities and may display discontinuities resulting in alerting bias when the number of data contributors changes. Burkom et al. obtained an improved alert rate by applying a provider-based regression method before using a

detection algorithm (Burkom et al. 2004), though such an approach requires knowledge of the number of currently participating data sources. Levin-Rector et al. also applied trend removal as one of their refinements to the historical limits method (Levin-Rector et al. 2015).

Once any preconditioning transformations are applied to the input data, most surveillance system alerting algorithms are combinations of baseline calculation, test statistic formulation, and thresholding. Figure 5.4 depicts the sequence of stages described in this section, with dashed boxes at the top for the operations of the previous section and at the bottom for the follow-up operations with alerting outputs.

Background estimation step

Following any preconditioning, input expected values are needed to enable recognition of the significantly unexpected, the statistical anomalies. The simplest estimate is a fixed baseline average, as computed in the Phase I step in industrial control chart development (Ryan 2008), but health surveillance data are typically too unstable to use long-term fixed averages and moreover, the underlying health data process cannot be halted for readjustment like a manufacturing process. Therefore, moving averages are often used, as in the CDC Early Aberration Reporting System (EARS) methods (Hutwagner et al. 2003). Surveillance data streams often contain yearly cycles, day-of-week patterns, or other systematic behaviors that may cause alerting bias, and multiple stratification and adjustment strategies may be applied to remove this bias. For yearly cycles, a simple and common adjustment is to take as the baseline period the days or weeks in the same season as the current data for each of the past several years. For example, in the historical limits method that monitors report counts from a current set of 4 weeks, the baseline period is the same 4 weeks and the immediately previous and ensuing 4-week periods, from each of the past 5 years (Stroup et al. 1993). Unkel et al. call this approach the simplest form of regression (Unkel et al. 2012). When monitoring daily syndromic counts for day-of-week effects, Tokars et al. successfully adjusted the baseline means by using total visit counts for the current day of week, and this adjustment proved more sensitive and robust than directly monitoring ratios of syndromic to total visits (Tokars et al. 2009). Developers have also extended baseline averaging with exponential baseline weighting, as in the exponentially weighted

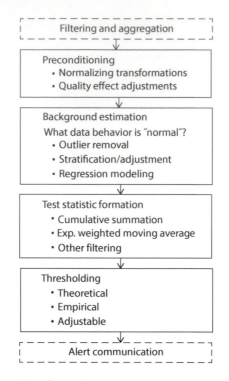

Figure 5.4 Steps in alerting algorithm formation.

moving average (EWMA) used by Stoto et al. before applying a CUSUM chart (Stoto et al. 2006). Burkom et al. applied generalized exponential smoothing to daily syndromic count data to obtain improved estimates over fixed-effects regression models (Burkom et al. 2007). The weighted averages have been used both to estimate the baseline and to combine the current test observation with recent observations in forming the test statistic.

Multiple authors have used regression models with added fixed, random, and auto-regressive effects to calculate expected values (Farrington and Andrews 2003; Reis and Mandl 2003; Brillman et al. 2005; Craigmile et al. 2007; Jackson et al. 2007; Fricker et al. 2008; Xing et al. 2011). The fixed effects have included indicator variables for day-of-week and for month or other baseline intervals, and continuous variables for total visits and for climatic measures like mean temperature. Craigmile et al. obtained improved estimates and more sensitive detection with a seasonally adjusted ARIMA plus fixed effects model (Craigmile et al. 2007). The advantage of all of these models over simple baseline averaging depends on the input time series behavior, and this behavior should be considered and reviewed by the surveillance system designer.

One of the most comprehensive and detailed models is the extension of the quasi-Poisson Farrington model published by Noufailly et al. (2013). This implementation is run every week on a database of more than 3300 distinct organisms at the Health Protection Agency of the United Kingdom, and the authors present an algorithm for applying the model to a variety of data scenarios.

Among alternative estimation approaches, Frisen discussed concerns with parametric models using analysis of six seasons of Sweden's ILI rate data in recommending a semiparametric method (Frisen et al. 2009). Hafen et al. presented a fully non-parametric approach based on seasonal trend decomposition that yielded low residuals relative to GLM modeling and to the direct averaging in the EARS methods (Hafen et al. 2009).

Test statistic formation

Given an observation x_t and an expected value u_t, the most commonly applied test statistic is the z-score ratio:

$$z_t = \frac{(x_t - u_t)}{s_t}, \qquad (5.1)$$

where s_t is a standard error intended as a normalizer to put the results on a common scale for threshold application. This expression is implicit in the EARS and historical limits methods, in which s_t is the standard deviation of the values in the moving baseline, a common practice. In regression methods, u_t is commonly taken to be the regression prediction and s_t is the standard error of regression or a more complex expression, depending on the model (Unkel et al. 2012).

However, the critical value in the test statistic need not be restricted to the most current observation x_t. Craigmile recommended testing optimal combinations of the most recent observations with "filter-based outbreak signature detection" (Craigmile et al. 2007). The most common ways to combine recent observations have been the adaptive versions of EWMA and CUSUM charts. The EWMA chart replaces x_t with a weighted sum of recent observations, with weights decreasing exponentially with observation age. For the basic CUSUM procedure, the test statistic is the upper sum

$$SH_j = \max(0,(z_t - k) + SH_{j-1}) \qquad (5.2)$$

where

- z_t is the running z-score
- 2k is the magnitude of anomaly to detect in units of the standard error
- the test statistic SH_j is initialized at 0 or a mean estimate and recursively updated

Thus, the CUSUM statistics does not necessarily weight deviations above expectations according to the observation age and thus does not require that observed values strictly increase at the outbreak onset. The EWMA and CUSUM charts often yield similar detection performance, and the choice depends on the time scale and the target signals expected from outbreaks of interest. The CUSUM is likely preferable for data fluctuations on a daily or more frequent scale. Generalizations of the EWMA averaging extend the exponential weighting idea to trends and cyclic effects that may cause regression errors, and an alerting algorithm based on Holt-Winters smoothing provided promising results (Elbert and Burkom 2009). Dorea et al. gave a recent discussion and performance comparison of EWMA, CUSUM, and Holt-Winters alerting methods using syndromic time series from veterinary laboratory test surveillance (Dorea et al. 2013a).

It is important to note that the test value x_t in the control chart implementations may be a regression residual or other derived prediction instead of a single or grouped observation. Mandel introduced the regression control chart in 1969, demonstrating advantages of using regression residuals rather than direct observations as control chart inputs (Mandel 1969). Fricker demonstrated substantial improvement by applying a CUSUM to regression residuals (Fricker et al. 2008).

For prospective monitoring, Farrington and Andrews observed that "a major difficulty with the regression approach is how to reduce the influence of base-line counts in weeks coinciding with past outbreaks" (Farrington and Andrews 2003). Indeed the influence of outbreaks is an obstacle for all detection methods with baseline updating. Very high values in the baseline bias the z-score ratio in two ways—they reduce the numerator by pushing up the expectation u_t, and they increase the denominator with an exaggerated variance. Both effects reduce the test statistic, so the net effect is a sensitivity reduction caused by the past outbreak (or data entry error). Farrington and Andrews implemented a statistical solution with reweighting to reduce confidence intervals exaggerated by outbreak effects. Other implementations have either ignored the problem, so that sensitivity may be reduced for a time interval after a large outbreak, or applied outlier removal methods, such as truncating values in the baseline to values at the alerting threshold (Burkom et al. 2008b).

Threshold determination

In a classical statistical hypothesis test, the null hypothesis is that an observed test statistic value is a random sample from an assumed distribution with a known probability density function, and the hypothesis is rejected if the probability of the observed test statistic is below a threshold value. In a public health monitoring context, rejection of the null hypothesis would trigger an alert with the intent to stimulate investigation of underlying cases as a possible outbreak. To derive threshold values that yield consistent, expected alert rates, developers have used Equation 5.1 and detailed normalizing transformations to achieve Gaussian-distributed algorithm output statistics. Indeed, the alerting threshold of three standard deviations above the baseline mean widely adopted for the EARS methods came from the fact that for a Gaussian variable with mean 0 and standard deviation equal to 1, the probability of a value greater than 3.09 is 0.001. Many users have found that the alert rates resulting from this threshold are inconsistent both in time and across data streams. Surveillance data streams are often count data, so Poisson distributions have been commonly used. However, the mean of a Poisson statistic is equal to its variance, and observed surveillance algorithm outputs are often *overdispersed*, i.e., with a variance exceeding the mean (often by a factor of 2 or higher), so quasi-Poisson or negative binomial distributions have also been used to derive distribution-based alerting thresholds.

Alternatively, many authors take an empirical approach to setting thresholds. This approach avoids testing algorithm output sets against theoretical distributions by pooling a large number of test statistic values using historical data. Quantiles derived from the pooled values are then used as thresholds. For example, if 5000 test statistic values are calculated and sorted, then a p-value of 0.001 would be assigned to the 5th highest value. For alerting, the developer is interested in accurate thresholds for low p-values, so for robust thresholds, large numbers of representative values are required. Moreover, a small number of outlier test statistic values caused by outbreak effects can distort empirical thresholds; in the example just given, if the threshold value is x, then 10 outliers from outbreak intervals would raise the empirical probability associated with a candidate threshold from 0.001 to 0.003. Thus, both theoretical and empirical approaches require careful analysis and ongoing inspection to obtain consistent background alert rates.

Practical threshold selection involves the trade-off between sensitivity and specificity, often defined as 1 minus the background alerting rate. For this discussion, assume that algorithm outputs are calculated from a large set of observations, some during target health events or outbreaks. For a fixed algorithm threshold value, we define the following:

True positives (TP) = Number of observations with alerts during target events

False positives (FP) = Number of observations with alerts, not during target events
True negatives (TN) = Number of observations without alerts, not during target events
False negatives (FN) = Number of observations without alerts during target events

By these definitions, sensitivity = TP/(TP + FN), specificity = TN/(TN + FP), and the false alert rate is (1 − specificity) = FP/(TN + FP). A more liberal alerting threshold generally provides greater sensitivity but also a lower specificity (i.e., more background alerts to investigate). A stricter threshold means lower sensitivity but fewer background alarms. Figure 5.5 gives a sample Receiver Operating Characteristic (ROC) curve, in which each marker gives the sensitivity and false alert rate of a distinct threshold. A practitioner may use such curves to choose a threshold with the most useful balance of sensitivity and alert rate.

An alternative performance measure is the Activity Monitor Operating Characteristic (AMOC) curve, similar to a ROC curve but with the modification that the ordinate indicates a timeliness score, not a detection probability. For example, this timeliness score may be defined as the median number of days from the start of an outbreak until the first alert has been observed during the outbreak. Because the goal of public health surveillance is to detect the onset of an outbreak as soon as possible, low values on an AMOC curve indicate good alerting performance, as in Figure 5.5 example. Methods for computing these in the surveillance context may be found in multiple sources (Buckeridge et al. 2005; Elbert and Burkom 2009; Lombardo 2015). Burkom et al. gave a larger set of measures (Burkom et al. 2015). In particular, the positive predictive value (PPV)

$$PPV = \frac{TP}{TP + FP} \qquad (5.3)$$

has practical importance for disease monitors because its reciprocal is the number of alerts expected before a true positive is found. However, TP is usually small, so this calculation requires an accurate count FP of false positives, and proving that an alert in historical data is false is typically difficult.

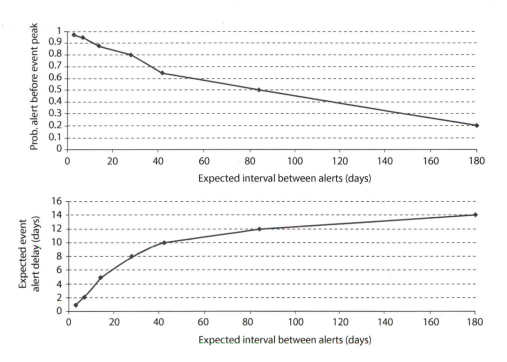

Figure 5.5 Sample adaptations of receiver operating characteristic and activity monitor operating characteristic curves. Markers correspond to different alerting thresholds and show the respective alert rates for each threshold with the corresponding detection probability (for ROC) or detection delay (for AMOC).

Component summary

The above discussion was an attempt to explain the components of a statistical alerting method to enhance understanding, selection, and adjustment of methods implemented in surveillance systems. An important takeaway idea is that effective statistical alerting depends on all of the steps in Figure 5.4, and the individual steps should be considered in evaluating detection performance rather than assuming that the problem lies with a control chart choice, regression model, or threshold. Substantial changes in sensitivity were shown to result from substitutions for the expectation and statistic formation steps and suggested that "recombinant" methods may yield improved performance (Murphy and Burkom 2008). In an article on improvements to the historical limits method, Levin-Rector et al. made refinements at multiple stages listed in Figure 5.4 (Levin-Rector et al. 2015). Their first refinement was to alter the inclusion case criterion in the filtering stage. They also reduced the number of monitored diseases to those for which early detection was plausible and

amenable to public health response. The second refinement was a regression adjustment to remove linear trends, and the third was outlier removal achieved with a rule to identify past outbreaks as outliers and replace them with expected values. Finally, they accounted for late reporting problems for selected diseases by recalculating the test statistic for 4 subsequent weeks. Their reported improvement in overall algorithm performance resulted from combining these refinements and illustrates the understanding of monitoring objectives, epidemiology of key outcomes, data quality, and statistical behavior required for alerting methods with practical utility.

DETERMINING SIGNIFICANT CLUSTERS IN SPACE AND TIME

The previous section focused on monitoring single time series for statistical anomalies that might be signals of health events of interest. If the data are available, there are many generalizations of health monitoring needs, including monitoring multiple syndromes or classifications of data that may overlap, monitoring the data organized by geographic subregion, and monitoring similar outcomes in multiple data sources of varying clinical specificity. The key considerations in monitoring multiple and distributed data streams have been outlined according to the surveillance needs and data availability of the monitoring institution (Burkom et al. 2005; Rolka et al. 2007; Frisen 2010). Unkel et al. summarized published efforts using multiple sources of evidence (Unkel et al. 2012). The remainder of this section describes the most popular monitoring application of distributed surveillance data, the search for significant clusters of cases in space and time.

The purely temporal methods of the previous section are most effective at outbreak detection if the data streams contain the effects of an outbreak without excessive masking by the customary case distribution. The perfect situation would be to monitor only the geographic region containing the outbreak over time intervals corresponding perfectly to the outbreak interval. However, the affected region and outbreak duration are unknown before the event, and monitored time series and spatial subdivisions are often dictated by available data streams and the location information that they contain.

Scan statistics provide a method to seek the optimal data subdivision to detect an event of interest. Purely spatial scan statistics are used to seek the optimal location and extent for data at a given time, and the spatiotemporal version is applied to seek the optimal location, extent, and time duration. Motivations for adopting these methods are strong; the epidemiologist needs to know the population-at-risk for outbreak investigation as soon as possible. Scan statistics offer the possibility of early detection in a reduced area for investigation. Instead of testing for anomalous levels or patterns in a specific data stream, cluster-detection methods seek anomalies in the spatial distribution of data. Rather than baseline time-series behavior, these methods require a baseline spatial pattern in the data.

An important consideration for evaluating these methods for a given data source is how well and how reliably the expected spatial data distribution can be estimated.

In particular, the free, downloadable program SaTScan originally developed by Martin Kulldorff for the National Cancer Institute has been widely adopted (Kulldorff 1997; Kulldorff et al. 2005). Developers have updated the software to keep pace

with user needs in a variety of applications, as reflected by the site bibliography (Kulldorff 2015). While the remainder of this section addresses concepts and issues derived from the use of SaTScan, many of them apply to other cluster detection methods as well.

Suppose that a total of N cases or visits are distributed over the entire monitored region, with each case assigned to a subregion. In SaTScan, to find purely spatial clusters, a set of grid points is taken as possible centers of case clusters; often the centroids of all of the data subregions are used for this purpose. For one of the grid points, candidate clusters are formed by testing the case counts of each member of a family of circles centered at that point, as shown in Figure 5.6. Such a circle may contain a single subregion or many subregions up to a preset fraction of the total number of cases or total region area. A test statistic is computed and stored for each such circle and then for families of circles centered at the other grid points as well. The cluster J^* whose test statistic $LR(J^*)$ has the maximum value obtained from all grid centers and all radii is considered the maximum likelihood cluster.

For every data set and each monitored test period, the cluster J^* with largest test statistic may always be found, but over the range of all spatial distributions, there is no analytical means to decide whether J^* merits an alert based on the magnitude of its statistic $LR(J^*)$. In the absence of a reference distribution, SaTScan empirically sets the statistical significance of the candidate maximum cluster J^* as a p-value by ranking $LR(J^*)$ against a set of other maximum likelihood ratios obtained using randomized simulations. The mth trial maximum $LR(J_m^*)$ is calculated from another sample of the N cases chosen randomly from the expected spatial distribution. The significance of $LR(J^*)$ then depends on its rank among the set of $LR(J_m^*)$ from the trial distributions m = 1, …, M. The p-value for the observed cluster J^* is then

$$p(J^*) = \frac{\text{rank}(J^*)}{M+1} \qquad (5.4)$$

For example, if the number of trials M is 999, the lowest possible p-value is 1/1000, achieved if $LR(J^*)$ is larger than any of the simulated trial maxima. The p-value is then compared to a preset significance threshold to determine significance.

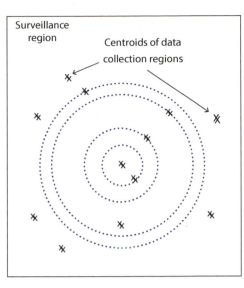

- *Form cylinders*: Bases are circles about each centroid in region; cylinder height is time for space–time clusters
- *Calculate statistic*: For event count in each cylinder relative to entire region, within space and time limits
- *Most significant clusters*: Regions whose centroids form base of cylinder with maximum statistic LR(J*)
- *But how unusual is it?* Repeat procedure with repeated simulated trials, rank LR(J*) among maxima of these to obtain significance for alerting decisions

Surveillance region
Centroids of data collection regions

Figure 5.6 Scan statistics concept.

Experience with a given data set is often required to set a practical threshold.

The spatio-temporal extension of this procedure adds the dimension of time, i.e., the number of time intervals for aggregating test cases in each candidate set of regions, as shown in Figure 5.6. In common practice, likelihood ratios for the candidate regions are stored and compared for cases from the current day, from the current and previous day, and so on back to some limit. Because of both epidemiological and run-time constraints, this limit is typically a small number of intervals.

The SaTScan software and variants in the literature include many modifications to this scheme to aid the user. The test statistic is usually taken to be a log likelihood ratio, and a Poisson log likelihood ratio is most often used for count data, but several options are available. Options exist for limiting cluster sizes, for elliptical cluster shapes, for covariate adjustments, for managing secondary clusters, and other practical modifications.

The health monitor who would use such a strategy for cluster detection should ask the following questions, to choose the method and appropriate options, and also to obtain useful output clusters:

- Are there case classification bias problems among subregions? For example, if syndromic definitions are applied differently, the significant clusters may be misleading.

- How stable is the spatial case distribution over time? What is a good, efficient way to estimate an expected distribution? Distributions inferred from baseline data are widely used. Census counts, eligibility/enrollment lists, and subregion modeling have also been tried (Kleinman et al. 2005).
- Do data from some subregions drop in and out of the distribution over time? False clustering may be reduced by ignoring problem subregions.
- Do day-of-week and seasonal effects exist in the data, and are they similar across subregions? Interaction between these effects and the spatial distribution may bias the clustering.
- Are there differences in late reporting problems across subregions? Resolving this issue may be more challenging than in the univariate case.
- How many total subregions are reasonably represented? Do a few subregions dominate the data?
- How sparse is the data set overall? Sparseness may affect choice of spatial estimation methods
- Is there a reason to expect noncircular disease clusters?
- Do resources exist to investigate significant clusters?

From the user point of view, Sherman et al. described the data preparation and analysis steps they used to search for clusters of individuals at high risk for diagnosis of late-stage colorectal cancer (Sherman et al. 2014). They found SaTScan useful for this purpose but reported a gap between the method's performance and their research needs. Their comments illustrate the remaining element of art as well as science in the practical use of scan statistics:

- Much of our analysis was underpowered and that no single method detected all clusters of statistical or public health significance
- The challenge is to identify areas in which the burden of disease can be alleviated through public health intervention
- Reliance on SaTScan's default settings does not always produce pertinent results…Some clusters were detected consistently but were not statistically significant by any method or at any aggregation or scale
- No single method detected all significant clusters but using an iterative, multimethod approach delivered varying results which leaves the researcher without an answer to this question: where should we target screening interventions?
- Many health researchers are unaware of the influence on results of the choice of method used for spatial analysis

One of the most appealing features of SaTScan is the limitation of excessive significant clustering because of the large number of candidate clusters tested. However, the user intending to use the prospective version of SaTScan to seek clusters on a daily or regular, indefinite basis should be aware of the work by Correa et al. summarizing and clarifying issues raised by several authors (Correa et al. 2015). They demonstrated that there is "no relationship between [the nominal significance level] α and the …. recurrence interval" used to adjust for multiple testing, which lead them to "strongly oppose the use of the scan statistic with the usual signal rules in the prospective context," though they deemed it "excellent" for retrospective analysis. They also cited other published results implying practical methods to achieve the desired effective significance level prospectively.

In summary, scan statistics offer valuable efficiency in seeking disease clusters of interest, though theoretical difficulties remain. For successful cluster determination, the user will need careful analysis of the geographic data distribution and quality of its spatial information, and the record filtering preparation described in the section "Data aggregation and filtering" is especially important.

REFERENCES

Berkelman, R.L. and J.W. Buehler. 1990. Public-health surveillance of noninfectious chronic diseases—The potential to detect rapid changes in disease burden. *Int. J. Epidemiol.* 19(3): 628–635.

Brillman, J.C., T. Burr, D. Forslund, E. Joyce, R. Picard, and E. Umland. 2005. Modeling emergency department visit patterns for infectious disease complaints: Results and application to disease surveillance. *BMC Med. Inform. Decis. Mak.* 5(4): 1–14.

Buckeridge, D.L., H. Burkom, M. Campbell, W.R. Hogan, and A.W. Moore. 2005. Algorithms for rapid outbreak detection: A research synthesis. *J. Biomed. Inform.* 38(2): 99–113.

Burke, D.S., J.M. Epstein, D.A. Cummings, J.I. Parker, K.C. Cline, R.M. Singa, and S. Chakravarty. 2006. Individual-based computational modeling of smallpox epidemic control strategies. *Acad. Emerg. Med.* 13: 1142–1149.

Burkom, H., Y. Elbert, J.M. Velasco, E.A. Tayag, and V.G. Roque, Jr. 2015. Analytic biosurveillance methods for resource-limited settings. *Johns Hopkins APL Tech. Dig.* 32(4): 11.

Burkom, H.S. 2007. Alerting algorithms for biosurveillance. In J.S. Lombardo and D.L. Buckeridge (eds.), *Disease Surveillance: A Public Health Informatics Approach.* Hoboken, NJ: Wiley-Interscience, pp. 143–192.

Burkom, H.S., Y. Elbert, A. Feldman, and J. Lin. 2004. Role of data aggregation in biosurveillance detection strategies with applications from ESSENCE. *Morb. Mortal. Wkly. Rep.* 53(Suppl.): 67–73.

Burkom, H.S., Y. Elbert, S.F. Magruder, A.H. Najmi, W. Peter, and M.W. Thompson. 2008b. Developments in the roles, features, and evaluation of alerting algorithms for disease outbreak monitoring. *Johns Hopkins APL Tech. Dig.* 27(4): 313.

Burkom, H.S., W.A. Loschen, Z.R. Mnatsakanyan, and J.S. Lombardo. 2008a. Tradeoffs driving policy and research decisions in biosurveillance. *Johns Hopkins APL Tech. Dig.* 27(4): 299–312.

Burkom, H.S., S. Murphy, J. Coberly, and K. Hurt-Mullen. 2005. Public health monitoring tools for multiple data streams. *Morb. Mortal. Wkly. Rep.* 54(Suppl.): 55–62.

Burkom, H.S., S.P. Murphy, and G. Shmueli. 2007. Automated time series forecasting for biosurveillance. *Stat. Med.* 26(22): 4202–4218.

Cates, W., Jr., J.C. Smith, R.W. Rochat, J.E. Patterson, and A. Dolman. 1978. Assessment of surveillance and vital statistics data for monitoring abortion mortality, United States, 1972–1975. *Am. J. Epidemiol.* 108(3): 200–206.

CDC Division of Viral Hepatitis. 2015. CDC DVH—Viral hepatitis statistics & surveillance. Centers for Disease Control and Prevention. Last Modified April 24, 2015, Accessed May 7, 2015. http://www.cdc.gov/hepatitis/Statistics/index.htm.

CDC Office of Public Health Preparedness and Response. 2015. Syndrome definitions for diseases associated with critical bioterrorism-associated agents. Centers for Disease Control and Prevention. Last Modified October 23, 2003, Accessed May 7, 2015. http://www.bt.cdc.gov/surveillance/syndromedef/.

Chanlekha, H. and N. Collier. 2010. A methodology to enhance spatial understanding of disease outbreak events reported in news articles. *Int. J. Med. Inform.* 79(4): 284–296.

Collier, N. 2012. Uncovering text mining: A survey of current work on web-based epidemic intelligence. *Global Public Health* 7(7): 731–749.

Collier, N., N.T. Son, and N.M. Nguyen. 2011. OMG U got flu? Analysis of shared health messages for bio-surveillance. *J. Biomed. Semant.* 2(Suppl. 5): S9–S10.

Conesa, D., M. Martinez-Beneito, R. Amoros, and A. Lopez-Quilez. 2015. Bayesian hierarchical Poisson models with a hidden Markov structure for the detection of influenza epidemic outbreaks. *Stat. Methods Med. Res.* 24: 206–223.

Conway, M., J.N. Dowling, and W.W. Chapman. 2013. Using chief complaints for syndromic surveillance: A review of chief complaint based classifiers in North America. *J. Biomed. Inform.* 46(4): 734–743.

Correa, T.R., R.M. Assuncao, and M.A. Costa. 2015. A critical look at prospective surveillance using a scan statistic. *Stat. Med.* 34(7): 1081–1093.

Craigmile, P.F., N. Kim, S.A. Fernandez, and B.K. Bonsu. 2007. Modeling and detection of respiratory-related outbreak signatures. *BMC Med. Inform. Decis. Mak.* 7: 28.

Dara, J., J.N. Dowling, D. Travers, G.F. Cooper, and W.W. Chapman. 2008. Evaluation of preprocessing techniques for chief complaint classification. *J. Biomed. Inform.* 41: 613–623.

Dawson, P., R. Gailis, and A. Meehan. 2015. Detecting disease outbreaks using a combined Bayesian network and particle filter approach. *J. Theor. Biol.* 370: 171–183.

Dorea, F.C., C. Dupuy, F. Vial, T.L. Reynolds, and J.E. Akkina. 2014. Toward one health: Are public health stakeholders aware of the field of animal health? *Infect. Ecol. Epidemiol.* Apr: 4.

Dorea, F.C., B.J. McEwen, W.B. McNab, J. Sanchez, and C.W. Revie. 2013a. Syndromic surveillance using veterinary laboratory data: Algorithm combination and customization of alerts. *PLOS ONE* 8: e82183.

Dorea, F.C., C.A. Muckle, D. Kelton, J.T. McClure, B.J. McEwen, W.B. McNab, J. Sanchez, and C.W. Revie. 2013b. Exploratory analysis of methods for automated classification of laboratory test orders into syndromic groups in veterinary medicine. *PLOS ONE* 8: e57334.

Edge, V.L., F. Pollari, G. Lim, J. Aramini, P. Sockett, S.W. Martin, J. Wilson, and A. Ellis. 2004. Syndromic surveillance of gastrointestinal illness using pharmacy over-the-counter sales. A retrospective study of waterborne outbreaks in Saskatchewan and Ontario. *Can. J. Public Health* 95(6): 446–450.

Elbert, Y. and H.S. Burkom. 2009. Development and evaluation of a data-adaptive alerting algorithm for univariate temporal biosurveillance data. *Stat. Med.* 28(26): 3226–3248.

Eysenbach, G. 2006. Infodemiology: Tracking flu-related searches on the web for syndromic surveillance. In *AMIA Annual Symposium Proceedings*, pp. 244–248.

Farrington, C. P. and Andrews, N. 2004. Outbreak detection: Application to infectious disease surveillance. In R. Brookmeyer and D.F. Stroup (eds.), *Monitoring the Health of Populations: Statistical Principles & Methods for Public Health Surveillance*, Oxford, U.K.: Oxford University Press, pp. 203–231.

Fricker, R.D., Jr., B.L. Hegler, and D.A. Dunfee. 2008. Comparing syndromic surveillance detection methods: EARS' versus a CUSUM-based methodology. *Stat. Med.* 27(17): 3407–3429.

Frisen, M. 2010. Principles for multivariate surveillance. In H.J. Lenz, P.T. Wilrich, and W. Schmid (eds.), *Frontiers in Statistical Quality Control*, Vol. 9 Heidelberg, Germany: Physica-Verlag, pp. 133–144.

Frisen, M., E. Andersson, and L. Schioler. 2009. Robust outbreak surveillance of epidemics in Sweden. *Stat. Med.* 28(3): 476–493.

German, R.R., L.M. Lee, J.M. Horan, R.L. Milstein, C.A. Pertowski, and M.N. Waller. 2001. Updated guidelines for evaluating public health surveillance systems: Recommendations from the Guidelines Working Group. *MMWR Recomm. Rep.* 50(RR-13): 1–35; quiz CE1–CE7.

Hafen, R.P., D.E. Anderson, W.S. Cleveland, R. Maciejewski, D.S. Ebert, A. Abusalah, M. Yakout, M. Ouzzani, and S.J. Grannis. 2009. Syndromic surveillance: STL for modeling, visualizing, and monitoring disease counts. *BMC Med. Inform. Decis. Mak.* 9: 21.

Hogan, W.R., G.F. Cooper, G.L. Wallstrom, M.M. Wagner, and J.M. Depinay. 2007. The Bayesian aerosol release detector: An algorithm for detecting and characterizing outbreaks caused by an atmospheric release of *Bacillus anthracis*. *Stat. Med.* 26(29): 5225–5252.

Hogan, W.R., F.C. Tsui, O. Ivanov, P.H. Gesteland, S. Grannis, J.M. Overhage, J.M. Robinson, and M.M. Wagner. 2003. Detection of pediatric respiratory and diarrheal outbreaks from sales of over-the-counter electrolyte products. *J. Am. Med. Inform. Assoc.* 10: 555–562.

Hulth, A., G. Rydevik, and A. Linde. 2009. Web queries as a source for syndromic surveillance. *PLOS ONE* 4(2): e4378.

Hutwagner, L., W. Thompson, G.M. Seeman, and T. Treadwell. 2003. The bioterrorism preparedness and response Early Aberration Reporting System (EARS). *J. Urban Health* 80(2 Suppl. 1): i89–i96.

Hyder, K., A. Vidal-Diez, J. Lawes, A.R. Sayers, A. Milnes, L. Hoinville, and A.J. Cook. 2011. Use of spatiotemporal analysis of laboratory submission data to identify potential outbreaks of new or emerging diseases in cattle in Great Britain. *BMC Vet. Res.* 7: 14.

Jackson, M.L., A. Baer, I. Painter, and J. Duchin. 2007. A simulation study comparing aberration detection algorithms for syndromic surveillance. *BMC Med. Inform. Decis. Mak.* 7: 6.

Jiang, X. and G.F. Cooper. 2010. A Bayesian spatio-temporal method for disease outbreak detection. *J. Am. Med. Inform. Assoc.* 17: 462–471.

Kleinman, K.P., A.M. Abrams, M. Kulldorff, and R. Platt. 2005. A model-adjusted space-time scan statistic with an application to syndromic surveillance. *Epidemiol. Infect.* 133(3): 409–419.

Kulldorff, M. 1997. A spatial scan statistic. *Commun. Stat. Theory Methods* 26(6): 1481–1496.

Kulldorff, M. 2015. SaTScan—Software for the spatial, temporal, and space-time scan statistics. Last Modified March 23, 2015, Accessed May 7, 2015. http://satscan.org/.

Kulldorff, M., R. Heffernan, J. Hartman, R. Assuncao, and F. Mostashari. 2005. A space-time permutation scan statistic for disease outbreak detection. *PLoS Med.* 2(3): 216–224.

Law, R.K., S. Sheikh, A. Bronstein, R. Thomas, H.A. Spiller, and J.G. Schier. 2014. Incidents of potential public health significance identified using national surveillance of U.S. poison center data (2008–2012). *Clin. Toxicol. (Phila.)* 52(9): 958–963.

Lescano, A.G., R.P. Larasati, E.R. Sedyaningsih, K. Bounlu, R.V. Araujo-Castillo, C.V. Munayco-Escate, G. Soto, C.C. Mundaca, and D.L. Blazes. 2008. Statistical analyses in disease surveillance systems. *BMC Proc.* 2(Suppl. 3): S7.

Le Strat, Y. and F. Carrat. 1999. Monitoring epidemiologic surveillance data using hidden Markov models. *Stat. Med.* 18: 3463–3478.

Levin-Rector, A., E.L. Wilson, A.D. Fine, and S.K. Greene. 2015. Refining historical limits method to improve disease cluster detection, New York City, New York, USA. *Emerg. Infect. Dis.* 21(2): 265–272.

Lewis, S.L., B.H. Feighner, W.A. Loschen, R.A. Wojcik, J.F. Skora, J.S. Coberly, and D.L. Blazes. 2011. SAGES: A suite of freely-available software tools for electronic disease surveillance in resource-limited settings. *PLOS ONE* 6: e19750.

Lombardo, B. 2015. *Disease Surveillance.* Hoboken, NJ: John Wiley & Sons, Inc.

Lombardo, J., H. Burkom, E. Elbert, S. Magruder, S.H. Lewis, W. Loschen, J. Sari, C. Sniegoski, R. Wojcik, and J. Pavlin. 2003. A systems overview of the Electronic Surveillance System for the Early Notification of Community-Based Epidemics (ESSENCE II). *J. Urban Health Bull. N.Y. Acad. Med.* 80(2): 132–142.

Magruder, S.F., S.H. Lewis, A. Najmi, and E. Florio. 2004. Progress in understanding and using over-the-counter pharmaceuticals for syndromic surveillance. *Morb. Mortal. Wkly. Rep.* 53(Suppl.): 117–122.

Mandel, B.J. 1969. The regression control chart. *J. Qual. Technol.* 1(1): 1–9.

Mandl, K.D., J.M. Overhage, M.M. Wagner et al. 2004. Implementing syndromic surveillance: A practical guide informed by the early experience. *J. Am. Med. Inform. Assoc.* 11: 141–150.

Marsden-Haug, N., V.B. Foster, P.L. Gould, E. Elbert, H. Wang, and J.A. Pavlin. 2007. Code-based syndromic surveillance for influenza like illness by International Classification of Diseases, Ninth Revision. *Emerg. Infect. Dis.* 13(2): 207–216.

Martinez-Beneito, M.A., D. Conesa, A. Lopez-Quilez, and A. Lopez-Maside. 2008. Bayesian Markov switching models for the early detection of influenza epidemics. *Stat. Med.* 27(22): 4455–4468.

Murphy, S.P. and H. Burkom. 2008. Recombinant temporal aberration detection algorithms for enhanced biosurveillance. *J. Am. Med. Inform. Assoc.* 15(1): 77–86.

Noufaily, A., D.G. Enki, P. Farrington, P. Garthwaite, N. Andrews, and A. Charlett. 2013. An improved algorithm for outbreak detection in multiple surveillance systems. *Stat. Med.* 32(7): 1206–1222.

Noufaily, A., Y. Ghebremichael-Weldeselassie, D.G. Enki, P. Garthwaite, N. Andrews, A. Charlett, and P. Farrington. 2015. Modelling reporting delays for outbreak detection in infectious disease data. *J. Roy. Stat. Soc. A: Stat. Soc.* 178(1): 205–222.

Okhusa, Y., M. Shigematsu, K. Taniguchi, and N. Okabe. November 2003–April 2004. Experimental surveillance using data on sales of over-the-counter medications—Japan. 2005. http://www.cdc.gov/mmwr/preview/mmwrhtml/su5401a10.htm.

Parker, R.A. 1989. Analysis of surveillance data with Poisson regression: A case study. *Stat. Med.* 8(3): 285–294; discussion 331–332.

Reis, B.Y., I.S. Kohane, and K.D. Mandl. 2007. An epidemiological network model for disease outbreak detection. *PLoS Med.* 4(6): 1019–1031.

Reis, B.Y. and K.D. Mandl. 2003. Time series modeling for syndromic surveillance. *BMC Med. Inform. Decis. Mak.* 3: 2.

Reis, B.Y., M. Pagano, and K.D. Mandl. 2003. Using temporal context to improve biosurveillance. *Proc. Natl. Acad. Sci. U.S.A.* 100: 1961–1965.

Rolka, H., H. Burkom, G.F. Cooper, M. Kulldorff, D. Madigan, and W.K. Wong. 2007. Issues in applied statistics for public health bioterrorism surveillance using multiple data streams: Research needs. *Stat. Med.* 26(8): 1834–1856.

Ryan, T.P. 2008. *Statistical Methods for Quality Improvement*, Chapter 8, 2nd edn., New York: John Wiley & Sons.

Shen, Y. and G.F. Cooper. 2009. Bayesian modeling of unknown diseases for biosurveillance. In *AMIA Annual Symposium Proceedings 2009*, pp. 589–593.

Sherman, R.L., K.A. Henry, S.L. Tannenbaum, D.J. Feaster, E. Kobetz, and D.J. Lee. 2014. Applying spatial analysis tools in public health: An example using SaTScan to detect geographic targets for colorectal cancer screening interventions. *Prev. Chronic Dis.* 11: E41.

Shmueli, G. and H. Burkom. 2010. Statistical challenges facing early outbreak detection in biosurveillance. *Technometrics* 52(1): 39–51.

Sniegoski, C.A. 2004. Automated syndromic classification of chief complaint records. *Johns Hopkins APL Tech. Dig.* 25(1): 68–75.

Sonesson, C. and D. Bock. 2003. A review and discussion of prospective statistical surveillance in public health. *J. Roy. Stat. Soc. A: Stat. Soc.* 166: 5–21.

Stoto, M.A., R.D. Fricker, Jr., A. Jain, A. Diamond, J.O. Davies-Cole, C. Glymph, G. Kidane, G. Lum, L. Jones, and K. Dehan. 2006. Evaluating statistical methods for syndromic surveillance. In A.G. Wilson, G.D. Wilson, and D.H. Olwell, (eds.), *Statistical Methods in Counterterrorism.* New York: Springer, pp. 141–172.

Stroup, D.F., M. Wharton, K. Kafadar, and A.G. Dean. 1993. Evaluation of a method for detecting aberrations in public health surveillance data. *Am. J. Epidemiol.* 137(3): 373–380.

Tokars, J.I., H. Burkom, J. Xing, R. English, S. Bloom, K. Cox, and J.A. Pavlin. 2009. Enhancing time-series detection algorithms for automated biosurveillance. *Emerg. Infect. Dis.* 15(4): 533–539.

Triple S-AGE. 2015. Fact Sheet 5: About data sources for syndromic surveillance. Triple S Assessment Towards Guidelines for Europe. Last Modified March 11, 2014, Accessed September 06, 2015. http://www.syndromicsurveillance.eu/Triple-S_FS5.pdf.

Unkel, S., C.P. Farrington, P.H. Garthwaite, C. Robertson, and N. Andrews. 2012. Statistical methods for the prospective detection of infectious disease outbreaks: A review. *J. Roy. Stat. Soc. A: Stat. Soc.* 175: 49–82.

van den Wijngaard, C., L. van Asten, W. van Pelt, N.J.D. Nagelkerke, R. Verheij, A.J. de Neeling, A. Dekkers, M.A.B. van der Sande, H. van Vliet, and M.P.G. Koopmans. 2008. Validation of syndromic surveillance for respiratory pathogen activity. *Emerg. Infect. Dis.* 14(6): 917–925.

Vial, F. and J. Berezowski. 2015. A practical approach to designing syndromic surveillance systems for livestock and poultry. *Prev. Vet. Med.* 120: 27–38.

Wallstrom, G.L. and W.R. Hogan. 2007. Unsupervised clustering of over-the-counter healthcare products into product categories. *J. Biomed. Inform.* 40: 642–648.

Warns-Petit, E., E. Morignat, M. Artois, and D. Calavas. 2010. Unsupervised clustering of wildlife necropsy data for syndromic surveillance. *BMC Vet. Res.* 6: 56.

Xing, J., H. Burkom, L. Moniz, J. Edgerton, M. Leuze, and J. Tokars. 2009. Evaluation of sliding baseline methods for spatial estimation for cluster detection in the biosurveillance system. *Int. J. Health Geogr.* 8: 45.

Xing, J., H. Burkom, and J. Tokars. 2011. Method selection and adaptation for distributed monitoring of infectious diseases for syndromic surveillance. *J. Biomed. Inform.* 44(6): 1093–1101.

Ziemann, A., T. Krafft, H. Brand et al. and Project Consortium Triple-S. 2012. Identifying good practice for syndromic surveillance in Europe—A comparative study based on site visits in eight countries. *Eur. J. Public Health* 22: 79.

6

Effective public health data visualization

NEIL F. ABERNETHY AND LAUREN N. CARROLL

INTRODUCTION

In the last 20 years, an increasing focus on the need for informatics and analytics in public health has resulted in a growing investment in information systems (Friede et al. 1993, 1995; Baker et al. 1995; Victor and Edberg 2005; Lopez and Blobel 2007; Khan et al. 2010; Reeder et al. 2012). This investment has generated a myriad of new tools for different public health activities and jurisdictions, including tools and systems developed by federal, state, and local governments, as well as research organizations (Driedger et al. 2007; Kothari et al. 2008; Lopes et al. 2010; Robertson and Nelson 2010; Schriml et al. 2010). Advances in electronic reporting and interoperability, computer technology, biotechnology (e.g., genetic sequencing), and other methods (e.g., social network analysis and geographic information systems) have put pressure on the informatics discipline and public health practitioners alike to translate these advances into common practice (Lopez and Blobel 2007;

Khan et al. 2010; Heymann and Brilliant 2011; Klompas et al. 2011). This pressure has been particularly acute for the surveillance and management of infectious diseases with pandemic or bioterrorism potential (Reis et al. 2007; Hills et al. 2008; Chen et al. 2010; Khan et al. 2010).

To characterize the variety of tools and analytical approaches developed for infectious disease control, in this chapter, we will review findings from studies utilizing informatics tools in public health, with a focus on platforms for information visualization. We assessed the landscape of these tools in terms of users' information needs and preferences, the features and system architectures of visualization tools, as well as considerations of usability and adoption. Due to the challenges of integrating, analyzing, and displaying public health data, particularly new types of data encountered in public health, we place a special emphasis on efforts to visualize geographic information systems (GIS), molecular epidemiology, and social networks.

Background

Since John Snow first plotted cholera cases on a map of London, graphs and visualizations have played important roles in epidemiology, supporting communication, aggregation, analysis, and use of data for hypothesis testing and decision making (Koch and Denike 2009; Karlsson et al. 2013). In the electronic age, computer-aided generation of charts, maps, and reports have enabled a further increase in the use of visualization tools to supplement individual-level clinical data and population-level statistics (Hills et al. 2008; Khan et al. 2010). Infectious disease burden in the population, whether measured for programmatic or outbreak management purposes, is now commonly analyzed in terms of geographic distribution, clinical risk factors, demographics, molecular and phylogenetic features, or sources of exposure such as social networks (Holmes 1998; Eubank 2005; Thacker et al. 2012; Hay et al. 2013). While routine features of public health reports include epidemic curves and choropleth maps, new visualization motifs such as social network graphs and phylogenetic trees have increasingly been used to characterize disease outbreaks (Abernethy 2005; Andre

et al. 2007). Indeed, a keyword search by year in PubMed highlights the increased reference to GIS, molecular epidemiology, and social network analysis in publications relative to all indexed PubMed publication (Figure 6.1).

Tools for these three types of complex data allow public health professionals and researchers to integrate, synthesize, and visualize information pertaining to disease surveillance, prevention, and control. The ability to track disease distribution with GIS tools has helped public health professionals and researchers alike to detect disease clustering, analyze spread of disease in communities and across territories, and predict outbreaks (AvRuskin et al. 2004; Gao et al. 2008; Castronovo et al. 2009; Dominkovics et al. 2011; Carpenter 2011). Surveillance of different strains of tuberculosis, influenza, and other diseases via characterization of molecular markers is commonly used to identify potential risk factors, pathogenicity, potential outbreaks, and prepare adequate interventions (Foxman and Riley 2001; Lowy and Miller 2002; Hollm-Delgado 2009; Arts and Weijenberg 2013; Carriço et al. 2013; Maccannell 2013). With the growth of network theory and the availability of modern computing, social network

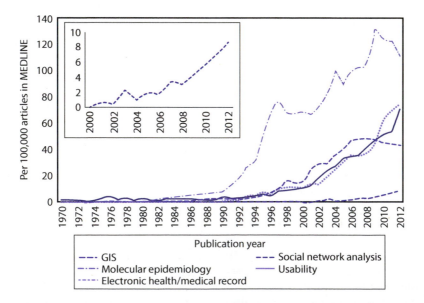

Figure 6.1 Increased reference to common complex data types. Keyword search for GIS, molecular epidemiology, and social network analysis in PubMed highlights the increase in these terms relative to all PubMed index articles. The frequency of other biomedical informatics terms (usability, electronic health record) is shown for comparison. Although the growth of social network analysis has been more recent, the inset shows that this concept has also experienced rapid growth in the published literature.

analysis and network-based epidemic models have been increasingly used to depict outbreaks and disease dynamics (Fitzpatrick et al. 2001; McElroy et al. 2003; Dewan et al. 2006; Morris et al. 2006), identify potential cases and focus control efforts by prioritizing contacts (Andre et al. 2007), and evaluate strategies to interrupt transmission (Morris et al. 2006; Basta et al. 2009; Polgreen et al. 2010). Together, these data types can tell a compelling story about disease risk factors and spread and transmission, and they can lead to more effective control measures and interventions.

However, this surge in surveillance capacity has produced more complex and disparate data, leading to new discussions about data sharing and interoperability, data confidentiality, and strategies for managing redundancies as well as incomplete data (Bishr 1998; O'Carroll et al. 1998; Hu et al. 2007; Lopez and Blobel 2007; Gao et al. 2008; Chen et al. 2010; Gesteland et al. 2012). For example, public health practitioners and researchers are faced with integrating diverse data sources such as mortality data (e.g., autopsy reports), clinical data (e.g., laboratory reports, immunization records), geographical data (e.g., address of work, residence, preschool), relationships (e.g., names of family, friends, partners), patient and pathogen genetics, medical imaging, travel plans, and timelines. Each of these types of information can be recorded, stored, accessed, evaluated, and displayed in many different systems and formats. Organizations are therefore challenged to maximize the potential of this flood of data to impact public health practice. Visualization tools have the potential to improve comprehension of these data by increasing the memory and processing resources available to users, reducing the search for information, enhancing the detection of patterns, and providing mechanisms for inference (Folorunso and Ogunseye 2008). However, visualization tools also risk misleading users due to misinterpretation or cognitive overload (Joyce 2009; Lê 2013).

As such, funders and developers of visualization tools encounter a range of challenges when designing new tools for public health data, generating a growing collection of tools as new ideas and approaches are explored. However, these tools are often developed in silos, limiting their use in practice (Fuller 2010). And despite the advances in public health informatics, many public health professionals still use visualization tools and data management systems that may no longer suit their

current needs (Pina et al. 2009; Khan et al. 2010; Reeder et al. 2012). By discussing the interactions between user information needs and preferences, system features and architectures, and usability and adoption considerations, we will address the entire life cycle of development and use of public health visualizations. Finally, we will explore commonalities among complex data types and underscore some of the challenges that lie ahead for novel visualization tool development.

SURVEYING APPROACHES TO VISUALIZATION IN PUBLIC HEALTH

This chapter explores the lifecycle of development and adoption of infectious disease visualization tools from conception to evaluation in practice. Infectious disease surveillance and control efforts encompass a wide variety of fields and require integration, synthesis, and analysis of information (Rolka et al. 2012; Thacker et al. 2012; Gorman 2013). Consequently, we surveyed diverse public health visualization literature from varied sources encompassing academia and public health practice. This survey covers the following topics:

1. Public health user needs and preferences for infectious disease information visualization tools
2. Existing infectious disease information visualization tools, including their architecture and features
3. Commonalities among complex data types
4. Usability evaluation efforts and barriers to the adoption of visualization tools

To gain a comprehensive understanding of the current landscape of these tools, we identified research articles published in English from January 1, 1980 to June 30, 2013. We included two broad classes of research articles: those discussing information needs for public health professionals and those explicitly describing visualization and mapping tools in the context of public health activities or usability studies. We reviewed on systems utilized in infectious disease epidemiology, and consequently excluded studies focused primarily on computer science, clinical medicine or research, organizational systems, and animal or ecological systems.

The approaches discussed in this chapter include descriptive reports, qualitative studies (e.g., interviews, focus groups), and usability studies, originating from U.S.-based and international journals. We organized approaches to visualizing public health data into six categories: information needs and learning behavior, tool architecture, user preferences, tool features, usability studies, and reports of implementation and adoption. These categories highlight the logical progression of novel tool development; note that these categories are not mutually exclusive. Summaries of findings in each category are described in the following sections.

INFORMATION NEEDS AND LEARNING BEHAVIOR

The types of information required by public health professionals have been studied in many contexts. The studies reviewed offer several insights about information seeking behavior among public health professionals. While the public health workforce is extremely diverse (Humphreys 1998; Walton et al. 2000; Lee et al. 2003; LaPelle et al. 2006; Revere et al. 2007; Turner et al. 2008) and public health information sources are often disparate and unstandardized (Humphreys 1998; Walton et al. 2000; Hu et al. 2007; Revere et al. 2007), several themes held constant. Public health professionals need timely access to current data from reliable, high quality sources (Centers for Disease Control and Prevention 2000; LaPelle et al. 2000, 2006; Revere et al. 2007; Kothari et al. 2008; Turner et al. 2008; Robinson et al. 2011). Furthermore, public health professionals need synthesized and collated data on relevant information such as best practices, effective prevention strategies or interventions, and evidence-based research, to name a few (Centers for Disease Control and Prevention 2000; LaPelle et al. 2006; Revere et al. 2007; Kothari et al. 2008; Ford and Korjonen 2012). Public health professionals gather information from colleagues, literature, and health departments (Lee et al. 2003; Revere et al. 2007; Turner et al. 2008; Twose et al. 2008; Robinson et al. 2011). However, multiple studies suggested that public health professionals are often unaware of available information resources and emphasized collaboration to improve search outcomes (Humphreys 1998; Walton et al. 2000; Fourie 2009; Ford and Korjonen 2012). Additional challenges associated with meeting information needs include external barriers (e.g., lack of time, sufficient staff), technological barriers

(e.g., inadequate equipment, lack of Internet access), internal barriers (e.g., stress, lack of confidence in ability to complete task, lack of training), and lack of trust in the information source (Humphreys 1998; Walton et al. 2000; Revere et al. 2007; Kothari et al. 2008; Turner et al. 2008; Twose et al. 2008; Fourie 2009; Robinson et al. 2011; Ford and Korjonen 2012). These studies suggested centralized access to reliable resources, as well as improved access to and delivery of timely information, as key to overcoming these barriers.

However, information needs specifically pertaining to information visualization tools have not been as well explored. Two studies explored the context in which participants learned about, used, and synthesized information from visualization tools through interviews and questionnaires with public health professionals (Robinson 2009; Robinson et al. 2011). The first highlighted the importance of prior knowledge and intuition to give context to the results, and demonstrated participants' frustration with tools that were not intuitive or were too awkward for regular use (Robinson 2009). The second study indicated that public health professionals spend less than 10 hours per month learning about new tools or methods for work and primarily learn about them from Internet, literature, conferences, and colleagues (Robinson et al. 2011). Participants wanted to know how the tool was developed and by whom (e.g., authors' names, fields of expertise, credentials, affiliations) as well as how the tool provided results. Additional studies also highlighted the importance of the users' perception of, and trust in, the tool's reliability as a potential learning barrier to new visualization tools (Bassil and Keller 2001; Kothari et al. 2008; Joyce 2009). In a study of user needs and preferences for visualization tools, 60% of users indicated they typically use more than one visualization tool for their visualization and analysis needs (Bassil and Keller 2001). This finding was supported in multiple studies wherein users indicated that no one existing tool or system met all their data needs (Revere et al. 2007; Turner et al. 2008; Joyce 2009; Robinson 2009). Further, studies indicated that users most commonly created static graphics, and many users relied on Microsoft Office suite (Bassil and Keller 2001; Joyce 2009; Robinson 2009; Robinson et al. 2011). Collectively, these findings indicate many users are interested in learning about new tools in a time-efficient manner and support an important relationship between user trust, tool credibility, and transparency.

Common concerns raised by these systems include cognitive overload and the misinterpretation of results. Some users voice concerns that data can be manipulated or unintentionally misrepresented due to confusion about how tools work or what type of graphics should be employed (Kienle and Müller 2007; Kothari et al. 2008; Joyce 2009). Cognitive overload, wherein a user is presented with more information than they are able to successfully process, was addressed in several studies. This highlights the challenge of displaying complex and large data sets without reducing usability, or reaching the technical limits of the platform or the cognitive limits of the user (Herman et al. 2000; Driscoll et al. 2011). Strategies to minimize cognitive overload were less defined, although Herman et al. (2000) suggested human-centered design as a means of improving data visualization interpretation.

The data sources available for a targeted use case often influence the architectural design of a visualization tool. The next section explores common architectures reported by the articles included in this survey.

ARCHITECTURE OF EXISTING TOOLS

We considered *architecture* to address the means by which a system was constructed in the software design sense, referring to the way in which system components fit together. Components may be individual classes in a software program or larger components, like a database management system, a web service, and the connections in between these components. Other features, such as interface design, operation workflow, functionality, features, visualization layouts, and analysis algorithms are often independent of underlying system architecture. These are covered later in the chapter.

Several articles in our survey made only cursory reference to system architecture. For example, some papers referenced use of specific components such as a particular management system, GIS, database, or statistical package (Green et al. 1998; Anselin et al. 2006; Blanton et al. 2006; Hurlimann et al. 2011; Porcasi et al. 2012; Sopan et al. 2012). Others alluded to particular architectural choices through discussion of other technical

issues, for example, the computational complexity of a statistical routine (Freifeld et al. 2008; Hurlimann et al. 2011). However, these references alone gave little insight into the structure of the system as a whole. Some of articles in this review contained more significant coverage of system architecture, including a discussion of the general architectural design in terms of the number and function of system tiers (Gao et al. 2008; Heitgerd et al. 2008; Yi et al. 2008; Dominkovics et al. 2011). This may reflect the purpose behind many such publications, which typically focused on the utility of design features for public health purposes or the challenges inherent in linking data to visualization tools. One publication, however, explicitly described the *structured application framework for Epi Info (SAFE)*, a set of application development guidelines to improve the software design and modularity of public health information systems developed using components from the Epi Info tool provided by the Centers for Disease Control and Prevention (CDC) (Ma et al. 2008).

Web-based systems, or systems having some web accessible components, were the delivery platform of choice in many cases (Blanton et al. 2006; da Silva et al. 2007; Hu et al. 2007; Freifeld et al. 2008; Gao et al. 2008, 2009; Heitgerd et al. 2008; Reinhardt et al. 2008; Yi et al. 2008; Dominkovics et al. 2011; Driscoll et al. 2011; Lewis et al. 2011; Sopan et al. 2012; Alonso and McCormick 2012; Ramírez-Ramírez et al. 2013). These were often intended to permit distributed access by public health staff, reduce software implementation costs, or expose public health information for public dissemination. As such, security and privacy was a frequently noted concern. However, only one article specifically discussed implementation of security protocols (Reinhardt et al. 2008). Others discussed methods for aggregating or otherwise de-identifying data (Yi et al. 2008; Sopan et al. 2012).

Total data volume, size of data transfer packets, or processing complexity in time or space were cited in a few studies (Atkinson and Unwin 2002; Gao et al. 2008, 2009; Dominkovics et al. 2011). These articles suggested the use of data warehousing and caching as possible approaches to address processing time related issues, noting that it takes time to calculate statistical values for use in infectious disease mapping. Several studies also mentioned cost as a major factor affecting architectural component choices (da Silva et al. 2007; Gao et al.

2008, 2009; Yi et al. 2008; Dominkovics et al. 2011). Presented solutions included using open source or free proprietary software, using free web resources like the Google Maps API (Google Maps 2015), and building modular, reusable components such as web services (Cook et al. 2007; Gao et al. 2008, 2009; Ma et al. 2008; Yi et al. 2008; Dominkovics et al. 2011). Overall, there is a trend away from stand-alone visualization systems, and toward modular, service-oriented architectures and web-based user interfaces.

USER PREFERENCES

User preferences highlight how users prefer to interact with a tool or system and can provide insights into possible sources of usability issues or adoption barriers. Studies of academic researchers and public health professionals indicated a preference for tools that help users evaluate disparate and complex high-quality data (McGrath et al. 2003; Hu et al. 2007; Joyce 2009; Robinson et al. 2011; Gesteland et al. 2012; Shneiderman et al. 2013), with the goal of improving comprehension and communication, as well as facilitating decision-making (Bassil and Keller 2001; McGrath et al. 2003; Hu et al. 2007; Joyce 2009; Robinson 2009; Koenig et al. 2011; Robinson et al. 2011; Gesteland et al. 2012; Karlsson et al. 2013; Shneiderman et al. 2013). Additionally, participants in qualitative and quantitative studies emphasized the importance of user-friendly, reliable tools, with high-quality online documentation, and easy access to the source code (Bassil and Keller 2001; Plaisant 2004; Hu et al. 2007; Kienle and Müller 2007; Kothari et al. 2008; Robinson et al. 2011). Users in a variety of settings raised concerns regarding interoperability of new and existing tools, data sharing, and data confidentiality (Plaisant 2004; Hu et al. 2007; Kienle and Müller 2007; Joyce 2009; Robinson 2009). Additionally, analysis of a survey conducted by Bassil and Keller (2001) indicated that users in academic settings are nearly twice as sensitive to the cost of a new tool as are users in industry. This finding is consistent with many studies exploring or advocating for open-source and web-based infectious disease visualization tools to overcome cost and resource barriers (Freifeld et al. 2008; Reinhardt et al. 2008; Yi et al. 2008; Driscoll et al. 2011;

Hurlimann et al. 2011; Lewis et al. 2011; Robinson et al. 2011; Alonso and McCormick 2012). Moreover, these preferences mirror key themes from previous sections, namely user trust, tool credibility, and transparency.

A host of studies highlighted user preferences for data abstraction, each with the underlying theme of making complex data digestible and useful for users. Users expressed a strong interest in dynamic, interactive graphics that allow them to review their data at different levels (e.g., population or individual level) (Herman et al. 2000; Bassil and Keller 2001; McGrath et al. 2003; Hu et al. 2007; Robinson 2009; Koenig et al. 2011; Gesteland et al. 2012; Karlsson et al. 2013; Shneiderman et al. 2013). With such a function, users felt they could incrementally explore the data to evaluate both the big picture and the finer details. In addition, users valued common interface features such as zoom, pan, search, filter, save, undo, and work history (Herman et al. 2000; Bassil and Keller 2001; Plaisant 2004; Hu et al. 2007; Kienle and Müller 2007; Kothari et al. 2008; Shneiderman et al. 2013). Users also showed interest in high-quality automated layouts and customizable features (e.g., color, size, shape) to facilitate understanding of the data (Herman et al. 2000; Bassil and Keller 2001; McGrath et al. 2003; Kienle and Müller 2007). Furthermore, some users demonstrated high interest in tools with multiple views or panels, enabling them to review their data from different perspectives (Herman et al. 2000; Bassil and Keller 2001; Plaisant 2004; Hu et al. 2007; Kienle and Müller 2007; Chui et al. 2011; Koenig et al. 2011; Gesteland et al. 2012; Upadhyayula et al. 2012; Shneiderman et al. 2013). In concert, users preferred easy navigation between views and synchronized browsing (e.g., monitor the same variable across panels) (Bassil and Keller 2001; Kienle and Müller 2007). The ability to layer data, particularly among GIS users, was a common request to facilitate understanding of interactions or risk factors that overlap with disease outcomes (Plaisant 2004; Hu et al. 2007; Kothari et al. 2008; Joyce 2009). Overall, these preferences emphasize the importance of discovery and information synthesis through iterative data exploration.

Such preferences guide the development of infectious disease visualization tools and can inform strategies for incorporating the tools into routine practice. The corresponding features and functions have the potential to help users discover complex or hidden patterns (Thew et al. 2011).

FEATURES OF EXISTING TOOLS

Having identified common information needs, system architectures, and user preferences, the following subsections explore existing tools and applications in more depth as they pertain to GIS, molecular epidemiology, and social network analyses. Each section also provides examples of common representations of GIS, molecular epidemiology, and social network data, respectively.

GIS

The development of increasingly sophisticated GIS has provided a new set of tools for public health professionals to monitor and respond to health challenges. These systems can help pinpoint cases and exposures, identify spatial trends, identify disease clusters, correlate different sets of spatial data, and test statistical hypotheses. Often, these analyses are aided by visualization and mapping of data, provided via web services or a user interface.

Our survey identified many approaches to delivering GIS functions based on various sources of public health data. Common functions among these studies and systems were geocoding (Rushton 2003; Blanton et al. 2006; Driedger et al. 2007; Yi et al. 2008; Hurlimann et al. 2011), integrating data sources (Blanton et al. 2006; Chen and MacEachren 2008; Fisher and Myers 2011; Hurlimann et al. 2011), and cluster detection (Rushton 2003; Reinhardt et al. 2008). Mapping of data was commonly achieved through dot maps (Figure 6.2a) (Nobre et al. 1997; Buckeridge et al. 1998; Green et al. 1998; Hadjichristodoulou et al. 1999; Blanton et al. 2006; da Silva et al. 2007; Driedger et al. 2007; Geanuracos et al. 2007; Hu et al. 2007; Reinhardt et al. 2008; Fisher and Myers 2011; Hurlimann et al. 2011; Lewis et al. 2011; ter Waarbeek et al. 2011; Thew et al. 2011; Alonso and McCormick 2012; Joshi et al. 2012b; Porcasi et al. 2012; Aimone et al. 2013), choropleth maps (Figure 6.2b) (Nobre et al. 1997; Green et al. 1998; Hadjichristodoulou et al. 1999; Anselin et al. 2006; Driedger et al. 2007; Geanuracos et al. 2007; Heitgerd et al. 2008; Fisher and Myers 2011; Thew et al. 2011; Gesteland et al. 2012; Joshi et al. 2012b;

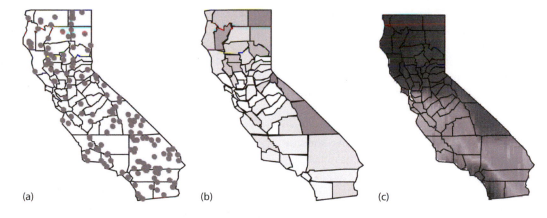

(a)   (b)   (c)

Figure 6.2 (a–c) Common geographic visualizations. A dot map (a) uses dots to represent a certain measure or feature displayed over a geographical map. They are often used to present the geographical distribution of various disease cases in infectious disease surveillance. This figure represents hypothetical infectious disease cases in the state of California. Each dot represents a specific disease case. These maps may help identify clusters of disease. In interactive tools, users may click individual cases or select subsets of cases to obtain further information. Individual level data is often aggregated in a choropleth map (b), which uses graded colors or shades to indicate the values of some aggregate measure in specified areas. This figure shows the incidence rate per 100,000 persons of cases from map (a). Differences in the incidence rates by county are indicated with different shades, with a darker color indicating a higher rate. Interactive choropleth maps allow selection of regions to obtain additional information. Individual or aggregate level data may be used to statistically derive a spatial risk gradient (c). Other visualization features may allow zooming/panning of maps, introduction of other map layers such as roads, or selection of color scales.

Upadhyayula et al. 2012; Aimone et al. 2013), and isopleth or gradient maps (Figure 6.2c) (Atkinson and Unwin 2002; da Silva et al. 2007; Driedger et al. 2007; Stevens and Pfeiffer 2011; Porcasi et al. 2012). Recurrent considerations cited within these papers included the privacy of public health data (Green et al. 1998; Geanuracos et al. 2007; Gao et al. 2008, 2009; Yi et al. 2008), the alignment of GIS analytics to users' needs (Buckeridge et al. 1998; Geanuracos et al. 2007; Thew et al. 2011; Joshi et al. 2012a,b; Porcasi et al. 2012), the motivations to make analysis services accessible, and the interoperability of systems/data (Driedger et al. 2007; Geanuracos et al. 2007; Gao et al. 2008; Yi et al. 2008). Since many GIS analytical services and geographic data are available through providers such as ESRI, Google, or the U.S. Census, GIS systems in our survey often utilize architectures based on these services and map data.

The systems reviewed were designed with various targeted users in mind. Two broad divisions of these were systems intended for public access using publicly available data and restricted systems intended for users with access to private public health data. In many cases, these systems cited the use of publicly available maps and cartographic data as a basis for spatial integration of other information (Blanton et al. 2006; Geanuracos et al. 2007; Chen and MacEachren 2008; Hurlimann et al. 2011; Sopan et al. 2012). Many systems utilize administrative geographic units as a basis to merge data across different health and population databases, for example, to calculate incidence rates based surveillance data and a population census. Other approaches may either map other sources into an internal data model (Freifeld et al. 2008) or to an ontology that supports data integration (Gao et al. 2008).

Visualization methods for GIS in public health focus on functions geared toward simplifying, integrating, or analyzing data in a spatial context. The simplest visualizations plot or aggregate spatial data to deliver static point or choropleth maps of individual or aggregate data, respectively. Many systems incorporate a temporal component, enabling either animation of data through time or restriction of the data displayed to a time window of interest (Freifeld et al. 2008; Reinhardt et al. 2008; Yi et al. 2008; Benavides et al. 2012). A step beyond mere display of information, some GIS or spatial statistical methods seek to perform kernel-based smoothing to estimate risk maps (Atkinson and Unwin 2002; Rushton 2003; Stevens and Pfeiffer 2011), visualize disease risk according to a statistical model (da Silva et al. 2007; Hu et al. 2007; Gao et al. 2008; Moore et al. 2008; Lewis et al. 2011; Maciejewski et al. 2011; Stevens and Pfeiffer 2011; Alonso and McCormick 2012; Porcasi et al. 2012), or compare one feature to another (Rushton 2003; Anselin et al. 2006; Geanuracos et al. 2007; Reinhardt et al. 2008; Aimone et al. 2013). While the ability to zoom and pan to navigate maps (Yi et al. 2008; Thew et al. 2011; Joshi et al. 2012b) is a common interactive feature enjoyed by users, more advanced systems contain interactive controls to enable users to retrieve information about selected items or regions, visualize the results of arbitrary queries (Yi et al. 2008), control visualization options, control temporal ranges of data returned (Freifeld et al. 2008; Yi et al. 2008), or link displays of data with alternate or comparative visualizations (Heitgerd et al. 2008; Yi et al. 2008).

Molecular epidemiology

Molecular epidemiology is concerned with understanding the distribution or clustering of genetic variants, strains, serotypes, or other molecular groupings of pathogens. In molecular epidemiology, relationships between isolates are often calculated and conveyed through phylogenetic trees or *dendrograms* (Figure 6.3). Visualization tools for molecular epidemiology often included phylogenetic analysis and visualization capabilities (Parks et al. 2009; Janies et al. 2011; Gopinath et al. 2013) and visualization of contextual data using connected graphs (Parks et al. 2009; Driscoll et al. 2011). The tools we reviewed were primarily designed to be accessed through the Internet (Macdonald et al. 2009; Parks et al. 2009; Driscoll et al. 2011; Gopinath et al. 2013). Most studies in our survey included the capability to integrate GIS or location-based data with genetic or serotype visualizations (Reinhardt et al. 2008; Macdonald et al. 2009; Parks et al. 2009; Grundmann et al. 2010; Schriml et al. 2010; Driscoll et al. 2011; Janies et al. 2011; Gopinath et al. 2013). Two of the tools were designed to produce visualization (KML) files for display in other GIS packages (Schriml et al. 2010; Janies et al. 2011), while other web-based tools made use of external GIS services embedded

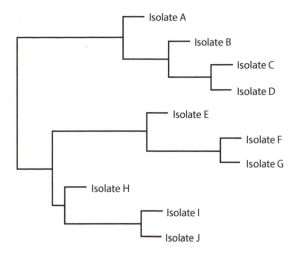

Figure 6.3 Dendrogram. A dendrogram, or phylogenetic tree, is a branching diagram or "tree" showing the evolutionary history between biological species or other entities based on their genetic characteristics. Species or entities joined together by nodes represent descendants from a common ancestor and are more similar genetically. This figure shows a hypothetical example of a rooted dendrogram, wherein the horizontal position of individuals represents the genetic distance from a specific progenitor. With the advancement of DNA sequencing technologies, phylogenetic trees have been used widely in infectious disease control to depict the genetic similarities and differences between strains and variants of a certain disease pathogen. Knowing whether infectious diseases occurring in different areas are from the same strain provides key information on the source of infection and how the disease may been transmitted. Interactive features of these visualizations may include the ability to collapse or color and label branches.

within the website, primarily Google Maps™, ESRI/ArcGIS or HealthMap (Macdonald et al. 2009; Grundmann et al. 2010; Driscoll et al. 2011).

Some tools were designed with specific organisms in mind, for example, staphylococcal (Grundmann et al. 2010) or influenza (Macdonald et al. 2009) infections. Driscoll et al. (2011) developed Disease View, a set of tools to understand host–pathogen molecular epidemiology. They demonstrated the use of this tool to analyze aspects of the *Vibrio cholerae* outbreak that occurred in the aftermath of the 2010 Haiti earthquake. These tools allow spatial views of molecular epidemiological properties associated with outbreaks, for example, showing sequence variation of genes associated with disease virulence between outbreak locations. Other tools were designed to accommodate multiple organisms or user-specified organisms (Parks et al. 2009; Janies et al. 2011; Gopinath et al. 2013). One such tool, designed specifically for geospatial surveillance of genomic characteristics of NIAID category A–C viral and bacterial pathogens, is GeMIna (Schriml et al. 2010). This tool collects curated

metadata relating to the diseases. Other views of the distribution of genotypes across a large geographic scale help to understand the relationship between the population biology and geography of a pathogen species (He et al. 2012). This is sometimes known as *phylogeography*.

As with GIS systems, data integration was a key component of the web-based tools, with all web-based tools incorporating access to or prepopulated with existing sets of data or metadata, including pathogen, isolate and sequence data. Several studies discussed approaches for integration of genetic and social network data (Lowy and Miller 2002; McElroy et al. 2003; Cook et al. 2007; Hollm-Delgado 2009; Zarrabi et al. 2012). In the absence of known exposures between cases, or in the case of ineffective contact investigations, molecular epidemiology or genomic approaches can identify potential members of an outbreak cluster. These studies showed social network data alongside genetic data using custom visualizations, but tools with the capacity to visualize the interplay of these data types systematically are still being developed.

Social network analysis

In addition to geographic and molecular epidemiologic data, networks of social contact or disease exposure are a third type of complex data that are increasingly being used to understand disease outbreaks. As shown in Figure 6.1, social network analysis as a field is growing relative to health literature as a whole; however, it is at an earlier stage than for the other two topics. In order to describe the use of social network visualizations for public health, we therefore considered a broader set of publications that often described visualizations of single outbreaks or analyses, in addition to those directly describing tools used to visualize outbreak networks. Nevertheless, these publications inform desiderata for visualizations of these networks, which in turn inform the features or design requirements such systems should consider. Applications of social network analysis in public health typically focus on routes of infection in communicable disease contact investigation; hence, most of the publications in our survey address this topic.

Among the systems and studies we reviewed, social network analysis was applied in a variety of ways. Common applications included risk stratification in contact tracing, identification of characteristics common among infected cases, visual communication or mapping of cases to improve understanding of outbreaks, and identification of potential transmission pathways between clustered cases (McElroy et al. 2003; Andre et al. 2007; Hansen et al. 2010). Among the considerations for data visualization addressed by these studies, several common features were observed: the use of shape, color, and graph position to convey information (McElroy et al. 2003; Viégas and Donath 2004; Andre et al. 2007; Cook et al. 2007; Hansen et al. 2010); the display of individual case features or identity; and the identification of important clusters or paths in the network (Andre et al. 2007; Cook et al. 2007; Hansen et al. 2010). In more advanced analyses, studies may seek to compare or estimate networks across other variables, such as including a temporal dimension in the study (McElroy et al. 2003; Viégas and Donath 2004; Cook et al. 2007; Hansen et al. 2010; Ramírez-Ramírez et al. 2013) (Figure 6.4); integrating geographic or location features (Viégas and Donath 2004; Cook et al. 2007; Hansen et al. 2010; Benavides et al. 2012; Ramírez-Ramírez et al. 2013), or identifying exposures via molecular epidemiology as discussed in the previous section.

Consistent with other findings from this survey, network analysis studies highlighted the importance of designing network visualizations that provide the right information to users without

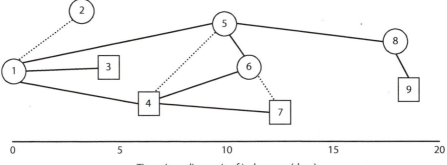

Time since diagnosis of index case (days)

Figure 6.4 Social network diagram. A social network is a graphical representation of social relations or exposures consisting of nodes (individuals within the network) and ties (relationships between individuals). Nodes are usually represented as points or other shapes while ties are represented by lines between the nodes. Differences in the shapes or lines of the diagram may be used to represent different characteristics of the individuals or the relationships. This figure shows a hypothetical example of a force-directed social networks diagram. Social networks analyses in infectious disease control have been gaining importance in the past decade. Examining these social relationships between disease cases and their secondary contacts may be beneficial to tracking the spread of infectious diseases within interconnected social networks. It is especially useful in identifying the index or source case and predicting which individuals are more likely to become infected and further infect others.

confusing them. These considerations took the form of discussions about information overload from complex graphs (Hansen et al. 2010), the inclusion of diverse user preferences for visualization (Viégas and Donath 2004; Hansen et al. 2010), and the importance of training to help users understand and utilize these graphics (Andre et al. 2007; Cook et al. 2007). Viégas and Donath (2004) and Hansen et al. (2010) studied non-standard network layouts and included user assessments to help evaluate how these could best be used. Although most publications discussed the use of networks in a disease control context, Andre et al. (2007), Cook et al. (2007), and McElroy et al. (2003) explicitly described how network visualizations could be used to aid decision-making via prioritization of resources or investigations. Other less common considerations for network analyses described in our survey include the use of repeated contacts as a heuristic for risk, studies of population mixing (Andre et al. 2007), the use of touch-screen interfaces to navigate networks (Hansen et al. 2010), the importance of aggregated data visualization options to prevent information overload (Hansen et al. 2010), and the use of simulation to augment missing data (Ramírez-Ramírez et al. 2013).

Mostly absent from these studies were visualization methods to help users understand network structures at an aggregate or summarized level, comparable to the choropleth map in GIS. Although visualizations like collapsed nodes, flow diagrams, and network metric distributions (such as node degree distribution) (Xia et al. 2013) have been used in other domains, these techniques may not yet be familiar interfaces for lay users, and hence have not been widely employed in tools for public health. As network data become increasingly integrated with GIS, molecular epidemiology, and other health indicators, evaluation of more diverse methods of network visualization consistent with end-user preferences, training level, statistical literacy, and cognitive ability will be needed.

USABILITY

The usefulness of a system is often used to describe a system's overall effectiveness. The concept of usefulness can be measured as a combination of utility and usability. Traditional system evaluation has focused on utility, determining whether an information system is able to meet the functional requirements of a user who wants to accomplish a specific set of work tasks. This is demonstrated in studies that evaluate information systems based on a strict set of functional metrics, such as accuracy and efficiency (Ives et al. 1983).

In addition to evaluating system functionality, it is becoming increasingly important to evaluate system usability. Some researchers have conducted usability evaluations to provide justification for the time and effort spent developing and deploying these complex tools (Ives et al. 1983). In addition, the intended benefit of many information systems is to facilitate interaction between users and data, and so usability itself is the primary measure of system usefulness (Roth et al. 2009). However, the features which improve the usability of one system cannot always be generalized to other systems, since different users may have different task-specific system requirements (Plaisant 2004; Robinson et al. 2011).

Even though specific design recommendations may not apply broadly across systems, studies cited common methods to reliably evaluate the usability of a system. These methods include the use of qualitative investigation techniques, such as participant observations, interviews, and workflow analysis (Kushniruk 2002; Robinson et al. 2005; Pina et al. 2009). Participant observations involve watching users as they perform their work, during which researchers have encouraged users to "talk aloud" during interactions with information systems. These observations have served as the basis for semi-structured interviews and focus groups used to obtain in-depth descriptions of user behavior (Kushniruk 2002; Robinson et al. 2005; Pina et al. 2009). Published studies also describe the use of interviews to highlight areas for further investigation, either by pinpointing particular aspects that a user does not like, or by uncovering new interactions that a user would like to see added (Robinson et al. 2005). In addition, observations and interviews have been combined with questionnaires containing Likert scale questions, asking users to rate their satisfaction with information systems (Hu et al. 2007).

However, study researchers acknowledged that efforts to simplify interactions between users and data may have the unintended consequence of limiting functionality (Robinson et al. 2011). For this reason, some researchers found it important to engage users in the design and development processes. This was accomplished by employing usability evaluation techniques in conjunction with participatory design methods, allowing feedback to be incorporated into the system throughout the development process (Kushniruk 2002; Robinson et al. 2005; Driedger et al. 2007; Driscoll et al. 2011). Researchers also expressed interest in studying user work behaviors over longer time periods (Plaisant 2004), an aspect which might be addressed by soliciting feedback during an ongoing participatory design process (Roth et al. 2009; Shneiderman et al. 2013).

IMPLEMENTATION AND ADOPTION

Barriers to adoption vary widely and are not mutually exclusive within a given organization or individual. System-level barriers, such as access issues (e.g., lack of Internet or finances) and lack of organizational support were significant barriers in organizations worldwide (Lee et al. 2003; Driedger et al. 2007; Geanuracos et al. 2007; Folorunso and Ogunseye 2008; Kothari et al. 2008; Turner et al. 2008; Yi et al. 2008; Joyce 2009; Driedger et al. 2010; Fisher and Myers 2011; Yan et al. 2013). Jurisdictions often struggle to share data due to lack of data standardization (e.g., data heterogeneity, missing data, lack of interoperability) and face data confidentiality concerns which collectively compound the already-complex task of monitoring diseases (Driedger et al. 2007; Hu et al. 2007; Gao et al. 2008; Kothari et al. 2008; Joyce 2009; Driedger et al. 2010; Fisher and Myers 2011; Hurlimann et al. 2011; Yan et al. 2013). Furthermore, user-level concerns may also result in adoption barriers. Confusion regarding how to create or use effective graphics and a lack of familiarity with the concepts in the tool could be substantial learning barriers (Folorunso and Ogunseye 2008; Turner et al. 2008; Fisher and Myers 2011). Fear of change and an interest in staying within one's comfort zone, in addition to a lack of trust and misconceptions about the use of the tool, may also prevent adoption of a valuable tool (Kienle and Müller 2007; Folorunso and Ogunseye 2008; Joyce 2009). Indeed, studies indicated that many users relied on other tools (e.g., Microsoft Office suite) because they felt that many existing tools were too complex and had a substantial learning curve (Driedger et al. 2007; Kienle and Müller 2007; Folorunso and Ogunseye 2008; Kothari et al. 2008; Yi et al. 2008; Fisher and Myers 2011;

Thew et al. 2011; Alonso and McCormick 2012; Yan et al. 2013).

Despite the potential for data visualization tools to monitor and aid control efforts for infectious diseases, such tools have had only limited adoption (Rushton 2003; Joyce 2009), and only one system was assessed for distribution (Harbage and Dean 1999). Usability studies and implementation projects are remarkably interdependent, as successful adoption often requires developers to re-design elements of the tool to further address the users' needs (Robinson et al. 2005; Driedger et al. 2007; Driscoll et al. 2011). The resulting iterative design process often helps users identify previously unexpressed or unknown information needs (Plaisant 2004), resulting in the need for subsequent usability studies. However, this process can be time consuming, and users may find alternative systems that meet their current needs before the tool is completed (Driedger et al. 2007, 2010). Moreover, existing tools are largely isolated to the jurisdictions and organizations that developed them and may be based on proprietary systems (Driedger et al. 2007; Hu et al. 2007). Such silos could prevent the widespread adoption of tools by other agencies or organizations.

While the specifics of adoption strategies may vary depending on the particular organization or agency and their needs, some common strategies emerged from the literature review. Several studies recommended ongoing user collaboration with the tool developers to ensure that the users' needs were heard early on in the project, and to create the opportunity for regular feedback (Robinson et al. 2005; Driedger et al. 2007, 2010; Kienle and Müller 2007; Kothari et al. 2008; Yi et al. 2008). Further, studies advocated for open source tools to reduce access barriers, particularly in low-resource settings (Anselin et al. 2006; Yi et al. 2008; Driedger et al. 2010; Fisher and Myers 2011). Integrating the tool into existing workflow was also recommended as a strategy to encourage users to regularly utilize the tool (Driedger et al. 2007; Kienle and Müller 2007; Folorunso and Ogunseye 2008; Pina et al. 2009; Roth et al. 2009; Fisher and Myers 2011). Additionally, providing adequate user training and education, as well as ongoing technical support, for staff was considered essential for successful adoption of a novel tool in many studies (Driedger et al. 2007, 2010; Geanuracos et al. 2007; Hu et al. 2007; Folorunso and Ogunseye 2008; Ma et al. 2008; Yi et al. 2008; Joyce 2009; Roth et al. 2009; Fisher and Myers 2011; Koenig et al. 2011; Robinson et al. 2011; Thew et al. 2011; Yan et al. 2013); effective user training may build the users' self-confidence in the use of the tool and encourage them to try the tool (Robinson et al. 2005; Driedger et al. 2010). In concert, these strategies may create an environment for sustained use.

CONCLUSION

In this chapter, we have assessed the current landscape of visualization tools developed for infectious disease epidemiology. We characterized these tools in terms of information needs and user preferences, features and system architectures of existing tools, as well as usability and adoption considerations. By focusing on visualizations of GIS, molecular or genetic, and social network data, we also explored similarities among these three types of increasingly common data types. The richness of the information offered by these data for communication and decision-making are counterbalanced by difficulties in displaying, interpreting, and trusting these data sources. In our survey of tools throughout their lifecycle from conception to development to sustained adoption, several themes and challenges emerged pertaining to both individual stages as well as broader topics. Despite the different scholarly approaches that inform public health visualizations and studies utilizing these visualizations, the following themes emerged: (1) the importance of knowledge regarding user needs and preferences; (2) the importance of user training and the integration of tools into routine work practices; (3) complications associated with understanding and use of visualizations; and (4) the role of user trust and organizational support in the ultimate usability and uptake of these tools. Another broad theme is that individual tools and data sets are rarely sufficient in and of themselves, even for local decision making. Therefore, interoperability of tools and the importance of data sharing and integration were important goals that should factor into the design of visualization tools.

The utility of visualization tools is constrained by the extent to which they address the information needs of users. Information needs are as complex and varied as the tasks performed by public health professionals. Consequently, developing information visualization tools to meet these needs is correspondingly complex. Indeed, developers have addressed information needs in a multitude of ways, resulting in the current diversity of data visualization tools, each serving as a case study for one approach to resolve these needs. Regardless of the task, users indicate that they needed timely access to reliable, high-quality information to perform their duties. Efforts to map users' queries of common data types (e.g., GIS, molecular epidemiology, and social networks) to meaningful visualizations have raised concerns regarding the potential for misinterpretation and cognitive overload due to the complexity of infectious disease data (Olsen et al. 1996).

Despite results from studies with users emphasizing the value of dynamic, interactive graphics to facilitate data exploration and abstraction, existing tools are largely still static. And while static graphics are extremely useful, pairing them with interactive features may give users more freedom to explore and learn from their data. Sophisticated data analysis and visualization systems, such as R (R Core Team 2013), SAS (SAS Institute 2013), and MATLAB® (MathWorks 2013) have traditionally enabled expert users to create hard coded (but rapidly adjustable) graphics using code. The increasing use of these platforms to create user-friendly, interactive, web-based versions of these visualizations through technologies such as scalable vector graphics (SVG), dynamic HTML (DHTML), and Shiny Inc. (2013) has the potential to greatly simplify users' access to interactive, web-based visualizations. The distinction between visualization tools requiring coding and online visualization tools is also somewhat blurred by the ability to embed fully functional data analysis and visualization within web applications, as has been done using RStudio (2013) to allow the use of R within the Centers for Disease Control and Prevention's BioSense surveillance system (Chester 2013).

Visualizations with interactive features or sophisticated visual elements may require sufficient rendering capability and user experience to maximize their potential. For example, to access an area of interest in a 3D representation, users will typically need to adjust other visual cues (e.g., rotate the graphic, change transparency, or depth queuing) (Herman et al. 2000). Koenig et al. (2011) explored visual perceptions among public health users in GIS environments and demonstrated a preference for a blue and red color scheme to represent health and morbidity, respectively. However, studies emphasized that color schemes and visual elements should be sensitive to multicultural users, users with color-blindness, and rendering limitations of existing systems (Bassil and Keller 2001; Hu et al. 2007; Koenig et al. 2011). These visual elements also contribute to data (mis) interpretation. Consequently, guidelines have been proposed for color schemes and visual elements to minimize the risk of misinterpreting the data. For example, use of single-hue color progression (e.g., white to dark blue) to show sequential data is more intuitive than spectral schemes (e.g., rainbow) that force users to assign arbitrary magnitudes to rainbow colors (Light and Bartlein 2004).

Together with utility (functional effectiveness), usability (perceived ease of use) is sometimes considered to be a core component of determining the overall usefulness of a system. This makes usability one of the dimensions that can contribute to the adoption of a new information system (Davis et al. 1989). Usability has been assessed by examining several dimensions including learnability, memorability, error prevention/recovery, efficiency, and user satisfaction (Nielson 2012). However, usability also varies depending on the specific information needs of an individual user, particularly because efficiency depends on the task being performed. This presents an interesting problem when trying to highlight best practices with regards to usability. After a system has been developed, usability evaluation techniques can be used to assess its overall usability. The evaluation can contain quantitative assessment of accuracy and time efficiency as compared to a previous system or suitable alternative, such as a spreadsheet or database. With a sufficient pool of users and clearly defined metrics, a usability evaluation can yield statistically significant results, although this is not necessarily meaningful when assessing qualitative aspects, such as user satisfaction and perceived learnability.

There has been relatively little research focused on the implementation phase of software tools in public health, and widespread implementation and adoption of data visualization tools in this field remains elusive. While substantial barriers exist, there are strategies to address many of them, including obtaining management support, providing ongoing user training support, and starting a pilot program to integrate the tool into existing workflow. However, with extensive variability in data management systems, needs, and attitudes, widespread adoption of a given tool is difficult task. For example, integrating the novel tool into a given workflow requires collaboration between agencies and organizations, qualified staff for observation and interview studies, and time. Due to the variability of organizational structure and workflow, the optimal implementation strategy may vary among public health sites and foci, limiting the desired widespread adoption. Consequently, implementation becomes a site-specific endeavor, rather than a one-size-fits-all task. The participatory design approach can increase the amount of exposure that users have to the system, allowing for a better approximation of usage habits over time and understanding of the users' needs. Obtaining management support and creating a pilot implementation project may benefit from theory-driven communication campaigns to raise interest and support. For example, the literature supports a highly variable knowledge of and support for data visualization tools among management and staff. Behavior change theories, such as the Stages of Change Model (Prochaska and DiClemente 1983) or the Diffusion of Innovations (Rogers 1995), may improve adoption rates by targeting messages to different populations based on their readiness and interest in adopting the novel tool.

Many studies highlight the importance of adequate and ongoing training for users, providing a possible avenue to explore in more depth to minimize the risk of misinterpretation as well as improve adoption. In a recent study, more than half of the participating public health professionals indicated they were likely to seek training in a variety of tasks, including data visualization, epidemic modeling, GIS, cluster analysis, and statistical modeling (Robinson et al. 2011). They also preferred a variety of training styles (e.g., task-oriented tutorials, user guides, and hands-on training). Such training opportunities may also improve the perceived transparency of the tool. Further, integrating user training time, cost of the tool, and support staff into site budgets may also encourage more consistent, trained use of the tool. An atmosphere supporting regular use of software tools can encourage users to spend more time learning about its features and functions while helping them become more savvy, creative, and comfortable with the tool (Robinson et al. 2005; Thew et al. 2011). Enhanced education in visual analytics and statistics is an unmet need in public health. For non-expert users, easy-to-use, "black box" visualization programs may disguise the limitations of data analysis. The desire for a system that allows users to query the data and receive results in plainly understood charts and language may undermine the very nature of complex data. Developers of public health visualization tools should endeavor to help users strike a balance between in-depth understanding of data and system usability.

Lastly, pragmatic constraints of widespread tool adoption, including funding considerations, jurisdictional constraints, as well as data sharing and confidentiality concerns, may prove more difficult to overcome. Public health organizations worldwide face technological and financial access barriers preventing them maximizing the potential of visualization tools for epidemiology. Finite funding streams often force organizations to adapt existing systems that may not best serve their needs. Further, jurisdictional constraints and data sharing concerns create information silos that can limit the utility of public health data. Best practices for development of visualizations and visualization tools should maximize the ability to share data, code, and analyses across these boundaries. The interoperability of tools and data thus goes hand-in-hand with the success of implementation and adoption.

Although this chapter portrays a range of important issues for visualization of public health data, systems or informatics needs assessments that have no associated publications on their visualization features (e.g., developed and used in practice only) were not readily available for our study. For example, a published evaluation of the Centers for Disease Control and Prevention EARS (Early Aberration Reporting System) focused chiefly on its aberration detection algorithms (Zhu et al. 2005), and consequently, the article was not included in this survey of visualization systems. Further, systems with access-controlled content could not be assessed in context with the other tools identified here. For example, the Centers for Disease Control and Prevention's Public Health Information Network (PHIN) and BioSense as well as the International Society for Disease Surveillance have non-indexed content

that the survey did not capture. Still, these systems face many of the same constraints as those discussed in this chapter: data standardization and quality in diverse jurisdictions, limitations of user knowledge and organizational capacity to implement the tool, as well as generation of accurate and easy-to-understand visualizations. Lastly, we focused on English articles for practical reasons, but by doing so, we may have excluded valuable contributions from teams around the world. However, our survey included English articles in journals worldwide.

Future directions

As data types and sources become increasingly large and complex, so too should the strategies to integrate disparate and often incomplete data into novel visualization tools. Concerns regarding data quality and accuracy are particular relevant for visualization tools as these tools can be limited by the inputted data. Discussions of current data limitations highlight issues of scale and uncertainty, accuracy of data sets for spatial and epidemic models used in tools, and the impact of residential address errors in geocoding, to name a few (Atkinson and Graham 2006; Zinszer et al. 2010; Tatem et al. 2011; Linard and Tatem 2012). In order to draw meaningful and accurate conclusions from the data, visualization tools should represent missingness and uncertainty clearly. For instance, a recent study demonstrated that participants interpreting graphics with missing data tended to misinterpret results, but with equal confidence in their interpretations as those viewing more complete graphics (Eaton et al. 2005). Similarly, geographic analyses are known to be sensitive to overestimation of rates in small populations, which often correspond to large, sparsely populated regions, resulting in visual biases in interpreting choropleth maps (Olsen et al. 1996). These results suggest that users may not be aware of the need for better representation of missingness and uncertainty, and studies to evaluate the best means of doing so are still in their infancy. Continuing research on visualization algorithms that account for missing and uncertain data is needed to overcome these hurdles.

Another important challenge for future developers of information visualization tools for public health is to focus not only on individual user needs and comprehension of graphics, but also to plan and develop these tools in the broader contexts of available data, existing algorithms/ services, team collaboration, and interorganizational and interdisciplinary needs. Too many software projects are developed as new information silos, resulting in redundancy of effort, failure to integrate data and tools, and challenges to training and adoption. Further, many existing systems (e.g., BioSense) are access-restricted, limiting their use in infectious disease epidemiology, and may not have completed (or shared) evaluations of their visualization features. Visualization tools of the future should be developed to be compatible with existing data formats and standards, and interoperable with each other. Future tools should also adapt to the increasing pressure to be open-access, allowing users from low-resource settings, academia, and industry to capitalize on the advances in surveillance and visualization technology. This level of interoperability could support more advanced features such as phylogeography (the study of genetic variation across geographic space), inference of person-to-person contact from molecular epidemiology, statistical cluster detection based on joint spatiotemporal and genomic data, integration of remote sensing and environmental data, and other tasks as users become increasingly savvy in their use of advanced analytical and visualization tools for public health.

ACKNOWLEDGMENTS

The authors gratefully acknowledge Margo W. Bergman, PhD, MPH and Kyle M. Jacoby, PhD for thoughtful review and comment.

REFERENCES

Abernethy, N.F. 2005. Automating social network models for tuberculosis contact investigation. Doctorate, Biomedical Informatics, Stanford University.

Aimone, A.M., N. Perumal, and D.C. Cole. 2013. A systematic review of the application and utility of geographical information systems for exploring disease–disease relationships in paediatric global health research: The case of anaemia and malaria. *Int. J. Health Geogr.* 12: 1.

Alonso, W.J. and B.J.J. McCormick. 2012. EPIPOI: A user-friendly analytical tool for the extraction and visualization of temporal parameters from epidemiological time series. *BMC Public Health* 12: 982.

Andre, M., K. Ijaz, J.D. Tillinghast, V.E. Krebs, L.A. Diem, B. Metchock, T. Crisp, and P.D. McElroy. 2007. Transmission network analysis to complement routine tuberculosis contact investigations. *Am. J. Public Health* 97(3): 470–477.

Anselin, L., I. Syabri, and Y. Kho. 2006. GeoDa: An introduction to spatial data analysis. *Geogr. Anal.* 38(1): 5–22.

Arts, I.C.W. and M.P. Weijenberg. 2013. New training tools for new epidemiologists. *Environ. Mol. Mutag.* 54(7): 611–615.

Atkinson, P.J. and D.J. Unwin. 2002. Density and local attribute estimation of an infectious disease using MapInfo. *Comput. Geosci.* 28(9): 1095–1105.

Atkinson, P.M. and A.J. Graham. 2006. Issues of scale and uncertainty in the global remote sensing of disease. In S.I. Hay, A. Graham, and D.J. Rogers (eds.), *Advances in Parasitology*, Vol. 62: *Global Mapping of Infectious Diseases: Methods, Examples and Emerging Applications*, pp. 79–118.

AvRuskin, G.A., G.M. Jacquez, J.R. Meliker, M.J. Slotnick, A.M. Kaufmann, and J.O. Nriagu. 2004. Visualization and exploratory analysis of epidemiologic data using a novel space time information system. *Int. J. Health Geogr.* 3(1): 26–36.

Baker, E.L., A. Friede, A.D. Moulton, and D.A. Ross. 1995. CDC's Information Network for Public Health Officials (INPHO): A framework for integrated public health information and practice. *J. Public Health Manage. Pract.* 1(1): 43–47.

Bassil, S. and R.K. Keller. 2001. Software visualization tools: Survey and analysis. Program Comprehension, 2001. In *Proceedings of the Ninth International Workshop on IWPC 2001.*

Basta, N.E., D.L. Chao, M.E. Halloran, L. Matrajt, and I.M. Longini, Jr. 2009. Strategies for pandemic and seasonal influenza vaccination of schoolchildren in the United States. *Am. J. Epidemiol.* 170(6): 679–686.

Benavides, J., B.C.P. Demianyk, S.N. Mukhi, M. Laskowski, M. Friesen, and R.D. McLeod. 2012. Smartphone technologies for social network data generation and infectious disease modeling. *J. Med. Biol. Eng.* 32(4): 235–244.

Bishr, Y. 1998. Overcoming the semantic and other barriers to GIS interoperability. *Int. J. Geogr. Inform. Sci.* 12(4): 299–314.

Blanton, J.D., A. Manangan, J. Manangan, C.A. Hanlon, D. Slate, and C.E. Rupprecht. 2006. Development of a GIS-based, real-time Internet mapping tool for rabies surveillance. *Int. J. Health Geogr.* 5: 47.

Buckeridge, D., L. Purdon, and The South East Toronto Urban Health Research Group. 1998. Health data mapping in Southeast Toronto: A collaborative project. In *Third National Conference GIS in Public Health*.

Carpenter, T.E. 2011. The spatial epidemiologic (r) evolution: A look back in time and forward to the future. *Spat. Spatiotemp. Epidemiol.* 2(3): 119–124.

Carriço, J.A., A.J. Sabat, A.W. Friedrich, M. Ramirez, and ESCMID Study Group for Epidemiological Markers (ESGEM). 2013. Bioinformatics in bacterial molecular epidemiology and public health: Databases, tools and the next-generation sequencing revolution. *Euro Surveill.* 18(4): pii=20382.

Castronovo, D.A., K.K.H. Chui, and E.N. Naumova. 2009. Dynamic maps: A visual-analytic methodology for exploring spatio-temporal disease patterns. *Environ. Health* 8(61).

Centers for Disease Control and Prevention. 2000. Information needs and uses of the public health workforce—Washington, 1997–1998. *Morb. Mortal. Wkly. Rep.* 49(6): 118–120.

Chang, W., J. Cheng, J. Allaire, Y. Xie, and J. McPherson. 2015. Shiny: web application framework for R. R package version 0.12.2.

Chen, H., D. Zeng, and P. Yan. 2010. Data visualization, information dissemination, and alerting. *Infect. Dis. Inform.* 21: 73–87.

Chen, J. and A.M. MacEachren. 2008. Resolution control for balancing overview and detail in multivariate spatial analysis. *Cartogr. J.* 45(4): 261–273.

Chester, K.G. 2013. BioSense 2.0. *Online J. Public Health Inform.* 5(1).

Chui, K.K.H., J.B. Wenger, S.A. Cohen, and E.N. Naumova. 2011. Visual analytics for epidemiologists: Understanding the interactions between age, time, and disease with multi-panel graphs. *PLOS ONE* 6(2). doi:10.1371/journal.pone.0014683.

Cook, V.J., S.J. Sun, J. Tapia, S.Q. Muth, D.F. Argüello, B.L. Lewis, R.B. Rothenberg, P.D. McElroy, and the Network Analysis Project Team. 2007. Transmission network analysis in tuberculosis contact investigations. *J. Infect. Dis.* 196(10): 1517–1527.

da Silva, F.A., H.F. Gagliardi, E. Gallo, M.A. Madope, V.C. Neto, I.T. Pisa, and D. Alves. 2007. IntegraEPI: A Grid-based epidemic surveillance system. *Stud. Health Technol. Inform.* 126: 197–206.

Davis, F.D., R.P. Bagozzi, and P.R. Warshaw. 1989. User acceptance of computer technology: A comparison of two theoretical models. *Manage. Sci.* 35(8): 982–1003.

Dewan, P.K., H. Banouvong, N. Abernethy, T. Hoynes, L. Diaz, M. Woldemariam, T. Ampie, J. Grinsdale, and L.M. Kawamura. 2006. A tuberculosis outbreak in a private-home family child care center in San Francisco, 2002 to 2004. *Pediatrics* 117(3): 863–869.

Dominkovics, P., C. Granell, A. Pérez-Navarro, M. Casals, A. Orcau, and J.A. Caylà. 2011. Development of spatial density maps based on geoprocessing web services: Application to tuberculosis incidence in Barcelona, Spain. *Int. J. Health Geogr.* 10(1).

Driedger, S.M., A. Kothari, I.D. Graham, E. Cooper, E.J. Crighton, M. Zahab, J. Morrison, and M. Sawada. 2010. If you build it, they still may not come: Outcomes and process of implementing a community-based integrated knowledge translation mapping innovation. *Implement. Sci.* 5(1). doi:10.1186/1748-5908-5-47.

Driedger, S.M., A. Kothari, J. Morrison, M. Sawada, E.J. Crighton, and I.D. Graham. 2007. Correction: Using participatory design to develop (public) health decision support systems through GIS. *Int. J. Health Geogr.* 6. doi:10.1186/1476-072x-6-53.

Driscoll, T., J.L. Gabbard, C. Mao, O. Dalay, M. Shukla, C.C. Freifeld, A.G. Hoen, J.S. Brownstein, and B.W. Sobral 2011.

Integration and visualization of host-pathogen data related to infectious diseases. *Bioinformatics* 27(16): 2279–2287.

Eaton, C., C. Plaisant, and T. Drizd. 2005. Visualizing missing data: Graph interpretation user study. In *Proceedings of the Human–Computer Interaction—Interact 2005*, Vol. 3585. Redlands, CA: ArcGIS Desktop, pp. 861–872.

Eubank, S. 2005. Network based models of infectious disease spread. *Jpn. J. Infect. Dis.* 58(6): S9–S13.

Fisher, R.P. and B.A. Myers. 2011. Free and simple GIS as appropriate for health mapping in a low resource setting: A case study in eastern Indonesia. *Int. J. Health Geogr.* 10: 15.

Fitzpatrick, L.K., J.A. Hardacker, W. Heirendt, T. Agerton, A. Streicher, H. Melnyk, R. Ridzon, S. Valway, and I. Onorato. 2001. A preventable outbreak of tuberculosis investigated through an intricate social network. *Clin. Infect. Dis.* 33(11): 1801–1806.

Folorunso, O. and O.S. Ogunseye. 2008. Challenges in the adoption of visualization system: A survey. *Kybernetes* 37(9/10): 1530–1541.

Ford, J. and H. Korjonen. 2012. Information needs of public health practitioners: A review of the literature. *Health Inform. Libr. J.* 29(4): 260–273.

Fourie, I. 2009. Learning from research on the information behavior of healthcare professionals: A review of the literature 2004–2008 with a focus on emotion. *Health Inform. Libr. J.* 26(3): 171–186.

Foxman, B. and L. Riley. 2001. Molecular epidemiology: Focus on infection. *Am. J. Epidemiol.* 153(12): 1135–1141.

Freifeld, C.C., K.D. Mandl, B.Y. Reis, and J.S. Brownstein. 2008. HealthMap: Global infectious disease monitoring through automated classification and visualization of Internet media reports. *J. Am. Inform. Assoc.* 15(2): 150–157.

Friede, A., H.L. Blum, and M. McDonald. 1995. Public health informatics: How information-age technology can strengthen public health. *Annu. Rev. Publ. Health* 16(1): 239–252.

Friede, A., J.A. Reid, and H.W. Ory 1993. CDC WONDER: A comprehensive on-line public health information system of the Centers for Disease Control and Prevention. *Am. J. Public Health* 83(9): 1289–1294.

Fuller, S. 2010. Tracking the global express: New tools addressing disease threats across the world. *Epidemiology* 21(6): 769–771.

Gao, S., D. Mioc, F. Anton, X. Yi, and D.J. Coleman. 2008a. Online GIS services for mapping and sharing disease information. *Int. J. Health Geogr.* 7(1): 8.

Gao, S., D. Mioc, X. Yi, F. Anton, E. Oldfield, and D.J. Coleman. 2009. Towards web-based representation and processing of health information. *Int. J. Health Geogr.* 8: 3.

Geanuracos, C.G., S.D. Cunningham, G. Weiss, D. Forte, L.M.H. Reid, and J.M. Ellen. 2007. Use of geographic information systems for planning HIV prevention interventions for high-risk youths. *Am. J. Public Health* 97(11): 1974–1981.

Gesteland, P.H., Y. Livnat, N. Galli, M.H. Samore, and A.V. Gundlapalli. 2012. The EpiCanvas infectious disease weather map: An interactive visual exploration of temporal and spatial correlations. *J. Am. Inform. Assoc.* 19(6): 954–959.

Google. Google Maps API. Accessed September 9, 2013. https://developers.google.com/maps/.

Gopinath, G., K. Hari, R. Jain, M.K. Mammel, M.H. Kothary, A.A. Franco, C.J. Grim, K.G. Jarvis, V. Sathyamoorthy, and L. Hu. 2013. The Pathogen-annotated Tracking Resource Network (PATRN) system: A web-based resource to aid food safety, regulatory science, and investigations of foodborne pathogens and disease. *Food Microbiol.* 34(2): 303–318.

Gorman, S. 2013. How can we improve global infectious disease surveillance and prevent the next outbreak? *Scand. J. Infect. Dis.* 45(12): 944–947.

Green, J., F.J. Escobar, E. Waters, and I.P. Williamson. 1998. Design and implementation of a geographic information system for the general practice sector in Victoria, Australia.

Grundmann, H., D.M. Aanensen, C.C. van den Wijngaard, B.G. Spratt, D. Harmsen, and A.W. Friedrich. 2010. Geographic distribution of *Staphylococcus aureus* causing invasive infections in Europe: A molecular-epidemiological analysis. *PLoS Med.* 7(1): e1000215.

Hadjichristodoulou, C., E. Soteriades, G. Goutzianna, M. Loukaidou, T. Babalis, M. Antoniou, J. Delagramaticas, and Y. Tselentis. 1999. Surveillance of brucellosis in a rural area of Greece: Application of the computerized mapping programme. *Eur. J. Epidemiol.* 15(3): 277–283.

Hansen, T.E., J.P. Hourcade, A. Segre, C. Hlady, P. Polgreen, and C. Wyman. 2010. Interactive visualization of hospital contact network data on multi-touch displays. In *Proceedings of the 2010 Mexican Workshop on Human–Computer Interaction*, Vol. 1, pp. 15–22.

Harbage, B. and A.G. Dean. 1999. Distribution of Epi Info software: An evaluation using the Internet. *Am. J. Prev. Med.* 16(4): 314–317.

Hay, S.I., K.E. Battle, D.M. Pigott et al. 2013. Global mapping of infectious disease. *Philos. Trans. Roy. Soc. B: Biol. Sci.* 368(1614). doi:10.1098/rstb.2012.0250.

He, X., H. Xing, Y. Ruan et al. 2012. A comprehensive mapping of HIV-1 genotypes in various risk groups and regions across China based on a nationwide molecular epidemiologic survey. *PLOS ONE* 7(10): e47289.

Heitgerd, J.L., A.L. Dent, J.B. Holt et al. 2008. Community health status indicators: Adding a geospatial component. *Prev. Chronic Dis.* 5(3): A96.

Herman, I., G. Melançon, and M.S. Marshall. 2000. Graph visualization and navigation in information visualization: A survey. *IEEE Trans. Vis. Comput. Graph.* 6(1): 24–43.

Heymann, D.L. and L. Brilliant. 2011. Surveillance in eradication and elimination of infectious diseases: A progression through the years. *Vaccine* 29: D141–D144.

Hills, R.A., W.B. Lober , and I.S. Painter. 2008. Biosurveillance, case reporting, and decision support: Public health interactions with a health information exchange. *Biosurveill. Biosecur.* 5354: 10–21.

Hollm-Delgado, M.-G. 2009. Molecular epidemiology of tuberculosis transmission: Contextualizing the evidence through social network theory. *Soc. Sci. Med.* 69(5): 747–753.

Holmes, E.C. 1998. Molecular epidemiology and evolution of emerging infectious diseases. *Brit. Med. Bull.* 54(3): 533–543.

Hu, P.J.-H., D. Zeng, H. Chen, C. Larson, W. Chang, C. Tseng, and J. Ma. 2007. System for infectious disease information sharing and analysis: Design and evaluation. *IEEE Trans. Inform. Technol. B* 11(4): 483–492.

Humphreys, B.L. 1998. Meeting information needs in health policy and public health: Priorities for the National Library of Medicine and the National Network of Libraries of Medicine. *J. Urban Health* 75(4): 878–883.

Hurlimann, E., N. Schur, K. Boutsika et al. 2011. Toward an open-access global database for mapping, control, and surveillance of neglected tropical diseases. *PLoS Negl. Trop. Dis.* 5(12): e1404.

Ives, B., Olson, M.H., and Baroudi, J.J. 1983. The measurement of user information satisfaction. *Commun. ACM* 26(10): 785–793.

Janies, D.A, T. Treseder, B. Alexandrov, F. Habib, J.J. Chen, R. Ferreira, Ü. Çatalyürek, A. Varón, and W.C. Wheeler. 2011. The Supramap project: Linking pathogen genomes with geography to fight emergent infectious diseases. *Cladistics* 27(1): 61–66.

Joshi, A., M. de Araujo Novaes, J. Machiavelli, S. Iyengar, R. Vogler, C. Johnson, J. Zhang, and C.E. Hsu. 2012a. A human centered GeoVisualization framework to facilitate visual exploration of telehealth data: A case study. *Technol. Health Care* 20(6): 457–471.

Joshi, A., M. de Araujo Novaes, J. Machiavelli, S. Iyengar, R. Vogler, C. Johnson, J. Zhang, and C.E. Hsu. 2012b. Designing human centered GeoVisualization application—The SanaViz—For telehealth users: A case study. *Technol. Health Care* 20(6): 473–488.

Joyce, K. 2009. 'To me it's just another tool to help understand the evidence': Public health decision-makers' perceptions of the value of geographical information systems (GIS). *Health Place* 15(3): 831–840.

Karlsson, D., J. Ekberg, A. Spreco, H. Eriksson, and T. Timpka. 2013. Visualization of infectious disease outbreaks in routine practice. *Stud. Health Technol. Inform.* 192: 697–701.

Khan, A.S., Fleischauer, A., Casani, J., and Groseclose, S.L. 2010. The next public health revolution: Public health information fusion and social networks. *Am. J. Public Health* 100(7): 1237–1242.

Kienle, H.M., and Müller, H.A. 2007. Requirements of software visualization tools: A literature survey. In *Fourth IEEE International Workshop on Visualizing Software for Understanding and Analysis (VISSOFT)*.

Klompas, M., M. Murphy, J. Lankiewicz et al. 2011. Harnessing electronic health records for public health surveillance. *Online J. Public Health Inform.* 3(3). doi:10.5210/ojphi.v3i3.3794.

Koch, T. and K. Denike. 2009. Crediting his critics' concerns: Remaking John Snow's map of Broad Street cholera, 1854. *Social Sci. Med.* 69(8): 1246–1251.

Koenig, A., E. Samarasundera, and T. Cheng. 2011. Interactive map communication: Pilot study of the visual perceptions and preferences of public health practitioners. *Public Health* 125(8): 554–560.

Kothari, A., S.M. Driedger, J. Bickford, J. Morrison, M. Sawada, I.D. Graham, and E. Crighton. 2008. Mapping as a knowledge translation tool for Ontario Early Years Centres: Views from data analysts and managers. *Implement. Sci.* 3: 4.

Kushniruk, A. 2002. Evaluation in the design of health information systems: Application of approaches emerging from usability engineering. *Comput. Biol. Med.* 32(3): 141–149.

LaPelle, N.R., R. Luckmann, E.H. Simpson, and E.R. Martin. 2006. Identifying strategies to improve access to credible and relevant information for public health professionals: A qualitative study. *BMC Public Health* 6: 89.

Lee, P., N.B. Giuse, and N.A. Sathe. 2003. Benchmarking information needs and use in the Tennessee public health community. *J. Med. Libr. Assoc.* 91(3): 322.

Lewis, S.L., B.H. Feighner, W.A. Loschen, R.A. Wojcik, J.F. Skora, J.S. Coberly, and D.L. Blazes. 2011. SAGES: A suite of freely-available software tools for electronic disease surveillance in resource-limited settings. *PLOS ONE* 6(5): e19750.

Light, A. and P.J. Bartlein. 2004. The end of the rainbow? Color schemes for improved data graphics. *EOS Trans. Am. Geophys. Union* 85(40): 385–391.

Linard, C. and A.J. Tatem. 2012. Large-scale spatial population databases in infectious disease research. *Int. J. Health Geogr.* 11. doi:10.1186/1476-072x-11-7.

Lopes, C.T., M. Franz, F. Kazi, S.L. Donaldson, Q. Morris, and G.D. Bader 2010. Cytoscape Web: An interactive web-based network browser. *Bioinformatics* 26(18): 2347–2348.

Lopez, D.M. and B. Blobel. 2007. Semantic interoperability between clinical and public health information systems for improving public health services. *Stud. Health Technol. Inform.* 127: 256.

Lowy, F.D. and M. Miller. 2002. New methods to investigate infectious disease transmission and pathogenesis—*Staphylococcus aureus* disease in drug users. *Lancet Infect. Dis.* 2(10): 605–612.

Lê, M.-L. 2013. Information Needs of Public Health Staff in a Knowledge Translation Setting in Canada. *J. Can. Health Librar. Assoc.* 34(1): 3–11.

Ma, J., M. Otten, R. Kamadjeu, R. Mir, L. Rosencrans, S. McLaughlin, and S. Yoon. 2008. New frontiers for health information systems using Epi Info in developing countries: Structured application framework for Epi Info (SAFE). *Int. J. Med. Inform.* 77(4): 219–225.

Maccannell, D. 2013. Bacterial strain typing. *Clin. Lab. Med.* 33(3): 629–650.

Macdonald, N., D. Parks, and R. Beiko. 2009. SeqMonitor: Influenza analysis pipeline and visualization. *PLoS Curr.* 1: Rrn1040.

Maciejewski, R., P. Livengood, S. Rudolph, T.F. Collins, D.S. Ebert, R.T. Brigantic, C.D. Corley, G.A. Muller, and S.W. Sanders. 2011. A pandemic influenza modeling and visualization tool. *J. Vis. Lang. Comput.* 22(4): 268–278.

MATLAB, Manual. 2012. The language of technical computing. The MathWorks, Inc. http://www.mathworks.com.

McElroy, P.D., R.B. Rothenberg, R. Varghese, R. Woodruff, G.O. Minns, S.Q. Muth, L.A. Lambert, and R. Ridzon. 2003. A network-informed approach to investigating tuberculosis outbreak: Implications for enhancing contact investigations. *Int. J. Tuberc. Lung Dis.* 7(12 Suppl. 3): S486–S493.

McGrath, C., D. Krackhardt, and J. Blythe. 2003. Visualizing complexity in networks: Seeing both the forest and the trees. *Connections* 25(1): 37–47.

Moore, K.M., G. Edge, and A.R. Kurc. 2008. Visualization techniques and graphical user interfaces in syndromic surveillance systems.

Summary from the Disease Surveillance Workshop, Sept. 11–12, 2007; Bangkok, Thailand. *BMC Proc.* 2 (Suppl. 3): S6.

Morris, M., S. Goodreau, and J. Moody. 2006. Sexual networks, concurrency, and STD/HIV. *Sexually Transmitted Diseases*, 4th edn. New York: McGraw-Hill.

Nielson, J. 2012. Introduction to Usability. Accessed September 10, 2012. http://www.nngroup.com/articles/usability-101-introduction-to-usability/.

Nobre, F.F., A.L. Braga, R.S. Pinheiro, and J.A.D. Lopes. 1997. GISEpi: A simple geographical information system to support public health surveillance and epidemiological investigations. *Comput. Meth. Programs Biomed.* 53(1): 33–45.

O'Carroll, P.W., M.A. Cahn, I. Auston, and C.R. Selden. 1998. Information needs in public health and health policy: Results of recent studies. *J. Urban Health* 75(4): 785–793.

Olsen, S.F., M. Martuzzi, and P. Elliott. 1996. Cluster analysis and disease mapping—Why, when, and how? A step by step guide. *Brit. Med. J.* 313(7061): 863–866.

Parks, D.H., M. Porter, S. Churcher, S. Wang, C. Blouin, J. Whalley, S. Brooks, and R.G. Beiko. 2009. GenGIS: A geospatial information system for genomic data. *Genome Res.* 19(10): 1896–1904.

Pina, J., A.M. Turner, T. Kwan-Gett, and J. Duchin. 2009. Task analysis in action: The role of information systems in communicable disease reporting. In *AMIA Annual Symposium Proceedings*.

Plaisant, C. 2004. The challenge of information visualization evaluation. In *Proceedings of the Working Conference on Advanced Visual Interfaces*.

Polgreen, P.M., T.L. Tassier, S.V. Pemmaraju, and A.M. Segre. 2010. Prioritizing healthcare worker vaccinations on the basis of social network analysis. *Infect. Control Hosp. Epidemiol.* 31(9): 893–900.

Porcasi, X., C.H. Rotela, M.V. Introini, N. Frutos, S. Lanfri, G. Peralta, E.A. De Elia, M.A. Lanfri, and C.M. Scavuzzo. 2012. An operative dengue risk stratification system in Argentina based on geospatial technology. *Geospat. Health* 6(3): S31–S42.

Prochaska, J.O., and C.C. DiClemente. 1983. Stages and processes of self-change of smoking: Toward an integrative model of change. *J. Consult. Clin. Psychol.* 51(3): 390–395.

R Core Team. 2013. *R: A Language and Environment for Statistical Computing.* Vienna, Austria: R Foundation for Statistical Computing.

Ramírez-Ramírez, L.L., Y.R. Gel, M. Thompson, E. de Villa, and M. McPherson. 2013. A new surveillance and spatio-temporal visualization tool SIMID: SIMulation of Infectious Diseases using random networks and GIS. *Comput. Meth. Prog. Biomed.* 110(3): 455–470.

Reeder, B., D. Revere, R.A. Hills, J.G. Baseman, and W.B. Lober. 2012. Public health practice within a health information exchange: information needs and barriers to disease surveillance. *Online J. Public Health Inform.* 4(3). doi:10.5210/ojphi.v4i3.4277.

Reinhardt, M., J. Elias, J. Albert, M. Frosch, D. Harmsen, and U. Vogel. 2008. EpiScanGIS: An online geographic surveillance system for meningococcal disease. *Int. J. Health Geogr.* 7: 33.

Reis, B.Y., I.S. Kohane, and K.D. Mandl. 2007. An epidemiological network model for disease outbreak detection. *PLoS Med.* 4(6).

Revere, D., A.M. Turner, A. Madhavan, N. Rambo, P.F. Bugni, A. Kimball, and S.S. Fuller. 2007. Understanding the information needs of public health practitioners: A literature review to inform design of an interactive digital knowledge management system. *J. Biomed. Inform.* 40(4): 410–421.

Robertson, C. and T.A. Nelson. 2010. Review of software for space-time disease surveillance. *Int. J. Health Geogr.* 9(1): 16.

Robinson, A. 2009. Needs assessment for the design of information synthesis visual analytics tools. In *IEEE International Conference on Information Visualization*, pp. 353–360.

Robinson, A., A. MacEachren, and R. Roth. 2011. Designing a web-based learning portal for geographic visualization and analysis in public health. *Health Inform. J.* 17(3): 191–208.

Robinson, A.C., J. Chen, E.J. Lengerich, H.G. Meyer, and A.M. MacEachren. 2005. Combining usability techniques to design geovisualization tools for epidemiology. *Cartogr. Geogr. Inform. Sci.* 32(4): 243–255.

Rogers, E.M. 1995. *Diffusion of Innovations*, 4th edn. New York: Free Press.

Rolka, H., D.W. Walker, R. English, M.J. Katzoff, G. Scogin, and E. Neuhaus. 2012. Analytical challenges for emerging public health surveillance. CDC's Vision for Public Health Surveillance in the 21st Century 61: 35.

Roth, R.E., A.M. MacEachren, and C.A. McCabe. 2009. A workflow learning model to improve geovisual analytics utility. In *Proceedings of the International Cartographic Conference*.

RStudio. 2013. RStudio: Integrated Development Environment for R, Boston, MA.

Rushton, G. 2003. Public health, GIS,and spatial analytic tools. *Annu. Rev. Public Health* 24: 43–56.

SAS. 2013. SAS Institute, Cary, NC.

Schriml, L.M., C. Arze, S. Nadendla et al. 2010. GeMInA, Genomic Metadata for Infectious Agents, a geospatial surveillance pathogen database. *Nucleic Acids Res.* 38 (Database Issue): D754–D764.

Shneiderman, B., C. Plaisant, and B. Hesse. 2013. Improving health and healthcare with interactive visualization methods. *Computer* 46(5): 58–66.

Sopan, A., A.S.-I. Noh, S. Karol, P. Rosenfeld, G. Lee, and B. Shneiderman. 2012. Community Health Map: A geospatial and multivariate data visualization tool for public health datasets. *Gov. Inform. Quart.* 29(2): 223–234.

Stevens, K.B. and D.U. Pfeiffer. 2011. Spatial modelling of disease using data- and knowledge-driven approaches. *Spat. Spatiotemp. Epidemiol.* 2(3): 125–133.

Tatem, A.J., N. Campiz, P.W. Gething, R.W. Snow, and C. Linard. 2011. The effects of spatial population dataset choice on estimates of population at risk of disease. *Popul. Health Metrics* 9. doi:10.1186/1478-7954-9-4.

ter Waarbeek, H., C. Hoebe, H. Freund, V. Bochat, and C. Kara-Zaitr. 2011. Strengthening infectious disease surveillance in a Dutch-German crossborder area using a real-time information exchange system. *J. Bus. Contin. Emer. Plan.* 5(2): 173–184.

Thacker, S.B., J.R. Qualters, and L.M. Lee. 2012. Public health surveillance in the United States: Evolution and challenges. *MMWR Surveill. Summ.* 61 (Suppl.): 3–9.

Thew, S.L., A. Sutcliffe, O. De Bruijn, J. McNaught, R. Procter, P. Jarvis, and I. Buchan. 2011. Supporting creativity and appreciation of uncertainty in exploring geocoded public health data. *Meth. Inform. Med.* 50(2): 158–165.

Turner, A.M., Z. Stavri, D. Revere, and R. Altamore. 2008. From the ground up: Information needs of nurses in a rural public health department in Oregon. *J. Med. Libr. Assoc.* 96(4): 335–342.

Twose, C., P. Swartz, E. Bunker, N.K. Roderer, and K.B. Oliver. 2008. Public health practitioners' information access and use patterns in the Maryland (USA) public health departments of Anne Arundel and Wicomico Counties. *Health Inform. Libr. J.* 25(1): 13–22.

Upadhyayula, S.M., S.R. Mutheneni, S. Kumaraswamy, M.R. Kadiri, S.K. Pabbisetty, and V.S. Yellepeddi. 2012. Filaria monitoring visualization system: A geographical information system-based application to manage lymphatic filariasis in Andhra Pradesh, India. *Vector Borne Zoonot. Dis.* 12(5): 418–427.

Victor, L.Y. and S.C. Edberg. 2005. Global Infectious Diseases and Epidemiology Network (GIDEON): A world wide web-based program for diagnosis and informatics in infectious diseases. *Clin. Infect. Dis.* 40(1): 123–126.

Viégas, F.B. and J. Donath. 2004. Social network visualization: Can we go beyond the graph. In *Workshop on Social Networks, CSCW*.

Walton, L.J., S. Hasson, F.V. Ross, and E.R. Martin. 2000. Outreach to public health professionals: Lessons learned from a collaborative Iowa public health project. *Bull. Med. Libr. Assoc.* 88(2): 165–171.

Xia, H., K. Nagaraj, J. Chen, and M.V. Marathe. 2013. Evaluating strategies for pandemic response in Delhi using realistic social networks. In *NDSSL Technical Report*.

Yan, W.R., L. Palm, X. Lu et al. 2013. ISS—An electronic syndromic surveillance system for infectious disease in rural China. *PLOS ONE* 8(4). doi:10.1371/journal.pone.0062749.

Yi, Q., R.E. Hoskins, E.A. Hillringhouse, S.S. Sorensen, M.W. Oberle, S.S. Fuller, and J.C. Wallace 2008. Integrating open-source technologies to build low-cost information systems for improved access to public health data. *Int. J. Health Geogr.* 7(1): 29.

Zarrabi, N., M. Presperi, R.G. Belleman, M. Colafigli, and A. De Luca. 2012. Combining epidiological and genetic networks signifies the importance of early treatment in HIV-1 transmission. *PLOS ONE* 7(9).

Zhu, Y., W. Wang, D. Atrubin, and Y. Wu. 2005. Initial evaluation of the early aberration reporting system—Florida. *Morb. Mortal. Wkly. Rep.* 54: 123–130.

Zinszer, K., C. Jauvin, A. Verma, L. Bedard, R. Allard, K. Schwartzman, L. de Montigny, K. Charland, and D.L. Buckeridge. 2010. Residential address errors in public health surveillance data: A description and analysis of the impact on geocoding. *Spat. Spatiotemp. Epidemiol.* 1(2–3): 163–168.

PART 2

Disease surveillance practice

7

The international health regulations in practice: Surveillance and a global community seeking health security

DAVID BRETT-MAJOR AND DENNIS FAIX

In 2005, during the aftermath of the severe acute respiratory syndrome (SARS) coronavirus epidemic, the persistence of outbreaks of avian influenza A (H5N1) and continued outbreaks of viral hemorrhagic fevers, the Member States of the World Health Organization (WHO) ratified a revised International Health Regulations (IHR 2005).

The IHR (2005) departed from narrow stipulations regarding ship quarantine and named threats in earlier versions in several ways. First, the Regulations sought to recognize that the most concerning health security threats might not be known, named, or understood at the outset. Second, they recognized that these threats might be biologic but also could be chemical, radiologic, or nuclear or have some other nature entirely. Third, they state that if both affected parties and those at risk are to meet these threats, they will share a vested interest in early warning and information sharing, cooperative risk assessment, and management. Finally, all signatories to the Regulations committed to their obligation to prepare themselves to be able to meaningfully participate in these early and cooperative activities.

Effective surveillance warns of threats and allows the adaptation of public health programming to meet an evolving concern or the initiation of public health programming to address a novel threat. The Regulations are a key way that these relationships are defined and reinforced internationally.

Influenza surveillance and research rests upon public health and research enterprises with more than 60 years of experience. While focused on influenza diseases, they function as a global mechanism for other emerging diseases. For example, this influenza network identified the SARS-CoV in 2003. Since the reemergence of highly pathogenic avian influenza H5N1 in 2003 and in particular the H1N1 pandemic in 2009, these enterprises and their countries reviewed and reorganized their respiratory disease surveillance systems under broad cooperative initiatives nationally and globally including the Pandemic Influenza Preparedness (PIP) Framework and the revised WHO pandemic preparedness plan: Pandemic Influenza Risk Management (PIRM) Framework.

THE REGULATIONS

The definitions and general structure of the IHR (2005) are built around the Regulations' traditional role in determining health impacts upon international traffic and trade (WHO 2008). Part II—Information and Public Health Response—opens with Article 5, Surveillance. Countries agree to

> ...develop, strengthen and maintain, as soon as possible but no later than five years from the entry into force of these Regulations for that State Party, the capacity to detect, assess, notify and report events....

The Regulations discuss the WHO's role in promoting this capacity as well as acting as a clearinghouse for reporting and risk assessment, the obligation of countries to monitor the situation with continued information sharing with the WHO, different ways information might move to the WHO such as through neighboring countries, information verification processes, and the relevance of cooperative risk management including deployed technical support. They outline ways that a public health emergency of international concern (PHEIC) might be determined and how a PHEIC leads to temporary measures.

For internationally active public health agencies and research houses, a particularly interesting feature of the Regulations is Article 46. The enhancing of laboratory capability at referral centers and increased attention to the importance of sample movement has remained a contentious issue. The Regulations state that countries should

> ...facilitate the transport, entry, exit, processing and disposal of biological substances and diagnostic specimens, reagents and other diagnostic materials for verification and public health response purposes under these Regulations.

Movements for increased affected country rights in sharing in the benefits of product development and international treaty around rights to biologic diversity complicate the conversations (Fidler 2013; Convention of Biological Diversity 2015a).

In part for these reasons, sample sharing has not occurred as fluidly as reporting of cases.

Countries continue to strive to achieve more and improved capacities identified through the WHO as critical to meeting their obligations under the Regulations. Predictable gaps exist between countries with readily available financial resources and human capital and those without. Of the 196 countries that are signatory to the Regulations, 118 requested extensions for attaining capacities to 2014. Eighty-one countries requested an additional 2-year extension to 2016. The WHO publishes progress on capacity attainment in the WHO Global Health Observatory (WHO 2015c).

The Regulations are an international legal document with many articles. Issues around them have spawned a myriad of monitoring, assessment, and guidance documents (WHO 2011a). Their practical use is much simpler. The Regulations simply affirm countries' interests in cooperative risk management while, when possible, allowing international traffic and trade to continue. In 2013, astute clinicians identified patients with atypical severe respiratory infection clinical courses and referred their specimens to laboratory-based surveillance systems. The relevant ministries of health and other stakeholders reported findings to WHO country offices. That triggered a cooperative risk assessment process in the countries and at the regional and global levels that led to the identification of, risk assessment and characterization of, and public health measures against avian influenza A(H7N9) and Middle East respiratory syndrome coronavirus (MERS-CoV). Within the WHO secretariat, there are staff and procedures in place to continue the conversation within the Organization and with the affected and other countries. This basic reporting accomplishes the key public health interest in the Regulations: warning, and when possible, early warning. It also allows the readying of further risk assessment and response mechanisms such as provision of technical assistance through the WHO Global Outbreak Alert and Response Network (GOARN), a partnership of public health agencies, academic institutions, and professional and academic networks as well as actions by other critical networks such as the WHO Global Influenza Surveillance and Response System (GISRS).

Annex 2 of the Regulations provides a simple flow chart (Figure 7.1) that depicts the initial

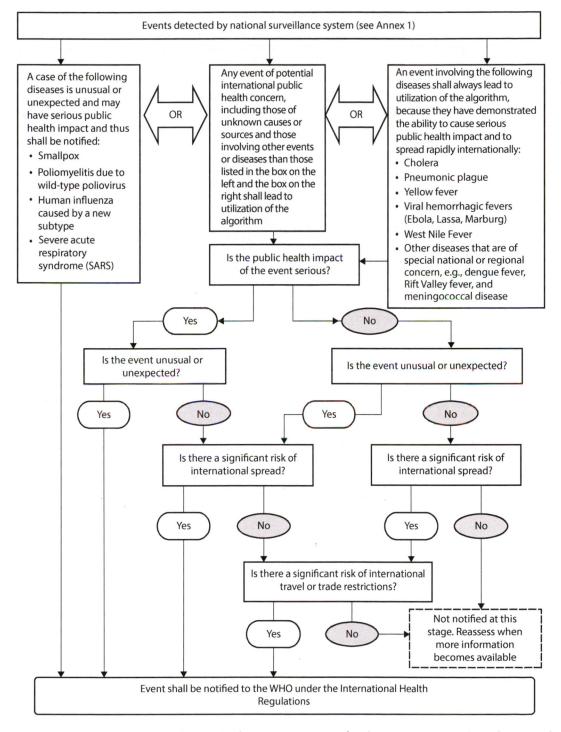

Figure 7.1 Annex 2, IHR (2005), the WHO, decision instrument for the assessment and notification of events that may constitute a PHEIC.

process and is meant to be used by countries as a decision instrument for initial reporting.

It and similar processes are used daily around the world for a myriad of events that never reach popular attention. However, like sample sharing, even data reporting has its challenges for countries and international actors. The H1N1 pandemic cost Mexico billions of dollars in tourism. Because of the Ebola virus disease (EVD) outbreak, West Africa currently is suffering even greater losses in tourism and, more critically for fragile, low-wage-labor–dependent economies, is experiencing the withdrawal of mining and other corporate concerns.

In the case of the influenza A(H1N1) pandemic, an Emergency Committee was convened under the authority of the Regulations in order to provide advice to the WHO Director General. When this occurs, the Regulations encourage, ultimately, a review committee and report on how all parties and the Regulations functioned during the crisis. The report on the H1N1 pandemic provides granular detail, praise, and criticisms on how the Regulations are used (WHO 2011c). It also spawned growth in influenza-specific systems. Similar reports might be expected in the wake of MERS-CoV and the 2014–2015 EVD outbreak in West Africa.

The H1N1 pandemic report had three summary conclusions.

1. The IHR helped make the world better prepared to cope with public-health emergencies. The core national and local capacities called for in the IHR are not yet fully operational and are not now on a path to timely implementation worldwide.
2. WHO performed well in many ways during the pandemic, confronted systemic difficulties and demonstrated some shortcomings. The Committee found no evidence of malfeasance.
3. The world is ill-prepared to respond to a severe influenza pandemic or to any similarly global, sustained, and threatening public-health emergency. Beyond implementation of core public-health capacities called for in the IHR, global preparedness can be advanced through research, reliance on a multisectoral approach, strengthened health-care delivery systems, economic development in low and middle-income countries and improved health status.

Progress in many of these areas has occurred since 2009. Nonetheless, although the details regarding capacity and threat and their impact in more recent outbreaks and health crises may be different, similar summary conclusions from the impending reviews are likely.

SURVEILLANCE SYSTEMS THAT CROSS BORDERS

The prototypical example for rapidly and widely moving health threats is pandemic influenza. Influenza viruses with pandemic potential are named threats in the Regulations and require reporting to the WHO (See Figure 7.1, referred to as "Human influenza caused by a new subtype"). The potential emergence of a novel influenza virus is carefully assessed by the members of the GISRS. This network of National Influenza Centers and referral laboratories was established in 1952. Through the Global Influenza Programme, it produces regular assessments of the state of seasonal influenza as well as more novel strains (WHO 2015c).

When the performance of the Regulations and international community was assessed after the H1N1 pandemic in 2009–2010, the Review Committee identified the importance of influenza infrastructure to meeting the pandemic threat. It also identified needs for growth, including in the area of sample sharing among laboratories and industry and increased benefit sharing with affected communities, in particular, access to vaccine. In 2007, shortly before that pandemic, work had begun on a PIP Framework (WHO 2011b). It was adopted in 2011 in the face of these and other influences.

In 2013, H7N9 emerged in China. The global influenza infrastructure acted swiftly. In addition to case reporting under the Regulations, because of these historic and more recent relationships, laboratory characterization and derivative testing and development related to vaccines and therapeutics also happened quickly (Kreijtz et al. 2013; Smith et al. 2013; Wang et al. 2013; Zhou et al. 2013). The way that H7N9 material moved between countries and across sectors can be reviewed through the PIP Framework's Influenza Virus Traceability Mechanism (IVTM), which can be accessed at http://www.who.int/influenza/pip/ivtm/en/.

A combination of a lower case count, different sample sharing dynamics, and intellectual property concerns by the affected country resulted in less progression of understanding of MERS-CoV in as limited a time. Nonetheless, initial reporting occurred under the Regulations, and larger impacts associated with international travel have been averted to date.

Both H7N9 and MERS-CoV were rapidly identified, characterized and tracked because of the complimentary and synergistic effects of astute clinician reporting, laboratory resources and indicator-based surveillance. One of the legacies of pandemic influenza preparedness has been Severe Acute Respiratory Infection (SARI) systems. Countries experienced with severe respiratory disease have developed protocol-based active and passive, laboratory-supported mechanisms designed to capture an emerging threat. In such systems, referred samples are tested for a predetermined range of potential pathogens. Often, a nonreferred sample of specimens also is tested. Similar systems exist for influenza-like illness in these same locations.

An example of a nonrespiratory-pathogen-focused surveillance system is the WHO's Extremely Dangerous Pathogen Laboratory Network (EDPLN) (WHO 2015c). This network coordinates national, regional, and global laboratory facilities to distribute diagnostic capacity and provide reference standards and referral services. These can be leveraged both for preparedness in at-risk areas and when suspicious events occur. These varied networks create a diverse and broadly applied system for threat detection and risk characterization. This also is true of the GISRS laboratories (Figure 7.2).

Other longitudinal disease programming also uses internationally communicated, indicator-based surveillance. The fight against polio typically has used mandatory reporting of acute flaccid paralysis as a surrogate marker to trigger investigation or assessment of control mechanisms. Influenza and polio rely on both syndromic and disease specific indicators. Global malaria, tuberculosis, and HIV programming relies upon systematic reporting on predetermined indicators, also available through the Global Health Observatory. On a global level, most other diseases do not have a timely indicator based surveillance, rather they are reported to the WHO annually on an aggregate level by country. At the local and country level, indicator-based systems exist in a variety of formats for a range of diseases selected by countries based on their own risk identification and prioritization. The specificity of these systems to disease and location provides great utility

at the local and country level, though challenges exist with regards to data compatibility, sharing, aggregation, and reporting across localities. Reports from these systems sometimes are collected during global and regional event-based surveillance.

Although indicator-based surveillance programming can detect some emerging threats, investigation of reports or situations that are not captured in this way sometimes are triggered through other means. The WHO, public health agencies, independent groups such as ProMED and increasingly countries and communities also engage in adaptive surveillance often referred to as event-based surveillance (WHO 2014a; International Society for Infectious Diseases 2015). Media monitoring, informal communications, observance of Internet trends, and, in some cases, informal text messaging all are assessed by event-based surveillance mechanisms. It is through these mechanisms that initial reports of diarrheal and hemorrhagic illness led to the Identification of the EVD outbreak in West Africa (Baize et al. 2014). ProMED is available to the public and open to anyone with an Internet connection. Related initiatives synthesize the direct reporting and event-based surveillance from ProMED and other sources into interactive maps, such as by HealthMap (2015). In contrast, the WHO, abiding by communication requirements of the Regulations, maintains a closed computerized web-based system for event-based surveillance and response known as the Event Management System. The WHO's Hazard Detection and Risk Assessment System (HDRAS) supports this effort by polling online available media reports for certain key words, similar to functions in ProMED.

Both indicator- and event-based surveillance systems are necessary to an event intelligence process that provides useful early warning against an emerging public health threat (Figure 7.3). Ideally, they are designed together to provide a cohesive strategy that applies resources based on the priorities of individual communities. Such cohesive planning to date is rare. The combination of existing public health programming infrastructures for disease-specific events like influenza and watch-like practices in the WHO and partner agencies serve a similar function until more cogent development occurs. Countries also have taken regional approaches with the WHO to make surveillance processes local but the results global (Andrus et al. 2010; Li and Kasai 2011). These efforts enhance cohesiveness and increase the

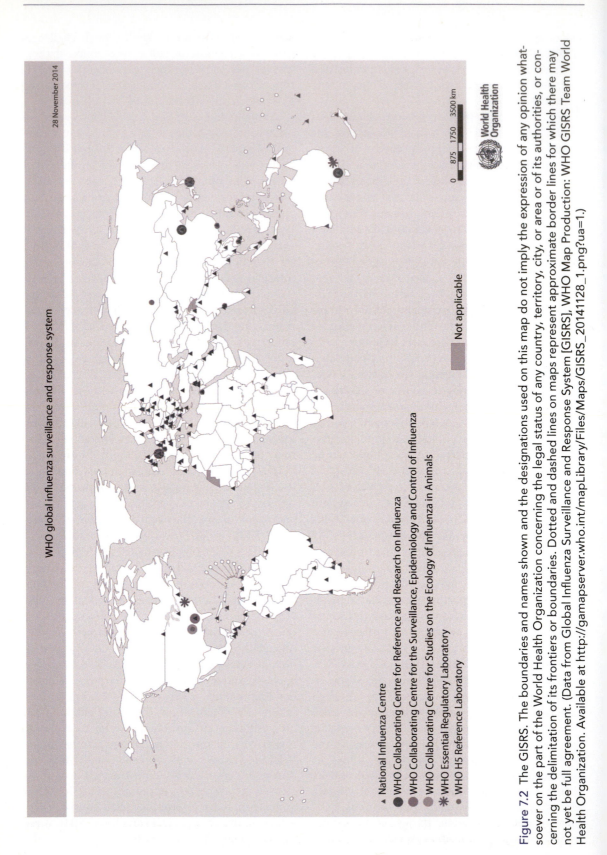

WHO global influenza surveillance and response system

▲ National Influenza Centre

● WHO Collaborating Centre for Reference and Research on Influenza

● WHO Collaborating Centre for the Surveillance, Epidemiology and Control of Influenza

● WHO Collaborating Centre for Studies on the Ecology of Influenza in Animals

✳ WHO Essential Regulatory Laboratory

• WHO H5 Reference Laboratory

Not applicable

0 875 1750 3500 km

World Health
Organization

Figure 7.2 The GISRS. The boundaries and names shown and the designations used on this map do not imply the expression of any opinion what-soever on the part of the World Health Organization concerning the legal status of any country, territory, city, or area or of its authorities, or con-cerning the delimitation of its frontiers or boundaries. Dotted and dashed lines on maps represent approximate border lines for which there may not yet be full agreement. (Data from Global Influenza Surveillance and Response System [GISRS], WHO Map Production: WHO GISRS Team World Health Organization. Available at http://gamapserver.who.int/mapLibrary/Files/Maps/GISRS_20141128_1.png?ua=1.)

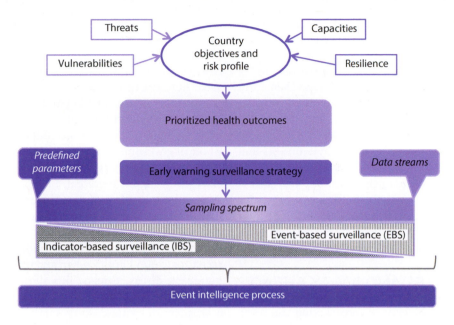

Figure 7.3 The spectrum of indicator- and event-based surveillance in early warning.

likelihood that efforts are aligned with community priorities as well encompass multisectoral resources (Quandelacy et al. 2011).

Disease surveillance programming based upon monitored indicators and event-based surveillance usually is predicated on the search for an acute change above noise in the detection system. In the past few years, the idea of the slowly evolving or indolent novel threat has entered the global health security consciousness in the form of antimicrobial resistance (AMR). While occasional spectacular identifications of resistance plasmids occur, they are the exception. In 2014, the WHO published a report on global surveillance for AMR (WHO 2014b). In his foreward, Dr. Keiji Fukuda, Assistant Director General for Health Security and Environment makes the following summary on AMR surveillance.

> One important finding of the report, which will serve as a baseline to measure future progress, is that there are many gaps in information on pathogens of major public health importance. In addition, surveillance of [AMR] generally is neither coordinated nor harmonized, compromising the ability to assess and monitor the situation.

He was speaking particularly of the under-addressed challenges of resistance in bacteria implicated in common infections. The report also touches on issues around gonococcal resistance as well as increasing drug resistance in malaria, human immunodeficiency virus (HIV) and tuberculosis (TB). Data was most available regarding Europe and the Americas. However, even in these relatively higher resourced regions, gaps exist. Potential root causes of these issues are not usual targets for indicator-based surveillance. Some of these causes are related to regulatory and counterfeit medication challenges, known to exist globally. In a regulatory and law enforcement cooperative project in Southeast Asia, up to one in three medications was out of acceptable range for active ingredient (Yong et al. 2015). This can result in pathogens being exposed to low levels of active ingredient, enough to promote resistance but not enough to clear the pathogen from a patient. This is a known challenge in high risk areas for emerging infection in Africa, as well (The Global Fund 2014). For now, indicators selected for surveillance programs focus on the existence of a disease and do not incorporate those related to risk, such as level of counterfeit drug in a region. *They target the existence of an issue, not the prediction of an issue developing.* This may be a growth area for indicator-based surveillance. A better focus on risk would facilitate improved prevention and mitigation measures regardless of the hazard of concern.

Event-based surveillance also could evolve toward considering risk for disease to a greater extent rather than only presence of disease. Event-based surveillance from some sources already is starting to do so. A search on "climate change" in ProMed yields occasional posts focused on risks ranging from ecosystem disturbance to human disease. However, alerts around changing food supply, population movement, civil unrest, and other predisposing factors for acute health events in communities remain uncommon. This also is true of National Focal Point (NFP) reporting under the Regulations, though some countries' NFP have reported and monitored proactively planned mass gatherings as well as civil emergencies.

CHALLENGES AND A WAY AHEAD

Several challenges exist to constructing and using cross-border surveillance. The countries that remain at highest risk of novel threats are often fragile with large resource needs. They may have challenging relationships with their neighbor countries and be loathe to acknowledge events. Lost trade or perceived vulnerability can be significant concerns. Economic loss is a powerful disincentive to information sharing. Early estimates are quite broad on the losses to mining revenue for countries in West Africa due to the EVD outbreak from 2014 to early 2015. They might be $4–$30 billion (The World Bank 2014). Even countries with more resources can suffer from the perceptions of others when experiencing a public health event. The decrement in Mexico's gross domestic product due to lost tourism as well as other factors during the H1N1 pandemic in 2009–2010 has been estimated to be more than $2.8 billion (Rassy and Smith 2013).

With rare exception already discussed here, there is a lack of timely, shared indicator-based disease surveillance at the international level. In the event of a novel threat—a previously unknown or under-appreciated emerging infectious disease—a regional or global level framework for syndromic surveillance would provide a base for rapid disease identification, response, and monitoring. The challenges of implementing such systems, as well as working through data compatibility and sharing issues, remain. In addition to the advance of disease-specific programming such as for influenza, the WHO has established a working group to begin addressing related implementation issues

for management of event response known as the Emergency Operations Center (EOC) network (WHO 2013). EOC activity is related to surveillance programming in that demands from an activated EOC organize the questions to be answered relevant to decision making and the conduits for data informing decision makers. Ideally, EOC and their operations are built around an all hazards, whole of government and society approach to risk management. The persons who staff an EOC in an emergency should represent all aspects of senior leadership, regardless of government sector. Also, non-governmental actors should be included. One way to exploit EOC in the context of surveillance systems is to exercise them in mock emergency scenarios around both known and unknown communicable disease threats. This allows disease and event-based surveillance programmers to develop a broader understanding of surveillance metrics which inform risk management actions.

The WHO secretariat has the challenging task of helping countries navigate their varied risks when public health events arise as well as both alerting and leveraging the global community, when appropriate. When countries lack the basic resources necessary to allow an alert and resilient health system, this task is significantly more challenging.

Each country's customs and laws regarding the collection and sharing of information also must be considered. In some instances, inside a single country differences in provincial laws have kept the national government from collating some information related to the public health response. Although Article 46 of the Regulations encourages sharing of biologic samples when appropriate to the response and allowed by local law, laws on regulations on this vary. For example, export of biothreat-infected samples from the United States is particularly challenging even among public health partners. Affected and at-risk countries and varied groups of stakeholders may have disparate views of the actual risk of a pandemic threat versus the intellectual property issues at stake including poverty and issues of benefit sharing among the affected populations. International conventions have come into play in these debates, including the burgeoning Convention on Biological Diversity, in particular the Nagoya Protocol (Convention on Biological Diversity 2015b).

These challenges must be overcome by continued success in building capacities such as those outlined under the Regulations. While adherence to the Regulations is important, helping stakeholders understand and take action on shared risks requires relationships and dialog. While some form for this dialog is outlined in the Regulations, these relationships are what is indicated across the articles.

In summary, the IHR (2005) takes a regulatory step toward a holistic view of what impacts public health and the kinds of cooperative relationships that should exist between affected and at-risk countries. This influences the ways that pre-existing and developing surveillance systems work together to provide early warning of emerging threats. Disease-specific systems work together with nonspecific early-warning systems to identify emerging public health threats. Early communication of potential events allows improved cooperative risk management.

CONFLICT OF INTEREST

The views expressed in this chapter are those of the authors and do not necessarily reflect the official policy or position of the Uniformed Services University of the Health Sciences, Department of the Navy, Department of Defense, nor the U.S. government. These views do not necessarily reflect those of the WHO or any other institution.

The authors have reported no conflicts of interest relevant to this chapter.

At least one author of this chapter is a U.S. military service member. This work was prepared as part of that author's official duties. Title 17 USC section 105 provides that "Copyright protection under this article is not available for any work of the U.S. government." Title 17 USC section 101 defines a U.S. government work as a work prepared by a military service member of the U.S. government as part of that person's official duties.

ACKNOWLEDGMENTS

The authors are grateful for the critical review of two senior professionals at WHO Headquarters. Dr. Wenqing Zhang, Head of the Global Influenza Programme, Pandemic Epidemic Diseases Department, Health Security and Environment cluster gave important input on the functioning of global influenza surveillance systems. Dr. Gilles Poumerol, Team Leader, IHR secretariat, Preparedness Surveillance and Response Operations, Global Capacities and Response Department, Health Security and Environment, the WHO. Public health response collaborations with the alert and response operations at the WHO regional offices and headquarters as well as country public health agencies have been critical.

REFERENCES

Andrus, J.K., X. Aguilera, O. Oliva, and S. Aldighieri. 2010. Global health security and the International Health Regulations. *BMC Public Health* 10(Suppl. 1): S2.

Baize, S., D. Pannetier, L. Oestereich et al. 2014. Emergence of Zaire Ebola virus disease in Guinea. *N. Engl. J. Med.* 371(15): 1418–1425.

Convention of Biological Diversity. 2015a. Convention of Biological Diversity. Accessed January 16, 2015. http://www.cbd.int/.

Convention on Biological Diversity. 2015b. The Nagoya protocol on access and benefit-sharing. Accessed February 10, 2015. http://www.cbd.int/abs/.

Fidler, D.P. 2013. Who owns MERS? The intellectual property controversy surrounding the latest pandemic. *Foreign Affairs*, June 6. http://www.foreignaffairs.com/articles/139443/david-p-fidler/who-owns-mers.

HealthMap. 2015. HealthMap. Accessed May 3, 2015. http://www.healthmap.org/en/.

International Society for Infectious Diseases. 2015. About ProMED mail. Accessed January 18, 2015. http://www.promedmail.org/aboutus/.

Kreijtz J.H., E.J. Kroeze, K.J. Stittelaar et al. 2013. Low pathogenic avian influenza A(H7N9) virus causes high mortality in ferrets upon intratracheal challenge: A model to study intervention strategies. *Vaccine* 31(43): 4995–4999.

Li, A. and T. Kasai. 2011. The Asia Pacific strategy for emerging diseases—A strategy for regional health security. *West. Pacific Surveill. Respon. J.* 2(1): 6–9.

Quandelacy, T.M., M.C. Johns, R. Andraghetti, R. Hora, J.-B. Meynard, J.M. Montgomery, V.G. Roque, Jr., and D.L. Blazes. 2011. The role of disease surveillance in achieving IHR compliance by 2012. *Biosecur. Bioterror. Biodef. Strat. Pract. Sci.* 9(4): 408–412.

Rassy, D. and R.D. Smith. 2013. The economic impact of H1N1 on Mexico's tourist and pork sectors. *Health Econ.* 22(7): 824–834.

Smith, G.E., D.C. Flyer, R. Raghunandan, Y. Liu, Z. Wei, Y. Wu, E. Kpamegan, D. Courbron, L.F. Fries, III, and G.M. Glenn. 2013. Development of influenza H7N9 Virus Like Particle (VLP) vaccine: Homologous A/Anhui/1/2013 (H7N9) protection and heterologous A/Chicken/Jalisco/CPA1/2012 (H7N3) cross-protection in vaccinated mice challenged with H7N9 virus. *Vaccine* 31(40): 4305–4313.

The Global Fund. 2014. Combatting theft and counterfeiting of medicines in West Africa. Accessed April 30, 2014. http://www.theglobalfund.org/en/blog/2014-06-26_Combatting_Theft_and_Counterfeiting_of_Medicines_in_West_Africa/.

The World Bank. 2014. The economic impact of the 2014 Ebola epidemic: Short and medium term estimates for West Africa. Accessed October 8, 2015. http://www.worldbank.org/en/region/afr/publication/the-economic-impact-of-the-2014-ebola-epidemic-short-and-medium-term-estimates-for-west-africa.

Wang, Y., Z. Dai, H. Cheng et al. 2013. Towards a better understanding of the novel avian-origin H7N9 influenza A virus in China. *Scient. Rep.* 3: 2318.

WHO. 2008. International Health Regulations (2005), 2nd edn. Geneva, Switzerland: World Health Organization.

WHO. 2011a. IHR key publications 2007–2012. Geneva, Switzerland: World Health Organization.

WHO. 2011b. Pandemic influenza preparedness framework for the sharing of influenza viruses and access to vaccines and other benefits. Geneva, Switzerland: World Health Organization.

WHO. 2011c. Strengthening response to pandemics and other public health emergencies: Report of the Review Committee on the Functioning of the International Health Regulations (2005) and on Pandemic Influenza (H1N1) 2009. Geneva, Switzerland: World Health Organization.

WHO. 2013. A systematic review of public health emergency operations centres. Geneva, Switzerland: World Health Organization.

WHO. 2014a. Early detection, assessment and response to acute public health events: Implementation of early warning and response with a focus on event-based surveillance. Geneva, Switzerland: World Health Organization.

WHO. 2014b. Antimicrobial resistance: Global report on surveillance 2014. Geneva, Switzerland: World Health Organization.

WHO. 2015a. Global Influenza Surveillance and Response System (GISRS). Accessed January 18. http://www.who.int/influenza/gisrs_laboratory/en/.

WHO. 2015b. International Health Regulations (2005) monitoring framework. Accessed January 17, 2015. http://www.who.int/gho/ihr/en/.

WHO. 2015c. WHO emerging and dangerous pathogens laboratory network (EDPLN). Accessed February 10, 2015. http://www.who.int/csr/bioriskreduction/laboratorynetwork/en/.

Yong, Y.L., A. Plançon, Y.H. Lau et al. 2015 Collaborative health and law enforcement operations on the quality of antimalarials and antibiotics in SouthEast Asia. *Am. J. Trop. Med. Hyg.* pii: 14-0574 (E-pub ahead of print, April 20, 2015).

Zhou, J., D. Wang, R. Gao, B. Zhao, J. Song, X. Qi, and Y. Zhang. 2013. Biological features of novel avian influenza A (H7N9) virus. *Nature* 499(7459): 500–503.

8

Possible solutions for sustainable surveillance systems

CHRISTOPHER L. PERDUE

Computer technologies have had a revolutionary effect on the ability of epidemiologists and other public health professionals to gather information about the populations they serve and conduct health surveillance, generally increasing the overall quality and timeliness of data as well as the awareness of "health events."* In high- and middle-income countries where health-related information systems—individual patient's medical and billing records, pharmacy systems, public websites and hotlines, local school attendance rosters, laboratory databases, among many others—have become ubiquitous, public health systems have found ways to leverage the collection of those data in central locations to conduct health surveillance activities and promote health security.† The World Health Assembly's International Health Regulations (2005) (IHR) require use of information technologies to enhance the ability of "State Parties" (the 196 signatory countries) to identify and communicate potential public health emergencies of international concern. The more quickly such notifications can occur and the better coordinated the rapid response to international outbreaks, the more likely it will be that public health authorities can prevent significant international spread of infectious diseases as well as reduce the impact on international travel and commerce resulting from any public health event. The recent Ebola virus outbreak that affected primarily Guinea, Sierra Leone, and Liberia (Centers for Disease Control and Prevention 2014b) highlights the persistent

---

* The phrase "health event" in this context should be interpreted very broadly to mean any apparent (real, false, or artifactual) change of, or threat to, the health of the population resulting from any type of natural, accidental, or intentional exposure.

† "Health security" in this context refers to the prevention, detection of, and response to public health threats (events) of any kind.

gaps that remain in many public health surveillance and response systems (Forrester et al. 2014).

Health information technologies can have a positive effect on routine and emergency public health activities. However, technological elements of a public health system require additional, specialized resources and a national commitment to sustainability. Scale-up from local pilot programs to national disease surveillance requires a plan that addresses adaptability and resiliency. This chapter will present a number of real-world case studies taken from peer-reviewed literature and the authors' personal experiences to outline models for successful scale-up and long-term sustainability of electronic disease surveillance systems without attempting to be prescriptive or normative.

Putting the horse before the cart, so to speak, a fundamental first step for any successful computer-based health surveillance system is to have available the human and administrative resources required to observe cases, collect data, and conduct analyses. In other words, there must be the essential elements of a good public health system in place before any attempt should be made at digitizing data. This is a significant challenge in parts of the industrialized and developing worlds where there still remain large gaps in health-care systems, as well as in the linkages between the health-care system and the public health system. Those problems often need to be solved beforehand, or at the very worst, concurrently. Many health information system projects starts as small pilots, but building out the digital aspects of the system to full scale must be concurrent with development of the health workforce, including the information technologists. This is a tenet that seems obvious but typically is not a part of the original technical specifications.

For any electronic disease surveillance system to function, there must be an operational public health system in place (i.e., following best practices as described by the World Health Organization) followed by a means to transfer data into a digital format. Health systems around the world are in varying states of development, and digital health data are either not widely available or not comprehensive enough to represent the population at risk. Though many efforts are underway to provide infrastructure, systems, and training for the creation of health information systems in general (World Health Organization 2015), it is a slow and complicated process constrained by the extraordinary costs associated with such technologies (when trying to reach full scale) and the low level of expertise available to manage complex computer systems at the district and sub-district levels. In lieu of a comprehensive health-care information (medical records) system that can serve individual patient's needs as well as be used for public health surveillance, it is also common to see parallel and (sadly) often uncoordinated efforts at national or subnational levels to conduct health surveillance in various forms.

The lack of coordination among public health stakeholders is a particularly difficult problem in the low- and middle-income countries where public health authorities and donor groups rarely work under a comprehensive national strategy for design and implementation. The authors can all point to personal experiences with different efforts occurring at different locations in the same country simultaneously without reference to a national health surveillance strategy. Site- or stakeholder-specific programs may target specific types of patient care, such as diagnosis and treatment of human immunodeficiency virus (HIV) infections and related care management; or they may be highly specific for epidemiologic data collection and not necessarily intended for individual patient care. The benefit of those systems and programs is not in question, but the resulting fragmentation in health-related "data streams" prevents simple redirection and aggregation using an (elusive) "integrative strategy" for the purposes of comprehensive health surveillance. At some point, the amount of effort required in such an attempt overwhelms the availability of resources. System design considerations and long-term commitments from the outset that support a strategy for scale-up and long-term sustainability are often lacking. This chapter will highlight some of those considerations through the use of case studies in order to raise awareness and hopefully show how smart (and adaptive) design and held-fast determination among the systems' stewards can allow electronic disease surveillance systems to grow into functional and indispensable elements of national and regional health security.

From the perspective of a public health practitioner trained in traditional epidemiologic methods, computerized data collection at the source is not necessary to conduct disease surveillance. This is especially true in smaller regions where human resources are sufficient to use paper-based data collection and transmission. In well organized systems, such paper-based surveillance for syndromes (influenza-like illness) or specific conditions (dengue fever) can greatly improve on the ability of epidemiologists to detect public health problems relatively early. However, small, subregional systems that are successful face the inevitable pressure to (a) expand to more sites, adding to the inherent logistical challenge, and (b) (almost infallibly today) attempt to devise a *de novo* strategy to introduces technology as a solution to the scale-up problem.

Ideally, a small, well planned pilot—referring now to the overlay of simple technology onto an already functional public health surveillance system—that has significant government buy-in and a relatively easy-to-use interface can be grown into a national electronic disease surveillance system simply by adding nodes and users. Careful attention to system design at the outset with monitoring and evaluation to demonstrate cost-effectiveness of the system would lead to further financial support and investment in the technological and human resource components needed to operate the system. Over time, enhancements to storage capacity, processor speed, and multi-user access control, along with aberration-detection software, could be implemented centrally (perhaps with an outwardly facing interface for public health professionals who are in the field) to augment the ability of the epidemiologists trained in traditional public health methodologies to identify and initiate investigation of abnormal cases.

In principle, such systems offer many benefits. In practice, the lives of epidemiologists can become much more complicated and drastically less productive because they lack sufficient training to utilize such systems efficiently, the system itself may not be very user-friendly, and they do not have resources available to trouble-shoot glitches as well as conduct end-user training, monitor the data feeds for accuracy, timeliness and completeness; and write the support contracts required to make improvements to the system. Learning new systems requires training, which can be time away from other duties; most epidemiologists and public health informaticists in the real world find themselves trying to build the rest of airplane (so to speak) as it begins its first runway attempt. Today, even marginally well designed technology systems will have reasonably affordable, accessible, and reliable components that encourage local adoption, championship, and sustainability. The ubiquity of powerful and adaptable computing resources often leads to the mistaken belief that creating an electronic disease surveillance system is simply a matter of consistent electricity and connection cables. Regardless of how inexpensive or accessible hardware and communication systems may be, or how user friendly the interface, there are typically two components at the heart of the system that cannot simply be replaced as needed: the database itself and the people who understand how to make the system work. This chapter, through several case studies, will explore those challenges and suggest a number of considerations for both data system design as well as strategic planning.

Epidemiologists are familiar with problems related to data quality, completeness, sensitivity, specificity, and comparability; but relatively few are familiar with data from a technological perspective; and fewer still are prepared to address the large-scale problems associated with information systems and a data architecture that will someday contain thousands, if not millions or billions, of records. Pilot projects are often relatively easy to start because of low cost of entry into modern technologies, including the availability of essentially free "open source" software solutions. Implementation plans commonly and appropriately take into consideration the immediate elements of human behavior, system performance requirements, equipment accountability, financing, government, local "ownership" of the system, and connectivity. Few, however, contain fully realized plans for managing the database, users, technological obsolescence, and unexpected requirements that will evolve over the following 5–10 years of the system's early life.

Case study #1: The Defense Medical Surveillance System

Christopher L. Perdue
United States Public Health Service
Washington, DC

The Defense Medical Surveillance System (DMSS) is a system that began large and has grown to be immense. This is not the kind of system that most epidemiologists anywhere would have access to, but it is a very useful example of the critical relationship between the epidemiologist and the technologist in an electronic disease surveillance system. The Armed Forces Health Surveillance Center (AFHSC) uses DMSS to conduct very large-scale health surveillance and epidemiologic studies on (primarily) the U.S. military active duty population. DMSS is composed of data feeds from a multitude of sources. Maintaining the orderly operation of that enormous data repository requires many highly trained staff members as well as data validation and normalization steps, the description of which goes well beyond the reach of this publication. Primarily used for non-acute health surveillance activities, DMSS can be used for certain types of outbreak detection as well as to inform the investigation of known outbreaks (Armed Forces Health Surveillance Center 2015).

The epidemiologists who use DMSS on a daily basis have a deep working knowledge of the information system in ways that outside epidemiologists do not. Changes to the ways in which data were collected over time, changes and inconsistent variations in the coding used by health-care systems throughout the world, changes to the military personnel system and the introduction of new data sources all factor into data retrieval and analysis. A technologist who is completely competent as a database administrator would not fathom the depths of those challenges initially, and those who are eventually appointed as senior epidemiologists have had 6 or more months on on-the-job training with extraordinarily detailed scrutiny over their study design and data handling.

DMSS highlights the critically important relationship between the technology team and the epidemiology team when building a system that will handle very large amounts of data. To ensure sustainability and successful scale-up, the implementation plan should involve one or more managing epidemiologists on the technology team. With a functional understanding of the relationship between technical components of the data system, especially the movement or transformation of data within the system, managing epidemiologists can serve as a critical linkage between the sciences of epidemiology and information. The epidemiologist does not necessarily need to be an informaticist to be effective, but the epidemiologist does need to learn to speak in the language of information technology. Ultimately, the lead technologists will also learn a significant amount of epidemiology and be able to more easily convey the impacts of data system problems on health surveillance. An interesting and relatively simple example of the convergence between epidemiology and information science is the assignment of the value "active duty" to service members in DMSS.

The U.S. military has long used a two-digit code to characterize the personnel status of service members and non-service members who are beneficiaries of the health-care system. service members are always 20, the first spouse of a service member is a 30 and the first child is a 01; other codes are used for other medical beneficiaries of other types. When prefixed to a person's Social Security Number and date of birth, each person is uniquely identified in the military health-care system.

In a variation of practice based on specific policies, the military services assign the designation "20" to new service members at respectively different points during their basic training. Prior to that point, those who are newly inducted have a different code that designates them as a "trainee." However, once a 20, always a 20, even after retirement when a former service member may continue to receive health-care benefits through the military system. Consequently, the epidemiologists who study the active duty component of the military must employ a series of positive and negative selection criteria in order to identify the correct population. Eventually, the military replaced the simple two-digit system with a more reliable and secure electronic identification number that does not contain the social security number (U.S. Department of Defense 2015). When that change went into effect, the informatics teams at AFHSC developed an algorithm to prevent person mismatches in longitudinal studies. When dealing with millions of health-care recipients over many decades, identifying the correct population is critical and requires that the epidemiologist have a very clear understanding of how the system gathers, transforms, and updates personnel data.

Complex situations can arise in smaller information systems. Counting (and unintentionally recounting) people and cases of influenza or other infectious diseases on a national scale over many years is a good example of a common problem among system of all sizes. The DoD solves this problem when assembling information from separate U.S. Army, Navy, and Air Force notifiable disease surveillance programs by combining health-care utilization and personnel data from DoD-wide systems, eliminating redundancy by using a reliable individual identification method.

PERSONAL IDENTITY AND DEMOGRAPHIC DATA

Uniquely identifiable data are critical for a successful health information system of any kind, including for a large-scale public health system. If a national identification system exists, then using those identifiers allows the public health system to identify unique cases as well as positively link cases to others. Without a national identification system, combinations of unique personal attributes can be used to identify each person. Sex, name, and date of birth are typical data elements that can help to identify a unique person, but in some locations, precise dates of birth are not kept, and names may be less unique than in other cultures. Biometric systems using fingerprints and/or photographs can substitute for unique identification numbers (UINs) but add other constraints related to power sources and equipment. Other

possibilities for creating unique identifiers can be explored. In particular, facts that a person may recall consistently over time (such as their place of birth, home town/district, or the name of a relative) where

RELATIVE* = Mother, father, oldest child, spouse
RELATIVE'S NAME = wxyz

… could be considered. Aside from identity itself, most other aspects of personhood can change over time. Therefore, the database should contain separate tables for identity plus the date of birth, place of birth, etc. that do not change; and demographic facts that could or will change. Importantly, and regardless of whether or not a person has a unique, nationally assigned identification number (NIN), each person must receive a UIN within the construct of the data system. Over time, NIN may be reused, and errors in data entry of the NIN itself will need to be corrected. The system-specific UIN links each person to their time-varying demographic data and allows demographic updates such as number of children, marital status, residence, etc. to be added periodically, leading to the potential for well informed temporal (longitudinal) and spatial studies. Unique personal identifiers (either UIN or NIN) are also critical for preventing redundant case counting and accurate rate estimates over time.

UIN are often numeric strings (there is no magic number, but 12 digits seems common), combinations of numbers and letters, or a combination of date-parts and a successive numeric sequence. Assigning UIN is a critical administrative functions that must be established early during the development of the database. The range of UIN must account for the potential size of the population and whether or not the UIN will be assigned

---

* Words in ALL CAPITALS are intended to represent the field name, though in some cases, those field names are not ideal for a database (e.g., a field name would never have an apostrophe or space). Words that follow the = sign represent potential values for that field, but not necessarily an exhaustive list of options.

centrally (possibly automatically), or locally using a distributed key. Discussion about the advantages and disadvantages of different types and models of UINs goes beyond the scope of this chapter, but suffice it to say that non-unique UINs can become extremely problematic over time.

Case study #2: Maryland state's electronic surveillance system for the early notification of community-based epidemics

Anikah H. Salim and Al Romanosky*
Office of Preparedness and Response
Maryland Department of Health and Mental Hygiene
Baltimore, Maryland

The Maryland Department of Health and Mental Hygiene (DHMH) was one of the first, large government jurisdictions to participate as a development partner in the use of computer-based technologies to enhance early detection of disease outbreaks and suspicious symptom patterns. The system, called Electronic Surveillance System for Early Notification of Community-Based Epidemics (ESSENCE), included data from the Washington, DC and Virginia Departments of Health when it was activated within hours following the September 11, 2001 terrorist attacks. Since then, the DHMH Office of Preparedness and Response (OP&R) has continued to support enhancement and evolution of the system.

Initially, selected health-care facilities submitted emergency department chief complaint data by facsimile to OP&R. Analysts reading the data categorized each chief complaint into one or more signs, symptoms, or

* Authors of this case study would like to acknowledge Sherry Adams, RN and Isaac Ajit, MD, MPH for their assistance on this study.

syndrome categories, which were then manually entered into the database by technicians. Today, data are automatically classified into one of 11 classic syndromes (influenza-like illness, febrile illness, gasteroenteritis, etc.) plus 148 "sub-syndromes" or associated signs and symptoms (cough, fever, dyspnea, headache, etc.) by free-text recognition software. Data are fed to OP&R electronically (via the Internet) from the originating record systems. The data in ESSENCE are maintained on a secure website that complies with federal standards for information privacy and public health uses.

Maryland's ESSENCE database also now incorporates nontraditional health indicators that are captured in near real-time with statewide coverage. Those sources include

- Poison Control Center calls
- Over-the-counter (OTC) medication sales (e.g., thermometers, fever medications, and cold/upper respiratory infection medications)
- School absenteeism reports
- Reportable disease data

All of Maryland's acute care hospitals and public school districts contribute to the ESSENCE data.

The ESSENCE system employs routine analysis of case counts according to established case definitions as well as ad hoc for novel case definitions created by the epidemiologist. The analysis of case counts using mathematic aberration detection methods is discussed elsewhere in this book, but being able to use the available data in novel ways is a critical feature of the Maryland system. Two valuable examples of that type of surveillance occurred in 2014–2015.

ENTEROVIRUS D68

Enterovirus (EV) D68 is one of over 100 non-poliovirus EVs that can cause mild to severe respiratory illnesses. Beginning mid-August of 2014, the United States experienced a nationwide outbreak of EV-D68 (Centers for Disease Control and Prevention 2014a). Through January 15, 2015, there were 1153 laboratory confirmed cases in 49 states and the District of Columbia, including Maryland (Centers for Disease Control and Prevention 2014c). To augment monitoring of EV-D68 across Maryland, epidemiologists in OP&R developed a specialized weekly surveillance report that was distributed through the DHMH Prevention and Health Promotion Administration.

ESSENCE data were used in the report to characterize respiratory illnesses in children aged 0–17 years. Respiratory syndrome chief complaints were compared week-by-week to the prior 2 years to create a historical context against which to evaluate current trends (Figure 8.1). Specific (subsyndrome) trends for cough (Figure 8.2), difficulty breathing (Figure 8.3), shortness of breath, and wheezing were also followed weekly to assess for unexpected increases that might represent clusters of EV-D68 cases. (The graphs for shortness of breath and wheezing were similar to the other two

sub-syndromes, and so are not included here.) The respiratory disease incidence expressed as a percentage of all chief complaints were mapped by county and compared to trends in school absenteeism to evaluate for potential geographic "hot spots." Ultimately, surveillance using ESSENCE during the 2014–2015 EV-D68 outbreak in the United States revealed no specific clusters of illnesses in Maryland, which served as important reassurance for the state public health officers that no special public health interventions were needed.

EBOLA VIRUS DISEASE

During the 2014–2015 outbreak of Ebola virus disease (EVD) in West Africa, DHMH again collaborated with the Washington, DC and Virginia Departments of Health, as well as the Tarrant County, Texas, Public Health Department, and the CDC BioSense 2.0 program to focus their surveillance program on the importation of EVD cases into Maryland. Data systems were queried for key words related to symptoms of EVD such as fever, hiccups, hemorrhage, nausea, and vomiting

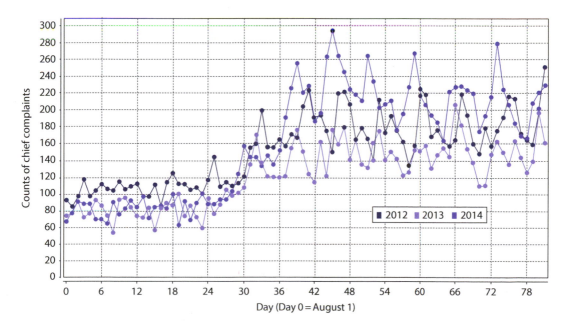

Figure 8.1 A multi-year comparison (2012, 2013, 2014 by calendar week) for respiratory syndrome diagnoses in children 0–17 years of age in Maryland.

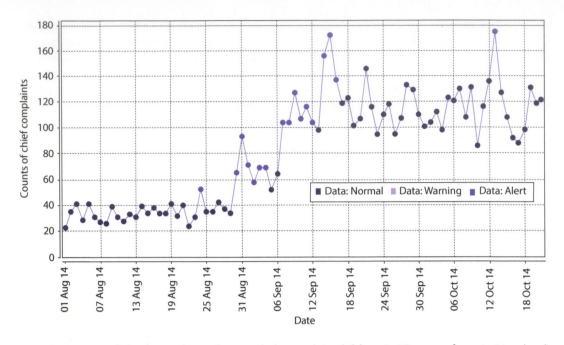

Figure 8.2 Counts of chief complaints for cough (by week in children 0–17 years of age in Maryland).

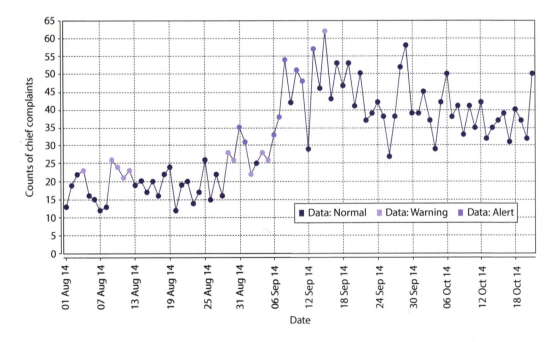

Figure 8.3 Counts of chief complaints for difficulty breathing (by week in children 0–17 years of age in Maryland).

(among others); along with self-reported international travel to affected countries (initially Liberia, Sierra Leone, and Guinea, and then Mali and Nigeria for a period of time); and literal references to the disease itself in the medical chief complaint (i.e., Ebola or EVD). The enhanced surveillance activities were repeated daily with appropriate follow-up by epidemiologists for highlighted cases (Figure 8.4).

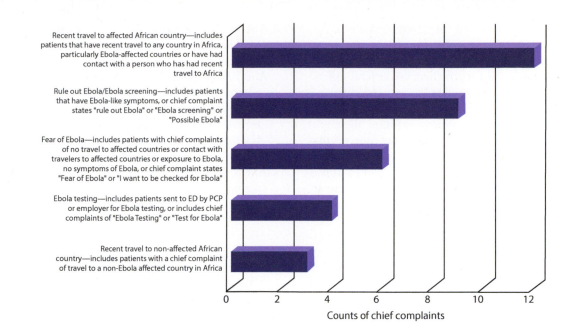

Figure 8.4 Counts of chief complaints in Maryland that met the local (administrative) case definitions for potential or perceived Ebola virus exposure (August 2015–January 2015).

Recent Travel to Affected African Country: Includes patients with a chief complaint of recent travel to Africa or one of the Ebola-affected African countries (Liberia, Guinea, Nigeria, Mali, Sierra Leone)

Rule Out Ebola/Ebola Screening: Includes patients that have Ebola-like symptoms, and/or chief complaints that state "rule out Ebola," "Ebola screening," or "possible Ebola"

Fear of Ebola: Includes patients sent to the ED by PCP, physician or employer for Ebola testing, or chief complaints with "Ebola testing" or "test for Ebola"

Recent Travel to Non-Affected African Country: Includes patients with a chief complaint of travel to a non-Ebola affected country in Africa

CASE DEFINITIONS

It is critical that disease surveillance systems provide the epidemiologists with an appropriate level of flexibility, and enough information about reported cases, to refine case definitions "on the fly" and to examine the relationships between elements of the case definition. A common inclination among surveillance system designers is to require a medical provider to select a single case type (syndrome) for each patient, whether or not they additionally require the provider to indicate some level of certainty (i.e., confirmed vs. suspected) about that diagnosis. Development and evolution of electronic disease surveillance systems such as ESSENCE highlight the extraordinary, long-term value of being able to access related data about the cases.

Similar to demographic data, case data must be conceptualized as being made of one-time values and time-dependent values. The date of diagnosis, the date of presentation, the initial impression by the provider, the data of onset, initial symptoms, etc., will never change, though such values may be updated or corrected when new information is obtained. The dates of follow-up visits, the dates that laboratory tests are completed, the dates that lab results are available, and the results of those tests, can occur multiple times during the handling of a case. Careful consideration must be given as to how to handle discreet (one-time) case data versus longitudinal case data.

An important characteristic of the case that often causes substantial confusion is whether or not the case is confirmed positive, probable, suspect, confirmed negative, unknown, or untested. Commonly, database designers unwisely attempt to capture these data values in a single field when there are several different concepts that need to be captured independently. It is critical to avoid creating a database that drives the invention of substantially more work in the field while, at the same time, results in data that are useful to the epidemiologists. This exercise may ultimately involve some changes to the workflow or data collection at the field sites, which can have both positive and negative impacts on data quality, completeness, and timeliness. The following are examples of possible laboratory descriptors:

SAMPLE TAKEN = Yes/no (on what date)*
SAMPLE TESTED = Yes/no (on what date)
TEST COMPLETE = Yes/no (on what date)
TEST RESULT = Variable values depending on the test
DIAGNOSIS = Positive X, negative X, unknown

DIAGNOSIS, as a discreet field, could be very useful when the TEST RESULT is a quantitative value. DIAGNOSIS would then contain the interpretation of that TEST RESULT according to published reference values and could be a calculated value assigned automatically when the TEST RESULT field is updated.

Another data element that often causes problems is "status" of the patient. Active, inactive, unknown, active but not under investigation, alive, deceased, lost to follow-up, refuses to be interviewed are all labels that describe the "relationship" between the case-patient and the epidemiologist (and possibly the database itself). Similar to TEST RESULT, attempting to capture the various "statuses" of a case in a single cell in a database will lead to tragedy. The following are suggestions for case-status descriptors:

CASE UNDER INVESTIGATION = Yes/no/ pending/unreachable/refused (by whom, started or attempted when)

* Phrases in parentheses represent additional data elements (fields) that are normally associated with the field in all capital letters and could be considered mandatory.

CASE LIVING = Yes/no/unknown (died from a cause that was the same as the diagnosis, on what date)
CASE DATA COMPLETE = Yes/no (by whom, on what date—the fact that the all of the epidemiologic data have been collected does not include pending laboratory tests, autopsy results, or supervisory review with a final case determination)
CASE STATUS = Open/closed (i.e., a supervisor has determined the case can be closed and requires no additional effort)

Case study #3: Peruvian military electronic disease surveillance system

Ricardo Hora
Biomedical Informatics Department
United States Naval Medical Research
Unit No. 6, Callao, Peru

Delphis Vera
Biomedical Informatics Department
United States Naval Medical Research
Unit No. 6, Callao, Peru

The Peruvian Medical Command (PMC) is responsible for the prevention, detection, and mitigation of communicable disease outbreaks in military populations. To strengthen its disease surveillance system, PMC has adopted electronic tools to ensure the availability of essential epidemiological data for cases diagnosed in central and remote military units. Following a cluster of eight malaria cases in 2001 in a military unit in the border area between Peru and Colombia, it was determined that real-time health surveillance and expert epidemiologic oversight for remote sites would require the use of modern information technologies.

Support from the United States Department of Defense (DoD) has played an important role in the successful establishment of Peru's military electronic disease surveillance tools. In 2002, DoD funded the development of software by a privately owned business that employed interactive voice response (IVR), online data entry through a browser-based form and text messages (short message service [SMS]) from deployed mobile phones (Soto et al. 2008). The IVR option allowed data entry from sites that had access to only a land-line telephone. With the emergence of new technologies, the Peruvian military opted to replace the original software with open-source alternatives that allowed greater local control and adaptability. Since its implementation, and with technical assistance from the U.S. Naval Medical Research Unit-6 (NAMRU-6), the electronic disease surveillance system resulted in significantly improved data collection and outbreak detection. Due to the Navy's successful experience, the Peruvian Army and Air Force transitioned into electronic disease surveillance in 2005 and 2009, respectively.

Because the tool was initially very successful in providing real-time epidemiological information to health officials, the PMC agreed to continue to explore new functionality and improved access to the health surveillance platform. Beginning in 2009, in collaboration with the Johns Hopkins University Applied Physics Laboratory (APL), PMC and the staff at NAMRU-6 developed and implemented a new, patent-free, open-source electronic disease surveillance tool based on the publicly available ESSENCE Desktop Edition and the Suite for Automated Global Electronic bioSurveillance.* The Peruvian Military Electronic Disease Surveillance System (PMEDSS) was installed in 2011 and has been in use among all military units since then. Like its predecessor, the newly developed PMEDSS tool uses IVR, web-based data entry and SMS.

PMEDSS is aligned with the disease notification policies issued by the Peruvian Ministry of Health. PMEDSS' stakeholders include reporting personnel, data analysts, and military authorities. Reporting personnel are individuals in each military medical facility who are assigned the responsibility to report specific health conditions according to standard operating procedures. Aggregated case counts are submitted once a week for all syndromes (including zero-counts); and individual reports for specified conditions (such as dengue fever or malaria) are submitted immediately (within the same day). In addition to submitting those routine reports, units' reporting personnel are

required to contact the central military surveillance office (in Lima) if they become aware of potential disease outbreaks.

The surveillance officers are military liaisons from each service detailed to the Biomedical Informatics Department at NAMRU-6 who assist units' reporting personnel with accurate data collection and reporting, monitor and follow-up on delinquent reporting units, coordinate outbreak response efforts, and analyze PMEDSS data to prepare reports that are sent to military authorities and other ministries. Military authorities use the information from PMEDSS to allocate resources and personnel during outbreak situations. NAMRU-6 has provided uninterrupted technical and logistical support the helps to ensure sustainability and long-term commitment from PMC. PMEDSS has proven extremely useful for electronic disease reporting and has shown high rates of acceptability among its end users. Similar, customized systems are being considered for the Ministries of Defense in Ecuador, Panama, and Nicaragua.

Case study #4: Syndromic surveillance systems in Europe (Triple-S Project)

Shraddha Patel
Applied Physics Laboratory
Johns Hopkins University
Laurel, Maryland

To date, several European countries have integrated syndromic surveillance into national surveillance programs (Hulth et al. 2009). In 2010, the Triple-S Project (Syndromic Surveillance Systems in Europe) was launched with the goal of increasing the European capacity for real-time or near real-time surveillance and monitoring of the health burden of expected and unexpected health-related events (Triple-S 2014; Triple-S Project 2011). The project was funded by the European Union and coordinated by the French Institute for Public Health Surveillance. It included 24 organizations from 13 countries. The project included conducting an inventory of the existing human and animal syndromic surveillance systems and initiatives in Europe, and

* http://www.jhuapl.edu/sages/.

determining if any gaps in coverage existed. The overall objectives of the Triple-S Project were (Trip-S Project 2010) as follows:

1. To provide member states, the European Centre for Disease Control and Prevention, and relevant bodies with an overview of the available systems of syndromic surveillance in Europe taking into consideration the different organizations of health systems in the countries of Europe.
2. To support harmonization of main data sources for morbidity syndromic surveillance.
3. To support the development and implementation of syndromic surveillance systems at a member state level according to the member states' needs and expectations.
4. To develop synergies between animal and human syndromic surveillance and promote dialogue and complementarity between syndromic surveillance systems, sentinel networks, and specific disease surveillance networks.

The objective was not to create a single European system but to review syndromic surveillance activities across member states. The Health and Consumer Directorate General of the European Commission, the European Centre for Disease Prevention and Control, WHO Regional Office for Europe, and the International Society for Disease Surveillance are members of the advisory board, which encourages exchange of practices across Europe and at the global level.

In October 2014, the Triple-S Project announced the first European guidelines for syndromic surveillance in human and animal health. The guidelines provide evidence-based recommendations and suggestions for each step of implementation, use, and assessment of a syndromic surveillance system. The guidelines also encourage a common understanding of the structure and utility of syndromic surveillance systems and seek to improve communications among European countries on critical public health threats (Hulth 2012).

Case study #5: Syndromic surveillance in Australia

David Muscatello
School of Public Health and Community Medicine
University of New South Wales
Sydney, New South Wales, Australia

Syndromic surveillance systems operating in Australia are best exemplified through the national influenza surveillance reports (Australian Government Department of Health 2015). The systems are mostly characterized by secondary use of prevailing health-care databases. Emergency Department surveillance for influenza-like illness is carried out in New South Wales, Western Australia, and the Northern Territory. Western Australia also monitors other syndromes including gastroenteritis and febrile rash (Government of Western Australia Department of Health 2008). General practice surveillance of influenza-like illness occurs through the national Australian Sentinel Practices Research Network (ASPREN) project and the Victorian Infectious Disease Reference Laboratory (VIDRL) influenza surveillance program. ASPREN monitors other conditions including gastroenteritis (School of Population Health and Clinical Practice 2015). Influenza-like illness is also monitored through the National Health Call Centre Network (Australian Government Department of Health 2014). Surveillance of excess influenza-attributable mortality using electronic death registration information is also conducted in New South Wales (Muscatello et al. 2008).

The FluTracking Internet influenza-like illness project covers all of Australia and monitors weekly Internet survey responses prompted by e-mail from over 10,000 participants recruited through advertising and word of mouth (Dalton et al. 2009; University of Newcastle et al. 2015).

NEW SOUTH WALES EMERGENCY DEPARTMENT AND AMBULANCE SURVEILLANCE

The state of New South Wales (NSW) has the most comprehensive near real-time, emergency service-based public health surveillance program in Australia. NSW is Australia's most populous state (7.5 million) and has its most populated metropolis, Sydney (4.8 million) (Australian Bureau of Statistics 2015). Its area is over 800,000 km^2 (310,000 miles^2) and while the population lives primarily on the coastal fringe, there are substantial numbers of populated remote localities (Geoscience Australia 2014).

Automated emergency department surveillance instituted by the NSW Ministry of Health has operated for almost 12 years and ambulance dispatch surveillance for at least 7. Electronic health-care surveillance was motivated by biopreparedness programs and mass gathering surveillance needs (Muscatello et al. 2005; Thackway et al. 2009).

The surveillance objectives are (New South Wales Ministry of Health 2010)

- To provide early warning of increases in disease activity in the population that may not be evident through other routine surveillance
- To provide situational awareness and supplement other information on trends in acute disease and injury in the NSW population
- To monitor syndrome epidemiology to assist the development and monitoring of prevention strategies for the causes of these syndromes

The near real-time surveillance database was implemented using open source software on computer servers housed in a state health data center. A PostgreSQL database is used to store and manage the incoming data. Customized programs written in the python programming language are used to manage data communications and database transactions. For emergency departments, the hospital patient management information system software vendors were engaged to implement alternative modes of data delivery; Health Level 7 (HL7) or batch feeds that could be scheduled at intervals of several hours. The mode of delivery was selected based on the preference or capability of the sending hospital or health service. The NSW hourly batch data feed of ambulance dispatch information was instituted by the New South Wales Ambulance Service (Muscatello et al. 2005; Thackway et al. 2009; Thomas et al. 2011).

As in 2013, 59 emergency departments representing approximately 84% of all emergency department activity in the state and all state ambulance emergency calls were included. This represents over 6000 emergency presentations and around 2500 ambulance responses each day (Liljeqvist et al. 2014; New South Wales Ambulance Service 2014; New South Wales Ministry of Health 2014; Centre for Epidemiology and Evidence 2015).

For emergency department presentations, a syndrome is allocated to the record if the primary provisional emergency department diagnosis falls within the group of related diagnoses defined in the surveillance system. The syndromes can be very broad or quite specific; for example, one syndrome is "all respiratory" and a subsyndrome is "influenza-like illness" (ILI). The diagnoses are recorded by clinicians in the patient information system at patient discharge from the emergency department. Three classification systems are used for recording diagnoses in the hospital databases: International Classification of Diseases (ICD) versions 9 or 10; or the Systematized Nomenclature of Medicine—Clinical Terminology (SNOMED CT) (Muscatello et al. 2005). As in 2014, there were 38 syndromes included in the system (Liljeqvist et al. 2014). SNOMED CT is the most common classification used in recent years (Mitchell et al. 2013). Problems recorded in the ambulance database are used to classify ambulance calls into syndromes (Thomas et al. 2011; Schaffer et al. 2012).

Use of syndromic groupings of problems rather than relying on specific diagnoses to identify clinically relevant cases is supported by an evaluation of emergency department diagnoses using discharge summaries from admitted patients as a reference. Loosening the precision of the case definition improved correlation to the discharge summary diagnosis (Liaw et al. 2012). Indeed, an evaluation of relying on emergency department diagnoses to trigger reporting of a meningococcal meningitis infection, a notifiable condition in Australia, showed that an emergency department diagnosis of meningococcal infection had poor sensitivity and positive predictive value compared with traditional clinical and laboratory reporting (O'Toole et al. 2010).

Systematic evaluations of syndrome time series for early warning generate mixed results. The surveillance time series for ILI presentations has been shown to respond around 3 days earlier to influenza activity compared with surveillance time series of laboratory-confirmed influenza infections (Zheng et al. 2007). Influenza-like illness and bronchiolitis emergency department time series respond independently to influenza and respiratory syncytial virus (RSV) activity, respectively (Schindeler et al. 2009). Monitoring emergency department presentations for cough does not appear to provide a time advantage to scheduled reporting of pertussis. Cough time series also respond to incidence of other pathogens including influenza and RSV and so lack specificity (Cashmore et al. 2013). The mental illness syndrome, a broad grouping, has good accuracy for surveillance of acute mental health problems collectively (Liljeqvist et al. 2014).

The automated surveillance reports are generated several times daily and include database information up to midnight on the previous day. They are delivered via a web server visible only to the state-wide intranet available to public health system personnel in the Ministry of Health and regional public health jurisdictions. For each syndrome and hospital or regional hospital grouping combination, three statistical control charts are calculated based on (Muscatello et al. 2005; Hope et al. 2008a, 2010) the following:

- A Shewhart-like (z-score) chart representing the number of standard deviations that the previous day's count differs from the average count for the same weekday in the previous 51 weeks, assuming the counts follow a Poisson distribution with the 51 week mean used to estimate the variance. This signals if the number of standard deviations (z-score) is positive and exceeds 5.
- A Shewhart-like chart representing the number of standard deviations that the most recent 7-day count differs from the average count for the previous 51 weeks,

again assuming the counts follow a Poisson distribution. This signals if the number of standard deviations (z-score) is positive and exceeds 5.
- A cumulative sum (CUSUM)-like chart representing the cumulative sum of the incremental change of the previous day's count relative to the same weekday in the previous week. The sum resets to zero if it falls below zero. It is adjusted according to both the mean level and the background variance of the syndrome counts over the previous year. This statistic provides a comparable index for all the syndromes being monitored and is dubbed the "index of increase." The signaling threshold is set to a value of 15.

The Ministry of Health surveillance team reviews the signals in the automatically generated daily reports; and if they assess the signal to potentially warrant further assessment by public health response personnel, they will issue a situation report using electronic mail. Response guidelines for regional public health units are published (New South Wales Ministry of Health 2010). Guidelines for response to situation reports relating to mental health or drug and alcohol problems are also published (New South Wales Ministry of Health 2012).

Applications of syndromic emergency department or ambulance information in New South Wales have included

- Monitoring and estimating the population impact of heat waves, natural disasters, and the pandemic of influenza A (H1N1)pdm09 (Hope et al. 2008b; NSW Public Health Network 2009; Schaffer et al. 2012)
- Mass gathering surveillance for the 2003 Rugby World Cup, the 2007 Asia Pacific Economic Cooperation forum, World Youth Day 2008, and the annual Tamworth country music festival (Muscatello et al. 2005; Thackway et al. 2009; Hope et al. 2010; Polkinghorne et al. 2013)
- Identifying or supporting the surveillance of emerging pathogens such as new or unusually pathogenic strains of norovirus or EV (Tu et al. 2007; Zander et al. 2014)

- Surveillance using automatic text classification or specific keyword matching in presenting problem and triage nurse narratives from emergency department or ambulance records (Muscatello et al. 2005; Thackway et al. 2009; Mitchell and Bambach 2015; Mitchell et al. 2015)
- Statistical control charts for surveillance (Sparks et al. 2010)
- Demonstration of the relationship between circulating influenza and febrile convulsions in young children (Polkinghorne et al. 2011)
- Surveillance of injury due to falls resulting in an ambulance call (Thomas et al. 2011)
- Evaluation of syndromic surveillance at the regional level (Hope et al. 2008a, 2010)
- Examining alcohol harms at the population level (Descallar et al. 2012; Gale et al. 2015)
- Assessing the epidemiology of out-of-hospital cardiac arrests leading to an ambulance call (Do 2013)
- Evaluation of the population impact of a rotavirus vaccination program on emergency department presentations for gastroenteritis (Davey et al. 2015)

New South Wales has also conducted syndromic influenza surveillance through its continuous population health survey program (Muscatello et al. 2011).

BUILDING SYSTEMS THAT LASTS

There are no specific roadmaps for developing and implementing electronic disease surveillance systems that will last far beyond their initial start-up period. Natalie Leon and colleagues provide an innovative framework for successful, and potentially sustainable, implementation of mobile phone-based technologies for health system data collection (Leon et al. 2012). That framework focuses on four key domains: stewardship, organizational factors, technological factors, and financial factors. Even after successful development, deployment and early implementation of a mHealth platform, the authors concluded that sustainability and long-term viability of the system remained unknown. Studies of long-term implementation projects are greatly

needed, and require followup, a prospect that itself requires substantial resources and commitment.

Anticipating the need to conduct substantial innovations beyond design and implementation are rarely included in a system's initial plan but represent a practical future for most systems because of unforeseeable obstacles involved in scale-up and the inexorably rapid pace of technological innovation independent of any one technology. Mobile phone and computing technologies change very quickly, and the need to consolidate or integrate technology programs at various levels of the government can require a highly agile capacity for reengineering if a system is to survive transformation. Planning for the system (in the broadest sense) to include the financial and administrative support that will allow for future redesign, reengineering, and innovation is a critical component of successful scale-up and sustainability. Small-scale pilot projects litter the public health landscape, and while some take root, too many others falter for lack of leadership and long-term technological support (among other things). The Peruvian military system is an example of one that survived the transformative forces that are inherent to digital technologies.

Lessons are out there to be learned, and serious efforts should be taken to coordinate with system owners to formally study the means through which technology systems successfully support public health, especially in the context of the developing world where there is little resiliency for failed investment. While not directly applicable to the unique aspects of a disease surveillance system, the work of a team of health informaticists and health-care specialists from Rome, Italy, provides another very informative example (Nucita et al. 2009). The Drug Resource Enhancement against AIDS and Malnutrition (DREAM) software supports that global health program as a platform for collecting, organizing, and analyzing health-care data generated in their multifaceted outpatient clinics. The published description of the computer-based information system highlights the value of investment in the capacity to evaluate and adapt to evolving technological and administrative challenges. In particular, the system has a centralized management structure that supports the field sites through training and reinforcement of accurate data entry. The central technology center also supports the integrity of the database and develops and deploys solutions that meet the needs of each of the clinical and laboratory centers. Impressively, the DREAM software is also capable of being switch easily into any of the languages (English, French, Portuguese, or Italian) that are used within the clinical network.

Another example of multi-stakeholder involvement to support a complex information system has occurred in the Philippines. The Department of Health in the Philippines, along with interagency partners, has developed a national disease surveillance program that brings together multiple data sources and methods. This national disease surveillance system is called the Philippines Integrated Disease Surveillance and Response Program (PIDSR) (Campbell et al. 2012; Buczak et al. 2014). PIDSR includes active electronic surveillance in the areas around Cebu City where a SMS-based mechanism is used to report case counts and monitor trends of disease. The integrated approach to public health surveillance has proven beneficial to the country's efforts to monitor alerts from real world threats such as MERS-CoV and Ebola. Moreover, it has served as a predictor for the impact of increased burden from ongoing dengue activity in the country. Additionally, the PIDSR provides a foundation for advanced analysis and training of field epidemiologists in rural parts of that diverse archipelago.

While the PIDSR system continues to grow and evolve, it serves as a model for how complex data and laboratory findings can inform and steer decision making at all levels of government to respond to a new threat. The Philippines faces unique and challenging concerns when it comes to identifying and monitoring disease activity among returning travelers. It leads the world in exporting health-care workers; well developed human resource systems employ thousands in the Middle East and elsewhere. As these health-care workers return home periodically, they introduce a new challenge to the Department of Health, as has been the case most recently

for both Middle Eastern respiratory syndrome coronavirus (MERS-CoV) and the Ebola virus. In the case of MERS-CoV, enhanced airport surveillance was put into place in the Philippines for both returning health-care workers and pilgrims attending the Hajj in Mecca. The enhanced disease surveillance activities involved work across multiple sectors and Presidential-level decision making in order to drive systematic response to imported cases. The process and lessons learned from such activities in the Philippines can and should be considered by all countries facing similar challenges with returning travelers, including well resourced countries.

Countries in the Asian-Pacific region have long collaborated on important public health challenges, coordinating to bridge the distances between population and transit centers, public health authorities and public health experts; and across complicated borders. One example of that, the Pacific Public Health Surveillance Network (PPHSN) was formed in 1996 and today is made up of 22 Pacific Islands and territories who participate as voluntary members (Roth et al. 2014; Secretariat of the Pacific Community 2015). Led jointly by the WHO Western Pacific Regional Office and the Secretariat of the Pacific Communities (SPC), this network has successfully streamlined disease surveillance, reporting and response. In fact, the PPHSN is something of a counterpoint to the focus of this book because as a "system," it is not centered on dissemination or replication of technological solutions (Kool et al. 2012). The partners in the Pacific Islands have based their health security collaboration on a strong, core epidemiologic data model, with the option to use available technologies for data collection. Computer-assisted interpretation of data is, however, a key feature that helps to highlight the value of judicious use of high-tech options. It also reinforces an earlier point from this chapter that no technological system can succeed without a strong foundation in public health essentials. The ability to rapidly and clearly communicate and share information remains a valuable tool in these geographically widespread and culturally diverse nations.

To date, no single formula for disease surveillance system planning has been shown to increase the likelihood that it can be successfully scaled up and sustained over time. Published works have identified key attributes that lead to increased local and national ownership, compliance with written operating procedures, accuracy and timeliness of data entry, and ultimately the detection of outbreaks. Experiences among the authors of this chapter argue that scale-up and sustainability are highly dependent on the early design of the system with growth and longterm use in mind. Designing the database to support complex analyses is important for the long-term, but this requirement must be balanced with the need for a system that is intuitive and acceptable to the users (and bears fruit quickly to secure a second round of funding). It may be reasonable to start with a relatively simple system and plan for the technology team to innovate and adapt the system to more sophisticated uses over time.

Longitudinal health surveillance systems have unique challenges due to the need to follow and characterize dynamic populations (and population-related data) and the wide variety of clinical case features that are important for disease surveillance, epidemiologic studies, and population health. The ongoing employment of an epidemiologist on the technology team (or some version of that concept) who can gain deeper understanding of the data system and its construction, will help to ensure that the system and subsequent data analyses are scientifically reliable. Reproducibility of results is an extraordinarily elusive quality of large information systems that relies on high data quality and consistency, especially when examining potentially small effects. Relatively small changes to a database can have ripple effects on data analyses that an epidemiologist who is well informed about the data system can detect and assist in repairing (or explain if those effects are simply unavoidable).

The ability to innovate is a quality that goes far beyond the initial design and installation of the database. The technology team must be empowered and equipped to evaluate new data system constructs (ideally through the use of a dedicated development environment) and then test those constructs with realistic data. Beyond the potential value of conducting better disease surveillance, exigent forces—technological, political, and financial—may drive the evolution of the system toward either sustainability or obsolescence. A system that seems perfectly suited today to support public health goals will survive only if the technology team can someday integrate old data (and database users) into new architectures. Such transformations should be seen as inevitability. Much more study is needed to understand the factors that enhance or curtail scale-up and sustainability of electronic disease surveillance systems, but it is difficult to ignore the need for epidemiologists and technologists to work together to find practical solutions to get better data faster.

ACKNOWLEDGMENT

The author of this chapter would like to acknowledge Rehka Holtry and Matthew Johns for their assistance on this chapter.

REFERENCES

Armed Forces Health Surveillance Center. May 15, 2015. DoD communicable disease weekly report, Silver Spring, MD. Retrieved May 15, 2015. http://www.afhsc.mil/documents/pubs/CommDz/comWeekly.pdf.

Australian Bureau of Statistics. 2015. 3218.0—Regional Population Growth, Australia, 2013–14 [Online]. c=AU; o=Commonwealth of Australia; ou=Australian Bureau of Statistics. Accessed June 3, 2015. http://www.abs.gov.au/ausstats/abs@.nsf/mf/3218.0/.

Australian Government Department of Health. 2014. National Health Call Centre Network [Online]. Australian Government Department of Health, Sydney, Australia. Accessed June 3, 2015. http://www.health.gov.au/internet/main/publishing.nsf/Content/national-health-call-centre-network-team-overview.

Australian Government Department of Health. 2015. Australian influenza surveillance report and activity updates [Online]. Canberra, Australian Capital Territory, Australia: Australian Government Department of Health. Accessed June 2, 2015. http://www.health.gov.au/flureport#current.

Buczak, A.L., B. Baugher, S.M. Babin et al. April 10, 2014. Prediction of high incidence of dengue in the Philippines. *PLOS ONE* 8(4): e2771.

Campbell, T.C., C.J. Hodanics, S.M. Babin et al. September 2012. Developing open source, self-contained disease surveillance software applications for use in resource-limited settings. *Biomed. Inform. Decis. Mak.* 12(99).

Cashmore, A., D. Muscatello, A. Merrifield, P. Spokes, K. Macartney, and B. Jalaludin. 2013. Relationship between the population incidence of pertussis in children in New South Wales, Australia and emergency department visits with cough: A time series analysis. *Biomed. Inform. Decis. Mak.* 13: 40.

Centers for Disease Control and Prevention. September 2014a. Severe respiratory illness associated with enterovirus D68—Missouri and Illinois, 2014. *Morb. Mortal. Wkly. Rep.* 63(36): 798–799.

Centers for Disease Control and Prevention. June 2014b. Ebola viral disease outbreak—West Africa, 2014. *Morb. Mortal. Wkly. Rep.* 63(25): 548–551.

Centers for Disease Control and Prevention. 2014c. Enterovirus D68. *Non-Polio Enteroviruses*. Atlanta, GA. Retrieved May 17, 2015. http://www.cdc.gov/non-polio-enterovirus/about/ev-d68.html.

Centre for Epidemiology and Evidence. 2015. Syndromic surveillance [Online]. New South Wales Ministry of Health, Sydney, Australia. Accessed June 6, 2015. http://www.health. nsw.gov.au/epidemiology/Pages/Syndromic-surveillance.aspx.

Dalton, C., D. Durrheim, J. Fejsa, L. Francis, S. Carlson, E.T. d'Espaignet, and F. Tuyl. 2009. Flutracking: A weekly Australian community online survey of influenza-like illness in 2006, 2007 and 2008. *Commun. Dis. Intell.* 33: 316–322.

Davey, H.M., D.J. Muscatello, J.G. Wood, T.L. Snelling, M.J. Ferson, and K.K. Macartney. 2015. Impact of high coverage of monovalent human rotavirus vaccine on Emergency Department presentations for rotavirus gastroenteritis. *Vaccine* 33: 1726–1730.

Descallar, J., D.J. Muscatello, D. Weatherburn, M. Chu, and S. Moffatt. 2012. The association between the incidence of emergency department attendances for alcohol problems and assault incidents attended by police in New South Wales, Australia, 2003–2008: A time-series analysis. *Addiction* 107: 549–556.

Do, A.C.M., D. Muscatello, and N. Rose. 2013. Epidemiology of out-of-hospital cardiac arrests, NSW, 2012: Time, place and person. Sydney, Centre for Epidemiology and Evidence, NSW Ministry of Health.

Forrester, J.D., S.K. Pillai, K.D. Beer et al. October 2014. Assessment of ebola virus disease, health care infrastructure, and preparedness—Four countries; Southeastern Liberia. *Morb. Mortal. Wkly. Rep.* 63(40): 891–893.

Gale, M., D.J. Muscatello, M. Dinh, J. Byrnes, A. Shakeshaft, A. Hayen, C.R. MacIntyre, P. Haber, M. Cretikos, and P. Morton. 2015. Alcopops, taxation and harm: A segmented time series analysis of emergency department presentations. *BMC Public Health* 15: 468.

Geoscience Australia. 2014. Area of Australia—States and Territories [Online]. Australian Government, Symonston, Australia. Accessed June 5, 2015. http://www.ga.gov.au/scientific-topics/geographic-information/dimensions/area-of-australia-states-and-territories.

Government of Western Australia Department of Health. 2008. Virus Watch homepage [Online]. Communicable Disease Control Directorate, Perth, Australia. Accessed June 2, 2015. http://www.public.health.wa.gov. au/3/487/3/virus_watch.pm.

Hope, K., D.N. Durrheim, D. Muscatello, T. Merritt, W. Zheng, P. Massey, P. Cashman, and K. Eastwood. 2008a. Identifying pneumonia outbreaks of public health importance: Can emergency department data assist in earlier identification? *Austr. NZ J. Public Health* 32: 361–363.

Hope, K., T. Merritt, K. Eastwood, K. Main, D.N. Durrheim, D. Muscatello, K. Todd, and W. Zheng. 2008b. The public health value of emergency department syndromic surveillance following a natural disaster. *Commun. Dis. Intell.* 32: 92–94.

Hope, K.G., T.D. Merritt, D.N. Durrheim, P.D. Massey, J.K. Kohlhagen, K.W. Todd, and C.A. D'Este. 2010. Evaluating the utility of emergency department syndromic surveillance for a regional public health service. *Commun. Dis. Intell.* 34: 310–318.

Hulth, A. August 2012. First European guidelines on syndromic surveillance in human and animal health published. *Euro Surveill.* 7(7): 670–681.

Hulth, A., G. Rydevik, and A. Linde. February 6, 2009. Web queries as a source for syndromic surveillance. *PLOS ONE* 4(2): e4378.

Kool, J.L., B. Paterson, B.I. Pavlin, D. Durrheim, J. Musto, and A. Kolbee. August 2012. Pacific-wide simplified syndromic surveillance for early warning of outbreaks. *Global Public Health* 7: 670–681.

Leon, N., H. Schneider, and E. Daviaud. 2012. Applying a framework for assessing the health system challenges to scaling up mHealth in South Africa. *BMC Med. Inform. Decis. Mak.* 12(123): 1–12.

Liaw, S.T., H.Y. Chen, D. Maneze, J. Taggart, S. Dennis, S. Vagholkar, and J. Bunker. 2012. Health reform: Is routinely collected electronic information fit for purpose? *Emerg. Med. Austr.* 24: 57–63.

Liljeqvist, H., D. Muscatello, G. Sara, M. Dinh, and G. Lawrence. 2014. Accuracy of automatic syndromic classification of coded emergency department diagnoses in identifying mental health-related presentations for public health surveillance. *BMC Med. Inform. Decis. Mak.* 14: 84.

Mitchell, R.J. and M.R. Bambach. 2015. Examination of narratives from emergency department presentations to identify road trauma, crash and injury risk factors for different age groups. *Health Inform. Manage. J.* 44: 21–29.

Mitchell, R.J., M.R. Bambach, D. Muscatello, K. McKenzie, and Z.J. Balogh. 2013. Can SNOMED CT as implemented in New South Wales, Australia be used for road trauma injury surveillance in emergency departments? *Health Inform. Manage. J.* 42: 4–8.

Mitchell, R.J., R. Grzebieta, and G. Rechnitzer. 2015. Capture and surveillance of quad-bike (ATV)-related injuries in administrative data collections. *Int. J. Inj. Control Safety Promot.* 1–9.

Muscatello, D.J., M. Barr, S.V. Thackway, and C.R. Macintyre. 2011. Epidemiology of influenza-like illness during Pandemic (H1N1) 2009, New South Wales, Australia. *Emerg. Infect. Dis.* 17: 1240–127.

Muscatello, D.J., T. Churches, J. Kaldor, W. Zheng, C. Chiu, P. Correll, and L. Jorm. 2005. An automated, broad-based, near real-time public health surveillance system using presentations to hospital Emergency Departments in New South Wales, Australia. *BMC Public Health* 5: 141.

Muscatello, D.J., P.M. Morton, I. Evans, and R. Gilmour. 2008. Prospective surveillance of excess mortality due to influenza in New South Wales: Feasibility and statistical approach. *Commun. Dis. Intell.* 32: 435–442.

New South Wales Ambulance Service. 2014. NSW ambulance year in review 2013–14 [Online]. Sydney, New South Wales, Australia: New South Wales Ambulance Service. Accessed June 6, 2015. http://www.ambulance.nsw.gov.au/Media-And-Publications/Publications.html.

New South Wales Ministry of Health. 2010. Public Health Real-time Emergency Dept Surveillance System (PHREDSS) public health unit response—NSW Department of Health [Online]. Sydney, New South Wales, Australia: NSW Ministry of Health. Accessed June 6, 2015. http://www0.health.nsw.gov.au/policies/gl/2010/GL2010_009.html.

New South Wales Ministry of Health. 2012. Mental health, drug and alcohol—Emergency Department and Ambulance monitoring—NSW Health [Online]. Sydney, New South Wales, Australia: NSW Department of Health. Accessed June 6, 2015. http://www0.health.nsw.gov.au/policies/gl/2012/GL2012_009.html.

New South Wales Ministry of Health. 2014. Annual report 2013–14 NSW Health [Online]. Sydney, New South Wales, Australia: New South Wales Ministry of Health. Accessed June 6, 2015. http://www.health.nsw.gov.au/publications/Pages/annualreport14.aspx.

NSW Public Health Network. 2009. Progression and impact of the first winter wave of the 2009 pandemic H1N1 influenza in New South Wales, Australia. *Eurosurveillance* 14: pii=19365.

Nucita, A., G.M. Bernava, M. Bartolo et al. September 2009. A global approach to the management of EMR (electronic medical records) of patients with HIV/AIDS in sub-Saharan Africa: The experience of DREAM software. *BMC Med. Inform. Decis. Mak.* 9(42).

O'Toole, L., D.J. Muscatello, W. Zheng, and T. Churches. 2010. Can near real-time monitoring of emergency department diagnoses facilitate early response to sporadic meningo-coccal infection?—Prospective and retrospective evaluations. *BMC Infect. Dis.* 10: 309.

Polkinghorne, B.G., P.D. Massey, D.N. Durrheim, T. Byrnes, and C.R. MacIntyre. 2013. Prevention and surveillance of public health risks during extended mass gatherings in rural areas: The experience of the Tamworth Country Music Festival, Australia. *Public Health* 127: 32–38.

Polkinghorne, B.G., D.J. Muscatello, C.R. Macintyre, G.L. Lawrence, P.M. Middleton, and S. Torvaldsen. 2011. Relationship between the population incidence of febrile convulsions in young children in Sydney, Australia and seasonal epidemics of influenza and respiratory syncytial virus, 2003–2010: A time series analysis. *BMC Infect. Dis.* 11: 291.

Roth, A., D. Hoy, P.F. Horwood et al. August 2014. Preparedness for threat of Chikungunya in the Pacific. *Emerg. Infect. Dis.* 20(8).

Schaffer, A., D. Muscatello, R. Broome, S. Corbett, and W. Smith. 2012. Emergency department visits, ambulance calls, and mortality associated with an exceptional heat wave in Sydney, Australia, 2011: A time-series analysis. *Environ. Health* 11: 3.

Schindeler, S., D. Muscatello, M. Ferson, K. Rogers, P. Grant, and T. Churches. 2009. Evaluation of alternative respiratory syndromes for specific syndromic surveillance of influenza and respiratory syncytial virus: A time series analysis. *BMC Infect. Dis.* 9: 190.

School of Population Health and Clinical Practice. 2015. The Australian Sentinel Practices Research Network (ASPREN) [Online]. University of Adelaide, Australia. Accessed June 2, 2015. https://www.dmac.adelaide.edu.au/aspren/asprenMISServlet?page=index.

Secretariat of the Pacific Community. May 4, 2015. Pacific Public Health Surveillance Network, Noumea, New Caledonia. Retrieved May 16, 2015. https://www.spc.int/phs/PPHSN.

Soto, G., R.V. Araujo-Castillo, J. Neyra et al. 2008. Challenges in the implementation of an electronic surveillance system in a resource-limited setting: Alerta, in Peru. *BMC Proc.* 2(Suppl. 3): S4.

Sparks, R., C. Carter, P. Graham, D. Muscatello, T. Churches, J. Kaldor, R. Turner, W. Zheng, and L. Ryan. 2010. Understanding sources of variation in syndromic surveillance for early warning of natural or intentional disease outbreaks. *IIE Trans.* 42: 613–631.

Thackway, S., T. Churches, J. Fizzell, D. Muscatello, and P. Armstrong. 2009. Should cities hosting mass gatherings invest in public health surveillance and planning? Reflections from a decade of mass gatherings in Sydney, Australia. *BMC Public Health* 9: 324.

Thomas, S.L., D.J. Muscatello, P.M. Middleton, and W. Zheng. 2011. Characteristics of fall-related injuries attended by an ambulance in Sydney, Australia: A surveillance summary. *New South Wales Public Health Bull.* 22: 49–54.

Triple-S Project. 2010. Triple-S objectives. Accessed May, 2015. http://syndromicsurveillance.eu/about-triple-s/objectives.

Triple-S Project. November 2011. Assessment of syndromic surveillance in Europe. *Lancet* 278(9806): 1833–1834.

Tu, E.T.V., T. Nguyen, P. Lee, R.A. Bull, J. Musto, G. Hansman, P.A. White, W.D. Rawlinson, and C.J. McIver. 2007. Norovirus GII. 4 strains and outbreaks, Australia. *Emerg. Infect. Dis.* 13: 1128.

U.S. Department of Defense. April 22, 2015. Identify theft concerns drive social security number program, Arlington, VA. Retrieved May 15, 2015. http://www.defense.gov/news/newsarticle.aspx?id=119841.

University of Newcastle, Hunter New England Health, and Hunter Medical Research Institute. 2015. Flutracking project [Online]. Accessed June 2, 2015. http://www.flutracking.net/Info/Contact.

World Health Organization. May 15, 2015. Public health surveillance, Geneva, Switzerland. Retrieved May 15, 2015. http://www.who.int/topics/public_health_surveillance/en/

Zander, A., P.N. Britton, T. Navin, E. Horsley, S. Tobin, and J.M. McAnulty. 2014. An outbreak of enterovirus 71 in metropolitan Sydney: Enhanced surveillance and lessons learnt. *Med. J Aust.* 201: 663–666.

Zheng, W., R. Aitken, D.J. Muscatello, and T. Churches. 2007. Potential for early warning of viral influenza activity in the community by monitoring clinical diagnoses of influenza in hospital emergency departments. *BMC Public Health* 7: 250.

mHealth and its role in disease surveillance

LAVANYA VASUDEVAN, SOMA GHOSHAL, AND ALAIN B. LABRIQUE

Disease surveillance, or the "continuous, systematic collection, analysis and interpretation of health-related data needed for the planning, implementation, and evaluation of public health practice," is a critical function of public health (World Health Organization [WHO] 2015a). Effective disease surveillance systems can help drastically minimize the duration and impact of an epidemic through early detection (WHO 2015a,b). In light of the global proliferation of connectivity and accessibility to mobile phones, mHealth, or the use of mobile information and communication technologies (ICTs) for the delivery of health information or services, is becoming a popular strategy in disease surveillance (National Institutes of Health [NIH] and Office of Behavioral and Social Sciences Research [OBSSR] 2015; WHO 2015b).

Within the spectrum of strategies encompassed by mHealth, the ability to leverage widespread ownership and access to mobile telephony offers an unprecedented method to quickly reach large numbers of people at relatively lower costs than previously possible (Labrique et al. 2013a,b; International Telecommunications Union [ITU] 2014; NIH and OBSSR 2015). A number of innovative mHealth strategies have emerged across health system layers that target populations or patients, health workers or providers, or more broadly, core health system functions such as supply chain management and event tracking (Leon et al. 2012; Labrique et al. 2013a; Roess et al. 2014). Mobile telephony's global reach—from near-ubiquitous ownership in urban centers to widespread access in remote, hard-to-reach villages—allows, at its most basic level, the dissemination of health information and access to timely data (ITU 2014). The ability to reliably and inexpensively communicate by voice or text, in the absence of traditional landline infrastructure, has been widely recognized as a critical "leapfrogging" technology that has helped overcome numerous barriers to rapid, appropriate health services in low-resource settings (Labrique et al. 2013a). More complex, integrated systems are also emerging in parallel that utilize the increased computing capacity of smartphones to enable sophisticated interventions such as point-of-care diagnostics or decision support (Labrique et al. 2013a; NIH and OBSSR 2015). As new strategies continue to be innovated and tested, increasing evidence suggests that mHealth can have a substantial impact on enhancing behavior change, improving data collection accuracy and efficiency, strengthening performance monitoring, building staff capacity, and enabling disease surveillance (Cole-Lewis and Kershaw 2010; Kallander et al. 2013; Agarwal et al. 2015; Kumar et al. 2013).

Disease surveillance is a multistep process that involves standardized reporting of health events throughout and between health systems; identifying trends and patterns in disease incidence; estimating speed of disease propagation and how many people are impacted; identifying vulnerable populations who are at greater risk for acquiring the disease; creating standardized case definitions based on the symptoms reported; and geolocating health events in order to properly ascertain the source of the disease (WHO 2015b,c). In public health emergencies, the swift identification and reporting of cases of an emerging disease shortens the time to mount a response, putatively allowing outbreaks to be effectively controlled. The capacity to collect and transmit data nearly instantaneously using mobile technologies offers tremendous advantages in identifying events as they occur, even in remote, low-resource settings (Yu et al. 2009; Gow et al. 2010; Lewis et al. 2011; Boyd 2012; Meier 2012; Rajatonirina et al. 2012; Githinji et al. 2013). Furthermore, the continued miniaturization of previously expensive, hospital-bound technologies such as ultrasounds, electrocardiography machines, and microscopes, combined with the increasing sophistication of smartphone technologies, has enabled field-ready equivalents of these devices to be deployed, allowing screening of large populations in their homes or communities. Examples include the AliveCor Mobile ECG (AliveCor Inc. 2015) that links to a smartphone to instantly detect heart conditions, and the MobiUS SP1 portable ultrasound machine (Mobisante 2015) that permits image viewing and sharing through a smartphone interface.

CHALLENGES IN EXTANT DISEASE SURVEILLANCE SYSTEMS

The purpose of disease surveillance systems is to collect and analyze information on the health of populations so that policy makers can prioritize and target timely and actionable services to areas of greatest need (WHO 2015a). There are several limitations inherent to extant disease surveillance systems that pose challenges to the efficient use of population-wide disease statistics for informing resource allocation and policies for disease management.

Timeliness of data

For health systems to mount an effective response to disease outbreaks, data on disease incidence available through surveillance efforts must be available to policy makers in a timely manner (WHO 2015c). Disease surveillance systems in many parts of the world are largely reactive, meaning that they tend to act in response to an epidemic or outbreak that has already occurred, instead of allowing intervention during the early stages of the epidemic when death and disability might be prevented or reduced through timely action (Nsubuga et al. 2010). These systems typically rely on inefficient paper-based methods for collection, transmission, and analysis of data on disease trends, potentially resulting in delays that necessitate greater investments in resources to combat outbreaks than if the outbreak had been identified earlier.

Quality and interoperability of data

Globally, disease surveillance systems differ drastically from country to country (Institute of Medicine [U.S.] Forum on Microbial Threats 2007; WHO 2015b). Varying reporting structures, differing data standards, and unstandardized case definitions make tracking global disease trends a challenging and complex task. Depending on the methods of data collection and the skill of individuals involved in reporting, data that are collected may contain missing records and incomplete information. This is especially true in situations where there is a heavy reliance on paper-based systems for data collection as inconsistencies and errors in data are difficult to detect and rectify as they occur (Labrique et al. 2013a).

Data integration

Many current disease surveillance systems are categorical and focus on one or more specific diseases or behaviors of interest, making it difficult for health agencies to capture and assess the overall health of a population and relative disease burdens (Institute of Medicine [U.S.] Forum on Microbial Threats 2007; Perry et al. 2007; Nsubuga et al. 2010). Categorical disease surveillance systems, when not integrated, result in duplications in data-collection efforts, inefficient allocation of resources, and poor coordination across disease control programs and laboratories (Nsubuga et al. 2010).

Geolocating data

Real-time geolocation of disease surveillance data allows health systems to track the intensity and spread of disease as it occurs. Such systems can monitor whether the number of reported cases in a particular geography is disproportionately higher than expected; whether there is geospatial clustering of a particular event; or whether there is a clustering of risk factors that may increase the likelihood of disease. Geolocating disease surveillance data is challenging and time consuming when traditional paper-based methods are used for data collection. A significant investment in time and effort is required to translate addresses or GPS coordinates from paper-based forms into maps displaying disease hotspots. Furthermore, maps created in this manner may quickly become outdated as the diseases spread.

mHEALTH FOR DISEASE SURVEILLANCE

mHealth strategies are already being harnessed to bridge the gaps in disease surveillance, either through the use of mobile electronic data collection platforms within extant systems, Internet, or citizen-sourced disease information, or via large integrated electronic surveillance systems that can help coordinate global responses to disease outbreaks (Yu et al. 2009; Gow et al. 2010; Lewis et al. 2011; Boyd 2012; Meier 2012; Rajatonirina et al. 2012; Githinji et al. 2013). Figure 9.1 illustrates the impact of mHealth systems within a typical disease surveillance workflow.

Electronic data collection platforms

mHealth systems for electronic data collection offer two critical advantages over traditional paper-based systems. First, they improve the timeliness of disease surveillance information. For instance, a syndromic surveillance system implemented in Madagascar to track malaria, influenza-like illness, and arbovirus infection using text messages allowed 86.7% of the data to be shared with the Ministry of Health within 24 hours (Rajatonirina et al. 2012). Second, mHealth systems allow field- or community-based health staff to be linked to supervisory support through collected data for real-time feedback and action. For instance, alerts are issued to community health workers using the International Institute for Communication and Development's (IICD) Ma Santé program in Mali and Senegal on the basis of malaria case reports collected via mobile phones, mobilizing resources on the ground to counter potential malaria outbreaks before they occur (IICD 2013). A multi-partner Real-Time Biosurveillance Program implemented in Sri Lanka and India allowed frontline health workers to collect data via mobile phones and reported back any patterns of suspected disease outbreaks to local health officials and regional health officials via Short Message Service (SMS) alerts (Gow et al. 2010). Thus, the timeliness of data and communication between frontline health workers and supervising officials can serve to accelerate and coordinate the health system's response to impending outbreaks. Electronic data collection platforms may also help improve data accuracy through automatic checks and display of error messages (e.g., when incomplete data are entered).

There are several open-source, customizable data collection platforms available globally that enable electronic data collection and transmission through a mobile phone interface. Software platforms such as Open Data Kit (Open Data Kit 2015) allow users to build and deploy forms on mobile phones. Other platforms such as Formhub (Modi Research Group 2015) provide additional back-end functionalities for the aggregation and visualization of collected data. Data from these systems can be imported into most standardized statistical software packages for advanced data analyses. DataDyne's Magpi (formerly known as EpiSurveyor; Magpi 2015) allows SMS and cloud-based data collection in low-resource settings.

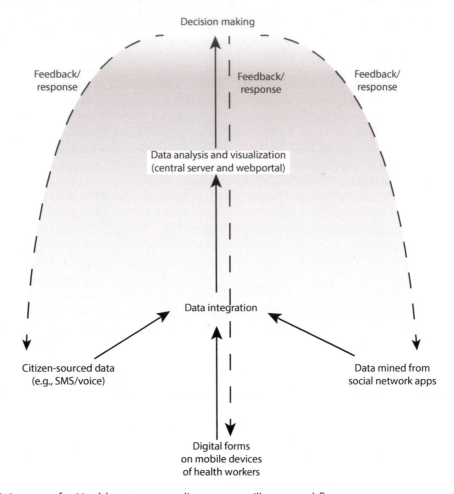

Figure 9.1 Impact of mHealth systems on disease surveillance workflow.

Magpi has been scaled to 25,000 users across the world, including organizations such as the World Bank, U.S. Centers for Disease Control (CDC), and the American Red Cross. Software platforms such as District Health Information Software 2 (DHIS2) allow the collection, aggregation, and visualization of data from mobile devices (HISP 2015). Data uploaded to DHIS2 can be geo-referenced and then visualized graphically using maps, tables, and figures.

RapidSMS (2015) is a free and open-source framework particularly created for mobile phone-based data collection (Boyd 2014). Users in the field can collect data through simple SMS messages that are then transmitted automatically to a central server for analysis and visualization. RapidSMS was deployed in Malawi to aid the National Integrated Nutrition and Food Security Surveillance System in overcoming delays and

the incompleteness of paper-based data (UNICEF 2009). Using this system, the frontline worker could be instantly notified if data suggested malnutrition in the patient so that any treatment or referrals could be prescribed on the spot (UNICEF 2009). In this context, RapidSMS lowered operational costs, reduced data entry errors, and was well received with the frontline workers (UNICEF 2009). RapidSMS is also used by facility- and village-based health teams in Uganda to provide Weekly Surveillance Reports (covering disease outbreaks and medicine stock information) to district health teams using SMS, as part of the mTrac initiative (UNICEF 2012). District health teams respond to disease reports or provide supportive supervision to resolve human resource management challenges (UNICEF 2012). During the 2012 Ebola and Marburg virus outbreaks in Uganda, mTrac was used to send SMS messages alerting health workers to the outbreak, the case definition (symptoms), isolation procedures, the location of the nearest isolation facilities, and the hotline to the national response team for reporting suspected cases (Berman 2012).

The national Malaria Consortium in Cambodia has developed a set of e- and mHealth tools to identify cases of malaria and track essential medical supplies at health facilities (Mellor 2013). Frontline health workers and local clinicians use mobile phones to instantly text central health facilities and alert them of possible or confirmed cases of malaria. This information is then used to coordinate the allocation and distribution of essential drugs to affected areas. Similarly, the International Center for Diarrheal Disease Research in Bangladesh has equipped local health facilities and frontline health workers with mobile phones in order to track cases of malaria (Haq 2013). The data are aggregated and analyzed in order to identify regions of Bangladesh with endemic malaria and target interventions, particularly to vulnerable populations in affected areas.

In Peru, health workers of the Cell-PREVEN project were equipped with mobile phones for reporting adverse health events among female sex workers taking metronidazole (Curioso et al. 2005). Rapid identification of adverse events through mobile phone-collected data, compared with the extant paper-based system of data collection, was hypothesized to improve medication adherence rates among the female sex workers, thereby reducing the likelihood of transmission of sexually transmitted diseases (Curioso et al. 2005). Within a 4-month period, 797 reports were submitted using this system, of which 60 reported at least one adverse event following metronidazole use. Furthermore, 30 SMS alerts were issued to team leaders, notifying them of the nature of adverse events (Curioso et al. 2005).

Internet or citizen-sourced disease surveillance data

Electronic diseases surveillance data need not be limited to information collected by health workers. Mining of data available on the web through search engines and social networks is increasingly being used to reveal health trends of populations (Ginsberg 2009; Collier 2012). The Global Public Health Intelligence Network (GPHIN) developed

by Health Canada in collaboration with the WHO uses search engines to crawl electronic media and discussion sites on the web for reports on diseases (WHO 2015b). In 2011, researchers were able to model the incidence of influenza in the United States using data mined from queries posed on the Google search engine (Ginsberg 2015). The methodology included searching for key words that were symptoms of influenza and watching the trends of the search queries by region over time.

Crowd sourcing, or community reporting of disease information through social media, can also serve as a quick and efficient way to predict disease trends and provide feedback on the quality and availability of health services. For instance, initiatives such as mTrac allow community members to report on service delivery challenges anonymously using an SMS hotline (UNICEF 2012). Ushahidi is a web-based platform that enables crowd sourcing of disease information by citizen journalists (Ushahidi 2015). In 2008, this system was used to map incidents of violence during the Kenyan elections. The web platform was wildly popular because safe havens were pointed out and lives were saved from the widespread violence (Tavaana 2015). Ushahidi was also used during the response to the earthquake in Haiti in 2010 to locate survivors and pinpoint possible clusters of disease (Meier 2012). Haitians were able to upload geo-referenced data on possible survivors or cases of cholera. Such information was used by the coordinating agencies on the ground to allocate emergency support and medicines (Meier 2012).

Animal disease surveillance systems

Mobile phones have also been used in the surveillance of diseases in livestock. The CDC developed a mobile phone-based surveillance system for animal diseases in conjunction with the Department of Animal Production and Health (DAPD) in Sri Lanka (Robertson et al. 2010). The goal of this system was to use emerging infections in animals to predict disease risks to humans. The study found improved timeliness and quality of surveillance data. The London International Development Centre (LIDC) also implemented a pilot project monitoring disease in livestock in Maasai, Kenya (LIDC 2015). Veterinarians in Maasai were equipped with GPS-enabled mobile phones to identify and report cases of diseases such as anthrax and East Coast Fever (ECF) in livestock.

The data were translated into maps so that other veterinarians and farmers could track the spread of disease. In addition, the mobile phone software was equipped with tutorials and educational information on how to identify signs of illness and steps in disease management.

FUTURE OF mHEALTH IN DISEASE SURVEILLANCE

The potential for the use of mHealth for disease surveillance—in data collection, analysis, and dissemination facilitating timely identification and coordinated response to outbreaks—is clear. However, the widespread use of these technologies for disease surveillance hinges on the development and use of common data standards that permit interoperability and data sharing across multiple subnational systems and, even, globally. It is critical to note that the mobile components of disease surveillance systems do not operate in isolation from the health systems they are being used to bolster. For optimal impact, a "systems" approach is required, where strengthening the other elements of the health delivery system is likely to yield greater impact. There are also logistical processes and requirements that must be taken into consideration. First, certain interventions may require a dependable network connection, whereas others may be able to operate "offline" for some periods of time. The levels of population access to mobile technology may inform the kinds of strategies appropriate for a particular context. The availability of local devices and networks with necessary capabilities required for the intervention, such as smartphones or high-speed Internet access, must also be considered. In many mHealth innovations, a "bring your own phone" model has been effective, reducing costs to the health system; this approach, however, also limits the sophistication of the intervention to simple text or voice functions, given the wide heterogeneity in available technologies. Such a strategy is particularly useful for interventions where crowd sourcing or obtaining feedback and suggestions from large groups of people in a short amount of time can help inform potential health interventions or target the distribution of limited resources within a community. Improved modeling methodologies and ability to predict outbreaks using automated active machine learning and prediction algorithms

will also become crucial in improving the response of disease surveillance systems as we increasingly begin to leverage "big data" through innovative wireless and sensor technologies.

REFERENCES

Agarwal, S., H.B. Perry, L.A. Long, and A.B. Labrique. 2015. Evidence on feasibility and effective use of mHealth strategies by front-line health workers in developing countries: systematic review. *Trop. Med. Int. Health* 20(8): 1003–1004.

AliveCor Inc. 2015. Last updated September 7, 2015. www.alivecor.com.

Berman, C. 2012. Leveraging mTrac to respond to disease outbreaks. Last updated September 7, 2015. http://www.mtrac.ug/blog/leveraging-mtrac-respond-disease-outbreaks.

Boyd, C. 2014. RapidSMS: Saving a life in 160 characters. *BBC*, November 18. Last updated September 7, 2015. http://www.bbc.com/future/story/20120803-saving-a-life-in-160-characters.

Cole-Lewis, H. and T. Kershaw. 2010. Text messaging as a tool for behavior change in disease prevention and management. *Epidemiol. Rev.* 32(1): 56–69.

Collier, N. 2012. Uncovering text mining: A survey of current work on web-based epidemic intelligence. *Global Public Health* 7(7): 731–749.

Curioso, W.H., B.T. Karras, P.E. Campos, K.K. Holmes, and A.M. Kimball. 2005. Design and implementation of Cell-PREVEN: A real-time surveillance system for adverse events using cell phones in Peru. In *AMIA Annual Symposium Proceedings*, Washington, DC, pp. 176–180.

Ginsberg, J., M.H. Mohebbi, R.S. Patel, L. Brammer, M.S. Smolinski, and L. Brilliant. 2009. Detecting influenza epidemics using search engine query data. *Nature* 457(7232): 1012–1014.

Githinji, S., S. Kigen, D. Memusi et al. 2013. Reducing stock-outs of life saving malaria commodities using mobile phone text-messaging: SMS for life study in Kenya. *PLOS ONE* 8(1): e54066.

Gow, G.A., N. Waidyanatha, and V.P. Mary. 2010. Using mobile phones in a real-time biosurveillance program: Lessons from the frontlines in Sri Lanka and India. In *2010 IEEE International Symposium on Technology and Society*, June, Wollongong, Australia, pp. 366–374. doi:10.1109/ISTAS.2010.5514617.

Haq, N. 2013. Cell phones can speed up malaria treatment in remote areas. *SciDev.net*. February 18. http://www.scidev.net/global/malaria/news/cell-phones-can-speed-up-malaria-treatment-in-remote-areas.html.

Health Information Systems Programme (HISP). 2015. University of Oslo, Last updated September 7, 2015. https://www.dhis2.org/.

Institute of Medicine (U.S.) Forum on Microbial Threats. 2007. *Global Infectious Disease Surveillance and Detection Assessing the Challenges—Finding Solutions, Workshop Summary*. Washington, DC: National Academies Press.

Institute of Medicine of the National Academies. 2007. Review of the DoD-GEIS influenza programs: Strengthening global surveillance and response. Last updated September 7, 2015. http://iom.edu/Reports/2007/Review-of-the-DoD-GEIS-Influenza-Programs-Strengthening-Global-Surveillance-and-Response.aspx.

International Institute for Communication and Development (IICD). 2013. Combating mother and child malaria mortality with mobiles. Last updated December 11, 2013. http://www.iicd.org/articles/combating-mother-and-child-malaria-mortality-with-mobiles.

International Telecommunications Union. 2014. The World in 2014: ICT facts and figures. Last updated September 7, 2015. http://www.itu.int/en/ITU-D/Statistics/Documents/facts/ICTFactsFigures2014-e.pdf.

Källander, K., J.K. Tibenderana, O.J. Akpogheneta et al. 2013. Mobile health (mHealth) approaches and lessons for increased performance and retention of community health workers in low- and middle-income countries: A review. *J. Med. Internet. Res.* 15(1): e17.

Kumar, S., W.J. Nilsen, A. Abernethy et al. 2013. Mobile health technology evaluation: The mHealth evidence workshop. *Am. J. Prev. Med.* 45(2): 228–236.

Labrique, A.B., L. Vasudevan, E. Kochi, R. Fabricant, and G. Mehl. 2013a. 12 Common applications and a visual framework. *Global Health Sci. Pract.* 1(2): 160–171.

Labrique, A., L. Vasudevan, L.W. Chang, and G. Mehl. 2013b. H_pe for mHealth: More 'Y' or 'O' on the horizon? *Int. J. Med. Inform.* 82(5): 467–469.

Leon, N., H. Schneider, and E. Daviaud. 2012. Applying a framework for assessing the health system challenges to scaling up mHealth in South Africa. *BMC Med. Inform. Decis. Mak.* 12: 123.

Lewis, S.L., B.H. Feighner, W.A. Loschen, R.A. Wojcik, J.F. Skora, J.S. Coberly, and D.L. Blazes. 2011. SAGES: A suite of freely-available software tools for electronic disease surveillance in resource-limited settings. *PLOS ONE* 6(5): e19750.

London International Development Centre. 2015. Maasai vets carry out disease surveillance of 86,000 animals with Google mobile phones. Last updated March 12, 2015. http://www.lidc.org.uk/node/80.

Magpi. 2015. Last updated September 7, 2015. http://home.magpi.com/.

Meier, P. 2012. Ushahidi—Haiti and the power of crowdsourcing. January 12. http://www.ushahidi.com/2012/01/12/haiti-and-the-power-of-crowdsourcing/.

Mellor, S. 2013. Moving towards malaria elimination developing innovative tools for malaria surveillance in Cambodia. September 12. www.malariaconsortium.org/pages/learning-papers.htm.

Mobisante. 2015. Last updated September 7, 2015. www.mobisante.com.

Modi Research Group. 2015. Last updated September 7, 2015. http://formhub.org/.

National Institutes of Health (NIH) and Office of Behavioral and Social Sciences Research (OBSSR). 2015. mHealth—Mobile Health Technologies. Last updated March 12, 2015. http://obssr.od.nih.gov/scientific_areas/methodology/mhealth/.

Nsubuga, P., W.G. Brown, S.L. Groseclose et al. 2010. Implementing integrated disease surveillance and response: Four African countries' experience, 1998–2005. *Global Public Health* 5(4): 364–380.

Open Data Kit. 2015. Last updated September 7, 2015. http:// opendatakit.org/.

Perry, H.N., S.M. McDonnell, W. Alemu, P. Nsubuga, S. Chungong, M.W. Otten, P.S. Lusamba-dikassa, and S.B. Thacker. 2007.

Planning an integrated disease surveillance and response system: A matrix of skills and activities. *BMC Med.* 5(January): 24.

Rajatonirina, S., J.-M. Heraud, L. Randrianasolo et al. March 2012. Short message service sentinel surveillance of influenza-like illness in Madagascar, 2008–2012. *Bull. World Health Organ.* 90(5): 385–389.

RapidSMS. 2015. Last updated September 7, 2015. http://www.rapidsms.org/.

Robertson, C., K. Sawford, S.L.A. Daniel, T.A. Nelson, and C. Stephen. 2010. Mobile phone-based infectious disease surveillance system, Sri Lanka. *Emerg. Infect. Dis.* 16(10): 1524–1531.

Roess, A., T. Gurman, S. Ghoshal, and S. Mookherji. 2014. Reflections on the potential of mHealth to strengthen health systems in low- and middle-income countries. *J. Health Commun.* 19(8): 871–875.

Tavaana. 2015. Ushahidi: From crisis mapping Kenya to mapping the globe. Last updated March 12, 2015. https://tavaana.org/en/content/ushahidi-crisis-mapping-kenya-mapping-globe.

The Johns Hopkins University Applied Physics Laboratory. 2014. SAGES: Suite for automated global electronic biosurveillance. Last updated October, 2014. http://www.jhuapl.edu/sages/.

UNICEF. 2009. 'RapidSMS' system for monitoring nutrition in Malawi gets Top Tech award. Last updated September 10, 2009. http://www.unicef.org/infobycountry/usa_51097.html.

UNICEF. 2012. mTrac is changing the face of health operations in Uganda. Last updated September 7, 2015. http://www.unicef.org/uganda/mTrac_article(1).pdf.

Ushahidi. 2015. How we work. Last updated March 12, 2015. http://www.ushahidi.com/services/how-we-work/.

World Health Organization. 2015a. Public health surveillance. Last updated March 12, 2015. http://www.who.int/topics/public_health_surveillance/en/.

World Health Organization. 2015b. Global infectious disease surveillance. Last updated March 12, 2015. http://www.who.int/mediacentre/factsheets/fs200/en/.

World Health Organization. 2015c. Integrated disease surveillance. Last updated March 12, 2015. http://www.who.int/csr/labepidemiology/projects/diseasesurv/en/.

Yu, P., M. de Courten, E. Pan, G. Galea, and J. Pryor. 2009. The development and evaluation of a PDA-based method for public health surveillance data collection in developing countries. *Int. J. Med. Inform.* 78(8): 532–542.

10

Global health and open source software (OSS): An example of legal considerations impacting technology and global health policy implementation

ERIN N. HAHN

INTRODUCTION

Over the past two decades, there have been significant changes in the fields of global health and information technology. In many ways, the law has not been adept at keeping up with the difficult ethical and policy questions presented by emerging diseases, or the pace of technology that has been developed or adapted to address these new challenges. The insidious spread of diseases such as HIV/AIDS, new strains of influenza, and most recently, Ebola, have underscored the need for international coordination to effectively respond to these threats. Meanwhile, rapid changes in information technology, and particularly in the field of public health informatics, have altered how we conduct disease surveillance and monitoring. Health data can now be collected from new sources (e.g., social media), combined with myriad other data sets, and analyzed to provide new insights (often referred to as "big data").

Although public health protections may have traditionally been developed and implemented at the local and national levels, it is now nearly impossible to separate them from the global context. Globalization has highlighted how public health issues can have far-reaching effects on most aspects of civil society, including national security, international development, economics, research, and human rights, to name a few. There has perhaps never been a time when the need for coordinated, international action supported by legal and policy solutions to encourage data and technology sharing has been greater. Indeed, the International Health Regulations (IHR) adopted by the member states of the World Health Assembly in 2005 created new requirements for information sharing and the development of capabilities to detect, assess, and respond to public health emergencies of international concern. Yet, to date, it is estimated that 80% of the countries have been unable to meet their obligations to implement IHR (Fischer and Katz 2013).

Some of the reasons cited for the inability to meet IHR obligations include inadequate financial and human resources, insufficient communication infrastructure for reporting public health emergencies to IHR focal points, and the lack of necessary equipment and supplies for detecting, reporting, and responding to public health events (World Health Organization [WHO] 2012). New tools developed to address global public health challenges are remarkable, but many proprietary software products are prohibitively expensive to buy, use, and maintain. However, the wide collection and use of big data in many publicly available open source software (OSS) applications (Google Flu Trends, HealthMap) demonstrates the power and potential usefulness of this information and the increasing acceptability of using these data for public health purposes. Global health initiatives can leverage the power of OSS to make public health tools accessible to diverse populations, including resource-limited settings that are often the hardest hit populations.

The purpose of this chapter is to discuss how law and technology can affect global health policy implementation, using OSS as a detailed example to highlight some of the issues. While there are many challenges associated with policy implementation of any kind, the focus here is addressing the specific issue of access to technology and how OSS may be useful in the global health context. A large portion of the chapter is dedicated to OSS licenses because use of OSS requires a better understanding

of what it is and how the licensing works. However, a basic overview of the framework for global health law is also included to provide useful background and to explain how some of its characteristics can make implementation and enforcement of policy difficult. Last, the chapter will provide some examples of how the use of OSS has influenced global public health crises such as the earthquake in Haiti and the Ebola epidemic in West Africa.

THE FRAMEWORK OF GLOBAL HEALTH LAW

Overview

The terms "global health law" or "international health law" refer to the body of law derived from various legal and policy instruments such as treaties, guidelines, and regulations that affect many aspects of global health. It is sometimes divided into "hard" and "soft" law to refer to binding law (treaties) and nonbinding instruments (negotiated codes or recommendations designed to influence or guide conduct) (Gostin and Sridhar 2014). Overall, global health law mainly falls within public international law, meaning its rules and regulations govern the conduct of countries and not individuals. Human rights law, an element of international law, does address individuals and non-state actors such as nongovernmental organizations (NGOs), but international law primarily covers the conduct between countries, so individual behavior is not easy to oversee or regulate.

International law did not traditionally address health issues, which were generally seen as a domestic matter. However, interest in international legal tools has increased as sovereign states have become less capable of addressing the threat of emerging diseases that spread quickly in a society that has become much more integrated. This interest may be based largely on economic and national security concerns; however, the notion of an individual's "right to health" does exist in international human rights law and also influences the development of legal safeguards (United Nations 1948). The *International Covenant on Economic, Social, and Cultural Rights*, which has been ratified by 163 countries and is considered binding international law, guarantees "the right of everyone to the enjoyment of the highest attainable standard of physical and mental health" and lists governmental obligations to ensure the individuals have access to treatment measures (United Nations 1976, Article 12). Prior to that, the WHO asserted this idea in Article 1 of its constitution, stating as its objective "the attainment by all peoples of the highest possible level of health" (WHO 1948). This right has been enforced through human rights cases in several countries.*

The WHO is the central international body for negotiating international agreements pertaining to health. It has the authority to create binding treaties as well as soft instruments such as recommendations and guidelines. While soft instruments are nonbinding, they often have political and legal significance and are sometimes considered part of international law, even if they cannot be enforced. Unlike other international bodies (the World Trade Organization, the United Nations), the WHO does not have the authority to enforce state compliance with any of the normative instruments it promulgates. In this sense, global health law is still managed at the national level, with states implementing treaties and regulations through the development of domestic law.

The lack of an enforcement mechanism is problematic because outside of political or diplomatic consequences, there is little leverage to influence state compliance. In cases where states have limited resource capacity or difficulty carrying out governance duties, there may be no leverage at all (arguably issues with IHR implementation are an example of this problem). However, some have made the case that soft instruments may be more effective than formal, legal mechanisms (Taylor et al. 2014).[†] The negotiation of nonbinding instruments can be achieved through a less stringent process, can be more quickly created or changed because ratification is not required, and can involve a variety of actors that impact global health, such as NGOs or communities and territories lacking formal statehood.

* Venezuela, India, South Africa, Canada, and Colombia, among others, have court decisions that have influenced public health policy based on human rights law. For a summary table of cases, see Gostin and Sridhar (2014).

† The authors cite the United Nations Declaration of Commitment on HIV/AIDS "among the most effective models of a nonbinding instrument in global health policy" (Taylor et al. 2014, p. 153).

IHR

The 2003 SARS outbreak demonstrated a need for mechanisms to achieve a better coordinated international response to public health crises. In response to this and the subsequent avian influenza outbreak of 2004, the World Health Assembly, the decision-making body of the WHO, adopted a revised version of the IHR in 2005. A main focus of the revised regulations was enhanced monitoring and reporting of international health threats. The regulations require countries to develop capabilities to conduct surveillance and reporting of internationally significant events and utilize a domestic public health law regime that balances human rights concerns with the need to monitor and intervene in public health crises of international concern. The WHO Director General has the power to declare an international health emergency, which occurred during the 2009 H1N1 pandemic and the Ebola epidemic in 2014.

Notably, the new regulations gave the WHO additional authorities to collect data and initiate rapid responses accordingly. Parties adopting the regulations had to commit to share information and to sustain the infrastructure needed to collect and assess the data. They also replaced a list of diseases that trigger notification with an algorithm that can assess public health threats as they emerge (Fischer and Katz 2013, p. 153). The IHR of 2005 were seen as offering "a foundation for a truly global disease detection and response network" (Fischer and Katz 2013, p. 153).

Despite the expanded scope of the IHR of 2005, they have not necessarily led to increased global disease detection and response, at least not in all areas. This outcome is largely due to the difficulty many countries have with implementation of national IHR frameworks. The IHR were designed to increase member states' ability to detect and respond to public health emergencies. However, many of the core capacities, e.g., surveillance, laboratory capacity, risk communication, and outbreak response require digital resources and infrastructure that many member states lack. For instance, the WHO Africa Region faces a number of threats from epidemic and pandemic-prone diseases, yet no member states had fully implemented their national IHR plans by the June 2012 deadline. Countries cited lack of detection and tracking resources and insufficient communication infrastructure for reporting public health emergencies to IHR focal points as some of the reasons (WHO 2012).

To date, 102 countries have requested a 2-year extension and were unable to implement their national IHR plans, many because of financial and human resource limitations. The broader adoption of OSS has the potential to improve the efficiency of IHR implementation, and therefore, global public health initiatives in general, because it provides a free, modifiable software option that can be altered to meet specific requirements for local governments and NGOs and shared and adapted for larger initiatives that may require extensive computing and information-sharing capabilities. Although IHR implementation requires more than just technology, particularly a national implementation plan that creates the structure for adopting the guidelines and the governmental infrastructure necessary to carry them out, technology using OSS can help solve part of the problem. There are several examples of successfully deployed OSS projects designed to improve IHR implementation. These are discussed more in the section titled "OSS and IHR Implementation."

UNDERSTANDING OPEN SOURCE

Open source and its related licenses are part of copyright law. The term "open source" generally refers to software that is made readily available by an individual or group for others to use, copy, or redistribute under a licensing agreement with very few restrictions. Anyone can use the software without having to pay royalties or negotiate a license agreement. Open source software is not a new creation, but it has been used with increasing popularity in large-scale commercial software projects in recent years. It has been called "the software that runs the Internet," referring to its significant use in the infrastructure of the Internet, such as the Apache web server, the Mozilla browser, and the Linux operating system (Dennis 2006). There are currently at least 50 different open source licenses, and they represent a unique approach to licensing when compared against licenses normally used in a commercial environment.*

---

* See the Open Source Initiative at http://www. opensource.org/licenses/alphabetical for a listing of licenses by name.

In the past several years, the field of mobile health or "mHealth" has exploded because of the ubiquitous nature of cellular telephones (Terry 2010). The field of mHealth is the practice of medicine and public health enhanced or supported by the use of mobile electronic devices. Many of these platforms or associated tools, whose primary users are those in the field of public health or clinical care, are purportedly open source. However, in a community that is generally not as savvy in information technology, the term open source is confusing and leaves many unanswered questions.

The purpose of the following sections is to provide an introduction to open source licensing and the main elements to consider when determining whether to use OSS or when selecting an open source license. They also provide background on copyright and the distinction between a copyright and a license, a discussion of the history of "open source" and "free software" (often consolidated as FOSS, or Free and Open Source Software), and an overview of commonly used licenses with strong user communities. Several myths related to the benefits and hazards of using open source licenses and OSS are discussed.

Background on copyright

Copyright is a form of intellectual property law and protects original works of authorship (U.S. Copyright Act, 17 U.S.C. § 101 *et seq.*). All software is subject to copyright law, and as soon as source code is created, no one but the author can use the code without explicit permission (Fontana et al. 2008). A copyright is how an author retains control over the work. Software copyright is "the exclusive legal right to control the rules for copying, modifying, and distributing a work of software" (U.S. Copyright Act, 17 U.S.C. § 101 *et seq.*). The person or organization that has the right to control the work is called the copyright holder. When the copyright holder permits others to use, modify, or distribute their software, they have granted a license. The license is the permission to use the software in some way—it can be an unconditional grant of permission that mirrors the rights of the copyright holder or a conditional grant that allows individuals to copy or use the software according to certain provisions. Open source licenses fall into both categories.

A general commercial copyright license usually protects the copyright holder's interests by placing restrictions on how the software can be used.

For example, a commercial software license usually prohibits the copying or modification of the software, mainly by distributing only the binary, or object code, that is machine readable. Open source software is governed by a license, but the license gives users more rights than a commercial license because the user gets access to source code and has the right to change the source code. The term "copyleft" was generated by the free software community and is the term for a condition of the license that ensures all modified versions of software can be copied, modified, or distributed in the same way as the original. By ensuring downstream users receive source code and permission to modify it, a copyleft license is said to keep code "forever free" (Fontana et al. 2008). Not all open source licenses have copyleft provisions, but many do. Despite what the name may imply, copyleft is still a license and is enforced by copyright law. Instead of withholding permission to copy or modify a work (as in the traditional sense of a copyright), copyleft uses copyright law to actually require that those permissions be granted.

It is important to note that an open source license is not the same as placing the software in the public domain. The terms of the open source license must be met and the copyright holder retains rights to the work. If the terms of the open source license are not met (e.g., the same licensing provisions are not applied to derivative works), the copyright has been infringed and the copyright holder has certain legal remedies (U.S. Copyright Act, 17 U.S.C. § 101 et seq.). No matter how permissive the open source license, the copyright holder's interests are protected. If software is released into the public domain, the author surrenders the copyright. Put another way, as soon as software code is created and saved, a copyright attaches to the work. Placing the software in the public domain relinquishes all rights associated with the work. It is not equivalent to granting a license because the author is not limiting or placing restrictions in any way on the use of the software. In fact, software placed in the public domain can be used, modified, and removed from the public domain by another user asserting copyright ownership.

Free versus open software

The terms "free software" and "open software" are often used interchangeably, and they are also frequently consolidated and referred to as Free and Open Source Software (FOSS). However, while a majority of software is both open and free, there are distinctions both in philosophy and in the licenses that fall within each category. The free software movement is, at its roots, about the users' freedoms, whereas open source focuses on making software better from a practical perspective by allowing access to the code for others to improve upon. The views may lead to the same outcome in how the software is treated from a copyright perspective, but the goals for getting there are slightly different.

The concept of free software began in 1984 with Richard Stallman, an MIT researcher (DiBona et al. 1999). Stallman was concerned computing would be dominated by a few powerful people if software were all proprietary. He considered software scientific knowledge that should be shared and distributed in order to further innovation in computer science. In 1984, he left MIT and began the GNU's Not Unix (GNU) project and the Free Software Foundation (FSF). One goal of the GNU project was the development of a freely available operating system that could run GNU software (DiBona et al. 1999).

The most important characteristic of free software is the underlying philosophy for why software should be free and what "free" means. The philosophy of free software is one that respects users' freedoms while benefitting society by promoting sharing and cooperation. The term "free software" is about freedom, not price. The distinction Stallman makes is free software is "free as in speech, not as in beer" (DiBona et al. 1999). A program is free if: you can run the program for any purpose; you have the freedom to modify the program (requiring access to the source code); you have the freedom to redistribute copies with or without a fee; and you have the freedom to distribute modified versions of the program so the community of software developers can benefit from improvements.* Note that the freedom to sell copies of software is permissible because "free" here does not refer to price so there is nothing prohibiting someone from generating revenue from free software, and the founders of the free software movement believed such revenue could ideally be used to generate new free software projects. However, in order to thwart businesses from co-opting free software for their exclusive commercial

* See also the Free Software Foundation at http://www.gnu.org/philosophy/free-sw.html.

use, Stallman created the GNU General Public License (GPL). The GPL license is discussed in detail later in this chapter.

Many software companies rejected the concept of free software in part because it seemed so fundamentally in conflict with having and furthering a commercial interest in a product. So, in 1997, a group of individuals came together to promote the concept of free software and created the term "open source" (DiBona et al. 1999). Using the term "open source" was a way to market the idea of free software by removing the economic context of "free" to make the idea more palatable to private companies. However, there are practical differences between free and OSS. While open source captures much of the spirit of GNU, it allows for provisions free software does not, such as the ability to mix proprietary software and OSS. The Open Source Initiative (OSI), an organization that provides oversight of the open source mission, refers to open source as "a development method for software that harnesses the power of distributed peer review and transparency of process. The promise of open source is better quality, higher reliability, more flexibility, lower cost, and an end to predatory vendor lock-in" (OSI 2015).

The OSI created the Open Source Definition (OSD), which has several distribution terms with which OSS must comply. According to OSI, software is open source if it meets the following criteria*:

1. *Free redistribution*: The license shall not restrict any party from selling or giving away the software as a component of an aggregate software distribution containing programs from several different sources. The license shall not require a royalty or other fee for such sale.
2. *Source code*: The program must include source code, and must allow distribution in source code as well as compiled form. Where some form of a product is not distributed with source code, there must be a well publicized means of obtaining the source code for no more than a reasonable reproduction cost preferably, downloading via the Internet without charge. The source code must be the preferred form in which a programmer would modify the program. Deliberately obfuscated source code is not allowed. Intermediate forms such as the output of a preprocessor or translator are not allowed.
3. *Derived works*: The license must allow modifications and derived works, and must allow them to be distributed under the same terms as the license of the original software.
4. *Integrity of the author's source code*: The license may restrict source code from being distributed in modified form *only* if the license allows the distribution of "patch files" with the source code for the purpose of modifying the program at build time. The license must explicitly permit distribution of software built from modified source code. The license may require derived works to carry a different name or version number from the original software.
5. *No discrimination against persons or groups*: The license must not discriminate against any person or group of persons.
6. *No discrimination against fields of endeavor*. The license must not restrict anyone from making use of the program in a specific field of endeavor. For example, it may not restrict the program from being used in a business, or from being used for genetic research.
7. *Distribution of license*: The rights attached to the program must apply to all to whom the program is redistributed without the need for execution of an additional license by those parties.
8. *License must not be specific to a product*: The rights attached to the program must not depend on the program's being part of a particular software distribution. If the program is extracted from that distribution and used or distributed within the terms of the program's license, all parties to whom the program is redistributed should have the same rights as those that are granted in conjunction with the original software distribution.
9. *License must not restrict other software*: The license must not place restrictions on other software that is distributed along with the licensed software. For example, the license must not insist that all other programs distributed on the same medium must be OSS.
10. *License must be technology neutral*: No provision of the license may be predicated on any individual technology or style of interface.

* The OSD is taken directly from the OSI's website at http://www.opensource.org/docs/osd.

Overview of commonly used licenses

In general, open source licenses can be broadly categorized into those that apply no restrictions on the distribution of derivative works* and those that do apply restrictions in order to ensure the code will always remain open/free. The former is also called an "academic license" and the purpose is to promote a public commons with unlimited use but no requirement to contribute back to the community (Turner 2006). The latter type of license is also referred to as a reciprocal or "share alike" license because it requires that any derivative work must retain the original license. Although there are licenses that exist outside of these categories, the licenses discussed below are grouped into one of these two categories, with the exception of the Mozilla license, which is characterized as a hybridization of both.

ACADEMIC OR NONPROTECTIVE LICENSES
The Berkeley Systems Distribution license

The Berkeley Systems Distribution (BSD) license is one of the least restrictive and most recognized open source licenses (Goldstein et al. 2004; Kennedy 2015).† The license was developed by the University of California at Berkeley and allows free use of the OSS including the ability to modify the software. The BSD license allows for redistribution and use of source code whether modified or not, as long as the source code retains the copyright notice and other notices regarding disclaimers of warranty and limitations on liability found in the license. The BSD license allows the software to be combined with proprietary software or modified and turned into proprietary software. The BSD allows derivative works to be released under a license other than

the BSD, hence there is no copyleft provision. The original BSD had a clause mandating attribution of contributors in advertising of the software. This clause has since been removed; however, users of code under the old version of the BSD license must be careful to comply with the advertising clause. A clause still exists prohibiting use of the copyright holder's name in any promotion of software (Table 10.1).

The Massachusetts Institute of Technology license

The MIT license is very similar to the BSD license and is often referred to as part of the BSD family of licenses. Like the BSD license, it permits reuse of open source code within proprietary software as long the MIT licensing terms are included in the proprietary software. The main differences between the MIT license and the BSD license is that the MIT license does not contain a clause prohibiting the use of the copyright holder's name in promotion of the software, and it places more emphasis on the user by emphasizing the right to "use, copy, modify, merge, publish, distribute, sublicense, and/or sell copies of the Software."‡

Apache

The Apache license was created by the Apache Software Foundation (ASF). Like the BSD and MIT licenses, the Apache license allows software to be used without any obligation to redistribute the source code of any of the derivative works. The main difference is that the Apache license provides a clause about patent licensing and termination. In addition to providing a patent clause, any modifications to the source code distributed under the Apache license must carry prominent notices that the files were changed.

Artistic

The Artistic license falls into the same category as the BSD, MIT, and Apache licenses in that it allows modified versions of Artistic software to be licensed independently, with some conditions. Version 1.0 was criticized by the FSF for being too vague, but version 2.0 is accepted by both the FSF and OSI. The Artistic license was the first open source

---

* Note that the term "derivative works" is defined by the U.S. Copyright Act and generally refers to a work based on one or more preexisting works. However, the Act does not specifically address derivative works in software so the law as it applies to open source software is not well established.

† See the Open Source Initiative, open source licenses by category, at http://www.opensource.org/licenses/BSD-3-Clause.

‡ See the MIT license, available at the Open Source Initiative at http://www.opensource.org/licenses/MIT.

Table 10.1 Commonly used open source licenses

License	Description
BSD	Very permissive, allows for redistribution and use of source code whether modified or not as long as source code retains the copyright notice and other notices regarding disclaimers of warranty and limitations on liability found in the license, software can be combined with proprietary software or modified and turned into proprietary software, allows derivative works to be released under a license other than the BSD (hence, there is no copyleft provision; see GPL below)
MIT	Very similar to BSD; main difference is that the MIT license does not contain a clause prohibiting the use of the copyright holder's name in promotion of the software
Apache	Like the BSD and MIT licenses, the Apache license allows software to be used without any obligation to redistribute the source code of any of the derivative works. The main difference is that the Apache license provides a clause about patent licensing and termination. In addition to providing a patent clause, any modifications to the source code distributed under the Apache license must carry prominent notices that the files were changed.
Artistic	It is in the same category as the BSD, MIT, and Apache licenses; it allows modified versions of Artistic software to be licensed independently, with some conditions; first open source license deemed enforceable under copyright law as opposed to contract law
GNU GPL	One of the most widely used licenses; first copyleft license, meaning it contains the requirement that all derived works must be distributed under the same license, i.e., it does not allow users to modify GPL programs and make them private or proprietary
Lesser GPL	Created to allow for the use of proprietary software with GPL software through the use of programming libraries (which is why it is sometimes referred to as the Library GPL); allows the proprietary software incorporated with GPL-licensed software through a library to be licensed independently from the GPL; represents a compromise between the strong copyleft nature of the GPL and more permissive licenses such as the BSD

license deemed enforceable under copyright law as opposed to contract law (*Jacobsen v. Katzer* 2008).

Mozilla

The Mozilla Public License (MPL) was originally created by Netscape, and version 1.1 is used by the Mozilla Application Suite, Mozilla Firefox, and other Mozilla software and has been adapted for use by other companies (Kennedy 2015). It combines aspects of the BSD and GPL licenses. It allows for commercial licensing of derivative works, and changes to source code covered under the license must be made freely available. Additions to source code that are not modifications and contribute to a larger work can be licensed under something other than MPL and do not have to be published. In this sense, the MPL is not a strong copyleft license like GPL. The license can be used to create a proprietary product where the MPL files must remain under that license, but other files or additions extending the work can be licensed under another open source license or in a closed source manner.

RECIPROCAL OR PROTECTIVE LICENSES

GNU GPL

The GNU GPL was written by Richard Stallman for the GNU Project and is the most widely used free software license. The license has been described as a manifesto because the license itself contains language about the freedom of software and the rationale behind the creation of the license (Kennedy 2015). It is the first copyleft license. As mentioned earlier, copyleft describes the requirement that all derived works must be distributed under the same license. Therefore, it does not allow users to modify GPL programs and make them private or proprietary.

The license takes a unique approach at guaranteeing freedom in that it uses restrictions in the license to protect users' rights to freely use software, as opposed to outlining what or how the license prohibits use. For example, it states:

> When we speak of free software, we are referring to freedom, not price. Our General Public Licenses are designed to make sure that you have the freedom to distribute copies of free software (and charge for them if you wish), that you receive source code or can get it if you want it, that you can change the software or use pieces of it in new free programs, and that you know you can do these things.
>
> *GNU GPL*

The GPL does not allow software licensed under a GPL to be combined with a proprietary program, because a proprietary program will not give a user as many rights as the GPL (fundamental to the notion of copyleft). Any software using a GPL must, when distributed, have the copyright notice published on each copy and the disclaimer of warranty and provide recipients of the program with a copy of the license. By modifying or distributing GPL software, a user is deemed to have accepted the terms of the GPL.

Lesser LGPL

The copyleft nature of the GPL and the concern that any code written in GPL incorporated into another program will require the second program to be licensed under GPL, no matter how small a portion of the code is originally GPL, led to the development of another license. The Lesser GPL (LGPL) was created to allow for the use of proprietary software with GPL software through the use of programming libraries (which is why it is sometimes referred to as the Library GPL). The LGPL allows the proprietary software incorporated with GPL-licensed software through a library to be licensed independently from the GPL. It is a compromise between the strong copyleft nature of the GPL and more permissive licenses such as the BSD. The LGPL allows GPL software to be linked to a non-GPL program whether or not it is free. In the case of programming libraries, the GPL software can be used by the library (and hence linked to other programs). Despite the fact

that the FSF created the LGPL, it does not encourage its use, mainly because with the exception of limited circumstances, it does not further the interests of free software developers.

Eclipse Public License

The Eclipse Public License (EPL) replaced a license called the Common Public License (CPL). It has weaker copyleft provisions than CPL had and it also has a patent clause. Additions to source code originally published under an EPL license can be licensed in another way as long as the additions to not constitute derivative works of the EPL-covered source code but act as "separate modules" of software (OSI 2015). Derivative works under EPL must also be licensed as EPL, which makes it a limited copyleft, a characteristic of the GPL license. However, the EPL requires that anyone distributing the work grant all recipients rights to any patents that may cover modifications. This patent clause is a restriction that is not compatible with GPL, so EPL and GPL works cannot be combined and legally distributed, but combined works using other licenses are permissible.

COMMON MISCONCEPTIONS ABOUT OPEN SOURCE LICENSES

Open source means free

This particular misunderstanding is perhaps the most common and is linked to the "free as in beer" way of thinking about free. Open source software is provided to users at no cost, but this does not mean implementing OSS is free of cost. While the software costs no money to download, which makes it accessible to a broader community of users, the assumption that there is no cost of ownership is faulty. For example, installation and integration of the software often requires technical expertise, and this cost can strain development budgets if the integration is complex. Maintenance of the code is another cost and requires the time of either in-house or external consultants. Moreover, the defining characteristic of open source is really the ability to access the source code, and not as much the fact that it is made available at no cost.

Open source has no copyright restrictions

As discussed previously, but worth emphasizing again here, providing software as open source does not mean the developer has relinquished their copyright. In fact, how a user is able to exploit the source code and restrictions on that use varies by license, each of which protects the rights and intent of the original author. Open source licenses are grounded in copyright law and the copyright holder gets to choose which rights are granted to other users.

Open source software is unreliable

There are two components to this myth. The first part is asserted on the basis that the software is unreliable because it is either produced by amateurs or circulated without being tracked for bugs or quality. The second part of the myth is that the software is unreliable in the sense that it is uniquely insecure because vulnerabilities in the code can be easily detected. As for the first assertion, and as discussed in the introduction of this chapter, large, commercial software projects use OSS, and there is a high level of demand for the use of OSS in many domains. Although the software is not necessarily tracked for quality, and the licenses may not assert warranties for fitness, some software projects do have managers tracking code. Moreover, the accessibility to a broad group of users is one of the reasons software is made open source, so others can improve upon the existing code. This logic speaks to the security issue as well. The transparency of OSS and the ability to improve upon the software are reasons many consider it more secure.

ENFORCEABILITY

The legal enforceability of open source licenses is a nuanced and developing area. The cases vary depending on the license at issue and the facts around which enforcement is sought. Given the philosophical underpinnings of OSS, it was not immediately clear whether certain contract elements, namely the exchange of consideration, could be met given the free nature of the license. There is a growing body of case law, but for purposes of this chapter, it is important primarily to note that open sources licenses are both enforceable under contract and copyright law.

The case of *Jacobsen v. Katzer* highlights the enforceability through both legal mechanisms. In *Jacobsen*, the court found that if a licensee breaches a condition placed on the license grant, the licensor's copyright has been infringed. The court also found that injunctive relief can be granted for open source licenses. Injunctive relief is relief granted by a court against an act or condition, as opposed to a grant of money damages. An example in this context may be an order to stop distribution of the software by those not complying with the license terms. This type of relief is particularly important in the open source community because monetary damages, which are typically sought in contract cases, may not be an available option as the software may have been distributed without profit. *Jacobsen* also confirmed that open source licenses do not lack consideration and can therefore be enforced under contract law.

BENEFITS AND LIMITATIONS OF OPEN SOURCE SOFTWARE

The open source model has been very successful and provides developers with many benefits. First, access to source code enables developers to improve on the code, create programs that are more interoperable, and perfect their own programs that they are using OSS to develop. It allows others to build on software in ways not envisioned by the original creators. This ability to access source code is, in part, due to the strong communities around many types of the open source licenses, which provide a large pool of code from which to work. Open source licensing provides developers who may not otherwise be able to pay for a program access to the source code, as most programs distributed under open source licenses are free. This is particularly important in the case of resource-limited countries that need access to similar software but do not have the means to pay for or sustain a proprietary software license. Most importantly, the broad rights granted a user through an open source license provide a huge benefit to users because they allow users to modify, use, or distribute the software, whereas commercial licenses are likely only distributed in a form that cannot be modified.

Despite the many benefits, users of OSS and those selecting an open source license must be aware of the distinctions between the types of licenses, no matter how seemingly small. A major consideration is whether the user wants derivative works to be proprietary, in which case a copyleft license would not be appropriate. Although there are various specialized licenses to address unique circumstances, if the developer wants to make the program open source to tap into the development community, he or she will want to pick a license under which developers can easily work and that is standard and widely used.

Although the accessibility of the software is a fundamental characteristic of open source, most licenses contain disclaimers concerning warranties and fitness for a particular purpose. Although there is no definitive evidence suggesting that OSS is of lesser quality than commercial software (as indicated above, some in fact argue the opposite), the licensee may have to accept risks that the software has major errors. Some initiatives are large enough to provide code monitoring and bug tracking, but this is not always the case. Also, the fact that numerous people are contributing to the code increases the likelihood that code infringing on intellectual property rights (here, perhaps certain copyright terms) is introduced. Most licenses disclaim all warranties, and it may be difficult to audit the code to determine which contributor or contributors may have violated the terms of the license. An open source project that has many authors, each of whom has a license on her work, makes determining who can enforce the copyright difficult, e.g., determining whether one owner can bring an action on behalf of all copyright owners or whether each must be found and joined in an action. However, the idea that OSS is more prone to claims of intellectual property infringement is generally not supported by fact, even though there have indeed been such claims against open source development projects and there will likely continue to be such claims. The existence of these claims alone does not support the conclusion that OSS is especially vulnerable. It does, however, emphasize the enforceability of open source licenses as legitimate intellectual property claims that can be brought before a court.

GOVERNMENT USE OF OPEN SOURCE SOFTWARE

Until recently, government use of OSS has been limited, but with the expansion of mobile and cloud computing, more agencies are adopting policies for using OSS on government-funded projects (Brodkin 2011). Some of the government's reluctance stems from the sensitivity of certain data and concerns about information assurance. However, because OSS goes through continuous peer review, some argue it is more secure than proprietary software (Brodkin 2011). In particular,

the Department of Defense (DoD) and NASA have embraced the use of OSS, with the latter agency being referred to as "the summa cum laude when it comes to open source" since using OSS to develop cloud computing networks (Brodkin 2011). The Department of Homeland Security (DHS) created the Homeland Open Security Technology (HOST) program to leverage the use of OSS in the development of technologies to support cyber security objectives (U.S. DHS 2015).

In a Department-circulated memorandum, DoD confronted many of the previously discussed misconceptions about OSS and stated that "there are many OSS [open source software] programs in operational use by the Department today, in both classified and unclassified environments" (DoD 2009). The memorandum specifically advises that as part of the market research federal agencies must conduct to procure property or services, OSS should be included in the research when it meets mission needs (DoD 2009). Moreover, it points out that many open source licenses allow the user to modify the OSS for use with no obligation to redistribute, therefore quelling the misunderstanding that DoD or any government agency would have to distribute the source code to the public, which would be prohibited on classified projects.* The memorandum underscores other benefits of using OSS, including the following:

- The ability to "respond more rapidly to changing situations, missions, and future threats" due to the unrestricted ability to modify source code.
- The identification and elimination of defects through the "continuous and broad peer review enabled by publicly available source code."
- The availability of the code for maintenance and repair by the government and its contractors (rebutting the notion that OSS comes with a limited or no warranty, and therefore, should not be used).
- The ability to reduce reliance on a particular vendor due to the use of OSS, which can be maintained by a variety of vendors.

* Note that the Memorandum does outline conditions under which the code should be distributed to the public, essentially stating that doing so must be in the government's interest; the government must be authorized to release the code; and public release cannot be otherwise restricted by law.

- Open source software may provide a cost advantage as it typically does not have a per-seat licensing cost.
- Open source software licenses allow wide dissemination of the software, which allows the agency to contribute to a collaborative software development environment, particularly one run by the Defense Information Systems Agency (software.forge.mil).

The work of DoD, NASA, and DHS will undoubtedly help set the trend for broader use of OSS by the government. However, the development of mobile technologies for the government is also stimulating increased use of OSS. Government-deployed mobile applications are an area of growth, and many agencies are interested in using mobile operating systems like Google's Linux-based Android for development (Brodkin 2011). Mobile health (mHealth) initiatives and the need for electronic processes to support health care (eHealth) provide particularly good examples of government use of OSS.

OPEN SOURCE SOFTWARE, AN mHEALTH/eHEALTH PERSPECTIVE

The growth of global and national mHealth and eHealth needs has spurred innovation in software development. As medical practitioners and health institutions are encouraged by the federal government to digitize patient information or reap efficiency and productivity benefits of digital information, a need for sophisticated tools has arisen.* In areas with limited resources but where cellular technology is prevalent and acquirable, mHealth solutions are able to move such communities into the digital age—whereas in prior years, they lagged and relied on inefficient paper-based workflows. Upon adopting information and communications technology (ICT)/digital solutions, monetary costs of licensing and maintaining proprietary software systems have been common challenges to these end users. Fortunately, the OSS paradigm has gained strong worldwide acceptance, and grassroots entities, researchers, and nonprofit institutions are on the frontier of developing innovative open source tools to fulfill user needs.

* See the Electronic Health Records Incentive Programs at https://www.cms.gov/EHRIncentivePrograms/.

Of a seven-project subset of active and widely used mHealth initiatives, the Apache 2.0, LGPL, and BSD licenses were used:

FrontlineSMS (LGPL), JavaRosa (Apache 2.0), ODK (Apache 2.0), RapidSMS (BSD), RapidAndroid (Apache 2.0), Ushashidi (LGPL), OpenXData (Apache 2.0).

The wide selection of OSS licenses equips project implementers with options to license their work depending on their preferences. Consequently, it is important for end users to evaluate licensing of a third-party tool before integrating it with their own projects to ensure that the license terms are not violated (Table 10.2).

Open source software and IHR implementation

The use of OSS has gained increasing popularity in large-scale commercial software and web-based projects. However, governments and NGOs charged with providing a variety of expected public services may benefit from OSS that mitigates the use of prohibitively expensive proprietary software. Although not all deficiencies can be solved with an information technology solution, many can. To the extent this type of solution requires software infrastructure, OSS can be used to dramatically reduce costs and make accessible software that would otherwise be too costly to procure.

As referenced earlier, IHR implementation has proceeded more slowly than anticipated, in part because of a lack of technical infrastructure, e.g., communications resources, among other things. However, countries may be able to comply with several of the IHR provisions concerning disease detection, tracking, and response with the assistance of OSS because it provides a lower cost option that can often be adapted to existing technology frameworks. Recently, the WHO partnered with the Centers for Disease Control (CDC) to strengthen integrated disease surveillance through global health security demonstration projects (Borchert et al. 2014). One demonstration project conducted in Uganda included the development of an outbreak response capability that detects suspected illness by priority pathogens (Borchert et al. 2014). The module uses text messaging to report to Uganda's District Health Information System (DHIS-2), which is an online, open source system for reporting

Table 10.2 Examples of OSS initiatives used in public health

License	Description	License used
Frontline Short Message Service (SMS)	Designed for grassroots NGOs in developing countries, it helps organizations overcome communication barriers by allowing users to send, receive, and manage SMS over a mobile network	LGPL
Java Rosa	Open source platform for data collection on mobile devices	Apache 2.0
Rapid SMS	Open source framework for dynamic data collection, logistics coordination, and communication that leverages basic SMS mobile phone technology	BSD
Suite for Automated Global Electronic bioSurveillance (SAGES)	Collection of modular, flexible OSS tools for electronic disease surveillance	Apache 2.0
RapidAndroid	A fully featured implementation of Rapid SMS, uses the mobile to act as a stand-alone appliance for SMS management	Apache 2.0
Ushahidi	Initiative that creates OSS for information collection, visualization, and interactive mapping	LGPL
ODK	FOSS of tools that help organizations author, field, and manage mobile data collection solutions	Apache 2.0
OpenXData	Open source data collection platform that supports low-cost mobile phones	Apache 2.0

national health data (Borchert et al. 2014). As part of the demonstration, the system was enhanced to accommodate real-time monitoring, and the text-messaging modules allowed specimen tracking. This is one example where fairly simple upgrades to an existing system leveraging OSS made significant improvements toward meeting IHR implementation criteria (Table 10.3).

While the Uganda project had as an objective improving IHR implementation, there are many other projects using OSS in resource-limited settings to meet urgent and emerging needs. These examples also serve to emphasize that utility of OSS in areas that may have many similar features to areas where IHR implementation is lacking. For instance, the role of OSS in disaster areas is now well documented.

Table 10.3 Recognized benefits of using OSS

Benefits of OSS	Description
Flexibility	Provides the ability to respond to changing situations and needs because of the unrestricted ability to modify source code
Increased reliability	Allows for the identification and elimination of defects through the continuous peer review enabled by publicly available source code
Vendor neutrality	Reduces reliance on a particular vendor because OSS can be maintained by a variety of vendors
Cost advantage	Provides a cost advantage because OSS typically does not have a per-seat licensing cost, and the software may be obtained for free (though implementation may not be free)
User support	Shares common characteristics across the tools available on the web, such as an open community, user and developer support threads actively managed by key contributors, living documentation, and third-party hosting of source code

OpenStreetMap (OSM) is a crowd-sourced mapping application that provided a detailed map of the areas hit by typhoon Haiyan in the Philippines within 3 days of landfall (Hern 2013). The Red Cross now uses OSS in all of its projects, OSM being one example, citing that OSS reduces or eliminates sustainment costs of software after the organization leaves an area. In addition, any software or data created by the Red Cross are released as open source (Robinson 2013). Prior to typhoon Haiyan, OSS was used to map the damage from the 2010 earthquake in Haiti. Most recently, several OSS tools are being used to track the Ebola outbreak in West Africa.

Challenges

Improving public health security through timely disease surveillance and information sharing will not be easy, even with OSS. Despite its cost-effective nature, data sharing for disease surveillance and response still requires both human and technical resources, even if the required resources are fewer. Beyond resources, there are often political barriers that must be overcome. Whenever data sharing is entertained, mistrust is frequently encountered because of concerns over how data will be used or even monetized by others. The agencies charged with carrying out public health mandates may face policy guidelines or restrictions on data use that can only be addressed through the appropriate administrative processes. On the other hand, the lack of guidelines or regulations can also create confusion about the extent to which data can be collected and used. Again, this is not a technical problem that OSS can address. In some instances, there are also cultural and ethical considerations to information sharing that are less evident but nonetheless important, e.g., the willingness of individuals to share they are HIV-positive and the potential social backlash that can occur if their information is compromised.

However, there are many methods for safeguarding information, which then has the potential to foster trust. And with improved trust among the many stakeholders in this field, a consolidated effort to address the global commons issue of public health security has a chance to succeed. These challenges exist, but once political and administrative hurdles are addressed, OSS can help tackle many of the technical challenges. Indeed, the more people understand the available technology and its many benefits, the more likely it is that the acceptability

of its use will increase. The more people understand about OSS and the variety of licensing options, the easier it will be to take full advantage of what OSS has to offer. OSS is not the sole answer to global public health issues. But, at this time when there is such a great need for technology and policy to come together to address some of the most daunting public health challenges, it offers much promise. It can and should be used to further international agreements and guidelines, such as the IHR, for which so much work has already been done.

ACRONYMS

ASF	Apache Software Foundation
BSD	Berkeley Systems Distribution
CDC	Centers for Disease Control
CPL	Common Public License
DHIS-2	District Health Information System
DHS	Department of Homeland Security
DoD	Department of Defense
EPL	Eclipse Public License
FOSS	Free and Open Source Software
FSF	Free Software Foundation
GNU	GNU's Not Unix
GPL	General Public License
HOST	Homeland Open Security Technology
ICT	Information and Communications Technology
IHR	International Health Regulations
LGPL	Lesser General Public License
MIT	Massachusetts Institute of Technology
MPL	Mozilla Public License
NGO	Nongovernmental Organization
OSD	Open Source Definition
OSI	Open Source Initiative
OSM	OpenStreetMap
OSS	Open Source Software
SAGES	Suite for Automated Global Electronic bioSurveillance
SMS	Short Message Service

REFERENCES

Borchert, J.N., J.W. Tappero, R. Downing et al. 2014. Rapidly building global health security capacity—Uganda demonstration project, 2013. *Morb. Mortal. Wkly. Rep.* 63(4): 73–76.

Brodkin, J. 2011. Nonprofit helps government expand open source software usage. *NetworkWorld.* June 27. Accessed

October 8, 2015. http://www.networkworld.com/article/2178694/windows/nonprofit-helps-government-expand-open-source-software-usage.html.

Dennis, K. 2006. Best legal practices for open source software: Ten tips for managing legal risks for businesses using open source software. *Mondaq*. Accessed October 8, 2015. http://www.highbeam.com/doc/1G1-143081381.html.

DiBona, C., S. Ockman, and M. Stone. 1999. *Open Sources, Voices from The Open Source Revolution*. Sebastopol, CA: O'Reilly Media.

Fischer, J.E. and R. Katz. 2013. Moving forward to 2014: Global IHR (2005) implementation. *Biosecur. Bioterr. Biodef. Strat. Pract. Sci.* 11(2): 153–156.

Fontana, R., B.M. Kuhn, E. Moglen, M. Norwood, D.B. Ravicher, K. Sandler, J. Vasile, and A. Williamson. 2008. A legal issues primer for open source and free software products, version 1.5.1. Software Freedom Law Center. Accessed October 7, 2015. http://www.softwarefreedom.org/resources/2008/foss-primer.html#x1-40002.

Goldstein, D.E., S. Ponkshe, and R. Maduro. 2004. *Analysis of Open Source Software (OSS) and EHRs: Profile in Increasing Use of OSS in the Federal Government and Healthcare*. Atlantis, FL: Medical Alliances Inc.

Gostin, L.O. and D. Sridhar. 2014. Global health and the law. *N. Engl. J. Med.* 370(18): 1732–1740.

Hern, A. 2013. Online volunteers map Philippines after Typhoon Haiyan. *The Guardian*. November 15. http://www.theguardian.com/technology/2013/nov/15/online-volunteers-map-philippines-after-typhoon-haiyan.

Jacobsen V. Katzer, 535 F.3d 1373 (Fed. Cir. 2008).

Kennedy, D.M. 2015. A primer on open source licensing legal issues: Copyright, copyleft, and copyfuture. Accessed March 24, 2015. http://www.cs.miami.edu/~burt/learning/Csc322.052/docs/opensourcedmk.pdf.

OSI (Open Source Initiative). 2015. Accessed October 7, 2015. http://opensource.org/.

Robinson, M. 2013. How online mapmakers are helping the red cross save lives in the Philippines. *The Atlantic*. November 12. Accessed October 8, 2015. http://www.theatlantic.com/technology/archive/2013/11/how-online-mapmakers-are-helping-the-red-cross-save-lives-in-the-philippines/281366/.

Taylor, A.L., T. Alfvenb, D. Hougendoblera, S. Tanakab, and K. Buseb. 2014. Leveraging non-binding Instruments for Global Health Governance: Reflections from the global AIDS reporting mechanism for WHO reform. *Public Health* 128(2): 151–160.

Terry, K. 2010. Mobile health: New cell phone-based technologies transform emergency care. *CBS Money Watch*. September 1. Accessed October 8, 2015. http://www.cbsnews.com/8301-505123_162-43841703/mobile-health-new-cell-phone-based-technologies-transform-emergency-care/.

Turner, S. 2006. Open source development for public health: A primer with examples of existing enterprise ready open source applications. In *Public Health Information Network Conference*. Accessed October 7, 2015. https://www.mendeley.com/profiles/stuart-turner1/.

United Nations. 1948. *Universal Declaration on Human Rights (UDHR)*. http://www.un.org/en/documents/udhr/.

United Nations. 1976. *International Covenant on Economic, Social, and Cultural Rights*. Office of the High Commissioner of Human Rights. Accessed October 8, 2015. http://www.ohchr.org/EN/ProfessionalInterest/Pages/CESCR.aspx.

U.S. Copyright Act, 17 U.S.C. § 101 et seq.

U.S. DHS (Department of Homeland Security). 2015. Cyber security division. Last published February 6. Accessed October 8, 2015. http://www.dhs.gov/science-and-technology/cyber-security-division.

U.S. DoD (Department of Defense). 2009. Memorandum, subject: Clarifying guidance regarding Open Source Software (OSS). Accessed October 8, 2015. http://dodcio.defense.gov/Portals/0/Documents/FOSS/2009OSS.pdf.

WHO (World Health Organization). 1948. Constitution. Accessed October 8, 2015. apps.who.int/gb/DGNP/pdf_files/constitution-en.pdf.

WHO. 2012. Implementation of IHR in the WHO Africa Region. Regional Committee for Africa, Report of the Secretariat. Accessed October 8, 2015. http://apps.who.int/gb/ebwha/pdf_files/WHA66/A66_16-en.pdf.

11

Role of mass gathering surveillance

SHRADDHA PATEL

The U.S. Centers for Disease Control and Prevention (CDC) defines "mass gathering" as a planned event in which a large number of people come together in a particular location for a specific purpose. Mass gatherings can be festivals, religious gatherings, sporting events, concerts, or political rallies and conventions. They can occur over different periods of time. Some last just a few hours like a music concert. Others are one-day events, such as the Super Bowl or a presidential inauguration. Still others extend over a period of days or weeks, such as the Hajj in Mecca, Saudi Arabia, the Olympic Games, or world cups. Mass gatherings are typically defined as events attended by more than 25,000 people (Arbon et al. 2001), but depending on local capacity to respond to an event, a smaller gathering could still be considered a mass gathering from a public health perspective.

Mass gatherings pose special challenges for health systems. The increase in population and population density, along with the potential for visitors from different nations, regions, and cultures, can increase the risk of spread of infectious disease among the visiting and local population. The greater number of people associated with mass gatherings can place a severe strain on the health-care system. When a health system is overwhelmed, the ability to detect, investigate, and respond to a problem is compromised. The CDC suggests that public health surveillance be implemented at mass gatherings to facilitate early detection of disease outbreaks and other health-related events and to enable public health officials to respond in a timely manner (Centers for Disease Control and Prevention 2006). The goal of public health at mass gatherings is to prevent or minimize the risk of injury or ill health and to maximize safety for participants, spectators, event staff and volunteers, and residents.

To effectively deal with the increased public health risks associated with mass gatherings, public health officials must enhance existing surveillance to rapidly identify public health concerns during the mass gathering, to communicate information about them, and to respond to them. Several types of surveillance systems can be used in mass gatherings: notifiable disease surveillance, sentinel site surveillance, injury surveillance, syndromic surveillance, and laboratory surveillance. Depending on the size and scope of the gathering, a combination of systems may be employed. No matter the type of system, technology plays a key role in implementing enhanced surveillance during mass gatherings. The articles in this chapter highlight recent mass gatherings around the world and describe the surveillance efforts for each.

In 2012, the city of Tampa, Florida, in the United States hosted the 2012 Republican National Convention, a 4-day political event, which drew about 40,000–60,000 people to the city. Along with the increased population in Tampa, officials were concerned about the potential for protests and civil unrest that had marked recent conventions, as well as the fact that the convention coincided with the start of the school year. Public health officials used emergency department (ED) data as the core of their surveillance efforts during the convention.

The Olympic Games are considered as the leading international sporting event, gathering thousands of athletes and millions of spectators from around the world. During the summer of 2012, England hosted the Olympic Games and the Paralympic Games, which represented a significant public health challenge to the host country. Preparations by major stakeholders, including the Health Protection Agency (HPA) and International Olympic Committee, began in 2009. Preexisting surveillance systems were enhanced, and new systems were introduced and in place before the summer of 2012. During the event, surveillance activities were "enhanced business as usual," including more frequent and comprehensive reporting.

Washington, DC, frequently hosts events that draw world leaders and other officials. These events are designated as National Special Security Events (NSSEs). The number of people in Washington, DC, increases substantially during the events, increasing the potential for large-scale terrorist activity or outbreak. Two such events are the 57th presidential inauguration, January 21, 2013, and the African Leaders Summit, August 4–6, 2014. In its role as the lead public health agency, the Washington, DC, Department of Health employed electronic data systems to perform enhanced public health surveillance during the events.

In the summer of 2014, Brazil was host to the Federation Internationale de Football Association

(FIFA) World Cup. The 32-day event was spread across 12 host cities and involved 32 teams from around the world. To improve the sensitivity of the national system of health surveillance, public health officials used participatory surveillance as a complementary data source to traditional systems. Participatory surveillance is rooted in crowdsourcing methods to gather data from the collective knowledge of social networks. The participatory surveillance strategy used for the World Cup incorporated both web and mobile platforms.

The 8th Micronesian Games took place in July 2014 in Pohnpei State, Federated States of Micronesia (FSM). The Micronesian Games are a quadrennial international multisport event that takes place in the Micronesian region of Oceania, a region centered on the islands of the tropical Pacific Ocean. The event drew athletes and spectators from various island states within Micronesia. All events took place on the island of Pohnpei. Health officials enhanced the existing syndromic surveillance during the Games by increasing the frequency of reporting, the number of syndromes to be reported, and the number of sentinel sites for data collection. A customized web-based data entry, analysis, and visualization application was used to create daily situation reports.

THE 2012 REPUBLICAN NATIONAL CONVENTION

DAVID ATRUBIN

Florida Department of Health–Hillsborough County

Tampa, Florida

The 2012 Republican National Convention (RNC) marked the first NSSE ever held in Florida. During the event, technology played an integral role in the Florida DOH in Hillsborough County's ability to conduct timely disease surveillance and provide situational awareness. Hillsborough County, the home of Tampa, Florida, has been conducting syndromic surveillance since shortly after the anthrax attacks in the fall of 2001. The county has used several syndromic surveillance systems over the last 13 years. Through the various iterations of these systems, the data sources, surveillance methods, and goals have evolved. As a result, the county's current ability to conduct syndromic surveillance is greatly enhanced compared with the time period shortly before the September 11, 2001, attacks.

When planning disease surveillance for a high-profile event like the RNC, it is imperative to tailor the surveillance efforts to the idiosyncrasies of the event. National political conventions are fairly short in duration, lasting only 4 days. These conventions draw a predominantly adult crowd, in terms of both the delegates and the staff working at the event. A changing population during an event can also affect the data; 40,000–60,000 people were expected to come to the Tampa Bay area for the convention, but, conversely, many Hillsborough residents planned to leave the area during this time. The 2012 RNC coincided with the start of the school year in Hillsborough County, which brought its own unique challenges to disease surveillance. Some recent political conventions have been marked by protests and civil unrest. All these factors needed to be accounted for in the biosurveillance methods that were used.

As many of our more traditional disease surveillance systems are too slow during an event of short duration, the ED visit syndromic surveillance served as the core of our biosurveillance efforts during the RNC. Hillsborough County was aided by complete participation by the 10 hospital EDs in the county (with the exception of the Veterans Affairs hospital). The numerous years of experience conducting syndromic surveillance and a system that allowed for easily customizable queries proved to be invaluable as well. Trained epidemiologists with significant experience in analyzing syndromic surveillance data and following up on important statistical anomalies and visits of interest were critical to the overall efforts during this event. Over half of the participating hospitals in Hillsborough County sent data every 2 hours (as opposed to once per day), thus providing near-real-time surveillance. This increased frequency of transmission is an enormous advantage when conducting biosurveillance for a high-profile event of relatively short duration.

The Florida DOH, on one previous occasion, requested that hospitals add a term to the chief complaint field to alert the DOH personnel that a particular visit is associated with a given event. Hospitals were asked to add the term "Haiti" to the start of the chief complaint after the 2010 earthquake in that country because the state was receiving Haitians in need of medical attention. A similar proposal to add "RNC" was discussed, but it was decided not to ask the hospitals to make a change to data that are primarily collected for hospitals' internal purposes. Differing opinions exist as to whether it is appropriate to ask hospitals to make such internal process changes, especially during times when there could be increased ED volume.

Without any data field specifically designating an ED visit as being related to the RNC, the zip code field in the syndromic surveillance data was used to look for increased visits from out-of-area visitors. Hillsborough County conducted specific analyses for ED visits by patients who normally reside outside the county. By looking for increased visits in this population, determining anything unusual in the visitors attending the RNC was possible. Adjusting statistical algorithms to reflect an increasing or changing population during an event deserves more attention as syndromic surveillance moves forward.

During disasters and some special events, the U.S. Department of Health and Human Services Office of the Assistant Secretary for Preparedness and Response will often deploy Disaster Medical Assistant Teams (DMATs) to provide medical treatment and triage to people associated with these events. Data are collected electronically at these sites. During the 2012 RNC, these data were sent every 15 minutes to our syndromic surveillance system for data analysis. Having DMAT syndromic surveillance data in near real time during an event of this magnitude was useful.

While electronic disease surveillance systems certainly showed their value during the 2012 RNC, traditional surveillance methods also played a vital role. Urgent care centers in the proximity of the RNC event venues were recruited and asked to collect data for each of their visits during the RNC. These data, collected on a paper form, were then faxed to the health department for analysis. Although it is certainly more labor intensive to ask questions specific to the event (e.g., "Are you here for the 2012 RNC?"), being able to do so provides obvious advantages over relying on data fields for which data are routinely collected. Working with the hotels hosting RNC visitors and daily telephone calls with our mosquito control personnel both enhanced our disease surveillance efforts during the event and strengthened relationships.

As we move forward with the provisions of "meaningful use" set forth in the American Reinvestment and Recovery Act of 2009, it is important that disease surveillance systems are useful for both routine and special event surveillance. Receiving data reliably and frequently (e.g., in real time or every 2 hours) is paramount to achieving these goals.

NATIONAL SPECIAL SECURITY EVENTS: ENHANCED DISEASE SURVEILLANCE IN THE DISTRICT OF COLUMBIA

SASHA MCGEE

District of Columbia Department of Health (DC DOH)

Washington, DC

Introduction

The September 11, 2001, terrorist attacks in New York, Pennsylvania, and the District of Columbia (DC, or the District) and the identification of powder containing *Bacillus anthracis* in envelopes mailed to news media companies and government officials in New York and DC in September and October of 2001 have led to heightened concern about bioterrorist activities in the United States. These events underscored the need for public health agencies to monitor and quickly respond to nonspecific health-related events and detect disease outbreaks. As the seat of the nation's capital, the District frequently hosts large-scale National Special Security Events (NSSEs), including the presidential inauguration, national rallies and protests, and memorial dedications. As the number

of persons in the District increases substantially during these events, an increased potential for targeted terrorist activity or the development of a large-scale outbreak exists. When the Secretary of Homeland Security designates an event as an NSSE, the Secret Service is mandated to serve as the lead agency for the design and implementation of the operational security plan (United States Secret Service 2014). During disasters and emergencies, the DC DOH serves as the lead District agency in providing assistance and resources to identify and respond to public health and medical care needs.

Advances in information technology have made it possible for DC DOH epidemiologists to rapidly and efficiently monitor health data by using electronic data systems. This chapter provides an overview of and describes our experience with using electronic data systems to perform enhanced public health surveillance during two NSSEs, the 57th U.S. Presidential Inauguration and the United States–Africa Leaders Summit (ALS).

Planning and implementation for enhanced surveillance

Planning and implementation activities for NSSEs often involve District agencies (e.g., the Fire and Emergency Medical Services Department, the Metropolitan Police Department, and the DC DOH), federal agencies (e.g., the Department of Defense, the Department of Health and Human Services, and the Secret Service), and regional health departments (typically the Maryland Department of Health and Mental Hygiene and Virginia DOH). Clear communication and collaboration among agencies is critical to ensure a coordinated response to any health emergency or threat that might arise. Depending on the scale and potential threats associated with the event, the DC DOH Health Emergency Preparedness and Response Administration (HEPRA) might set up a Health Emergency Coordination Center (HECC) to support public health and medical service activities. The HECC is a facility in which representatives from each participating jurisdiction or agency gather to coordinate their resources in support of an event (Federal Emergency Management

Agency Emergency Management Institute 2014). The HECC ensures timely situational awareness for collaborating agencies and allows DC DOH epidemiologists to gain a comprehensive view of health-associated incidents through the data collected from other agencies.

Enhanced biosurveillance methods and tools

Our goals when performing enhanced surveillance are as follows: (1) to identify unusual or suspicious occurrences of a health outcome or an increase in the frequency of an outcome and (2) to rapidly initiate measures to protect the public from morbidity or mortality if a potential threat is identified. DC DOH epidemiologists leverage multiple standard surveillance systems to perform enhanced surveillance during an NSSE. One such system is the Electronic Surveillance System for the Early Notification of Community-based Epidemics (ESSENCE).

ESSENCE was developed by the Johns Hopkins University Applied Physics Laboratory and the Department of Defense in collaboration with public health officials from DC, Maryland, and Virginia. ESSENCE uses Microsoft® SQL Server databases (Microsoft Corporation, Redmond, WA) and Java web applications. The system's purpose is to identify illness clusters early, before diagnoses are confirmed and reported to public health agencies (i.e., syndromic surveillance) (Henning 2004). ESSENCE compiles ED electronic health data from acute care hospitals, over-the-counter pharmaceutical sales data from participating pharmacies, and poison control center data. Aggregate data from DC, Maryland, and Virginia hospitals are displayed on the Aggregated National Capital Region (ANCR) ESSENCE website. ESSENCE and ANCR ESSENCE are secure applications that are accessible only to authorized users.

ANCR ESSENCE parses the chief complaint free text data transmitted from EDs and groups them into predefined or user-defined syndrome and subsyndrome categories. Each syndrome or subsyndrome is defined by a specific set of search criteria associated with Boolean operators. Patient data are assigned to a given syndrome or subsyndrome by means of queries of the chief complaint text data. The syndromes include symptoms associated with botulism (referred to as botulism-like illness), fever, gastrointestinal (GI) disease, hemorrhagic illness, localized lesion, lymphadenopathy, neurological disease, rash, acute respiratory diseases, severe illness or death, and others. Subsyndromes are more specific, and those that are predefined in the system include symptoms associated with influenza (influenza-like illness) and trauma. The system allows sharing of queries with other ANCR ESSENCE users as needed. Additional data fields extracted from ED records include age, sex, and jurisdiction information (e.g., Maryland or Virginia). ED data are displayed by ANCR ESSENCE in real time, but the frequency of data transmission varies by hospital.

ANCR ESSENCE uses various automated algorithms to detect and generate alerts when an unusually high number of cases of a syndrome or subsyndrome are identified on the basis of historical data. Public health officials begin reviewing ANCR ESSENCE data 2 weeks before the start of an NSSE to capture baseline data on the frequency of each syndrome or subsyndrome. These baseline data improve our capacity to more fully detect unusual or suspicious occurrences or increased frequency of a syndrome or subsyndrome that occurs during NSSEs. Data review consists of examining graphs of time series trends and the individual records from the query results. If a potential unusual occurrence or frequency of a syndrome or subsyndrome is identified, the ED where the patient was treated is contacted to collect additional clinical information. ANCR ESSENCE data are reviewed until 2 weeks after the NSSE to capture illnesses that might develop days after the initial exposure (e.g., measles, hepatitis A).

HC Standard® (Global Emergency Resources 2014) is an additional system that the DC DOH uses to collect health data during NSSEs. HC Standard is an Internet-based, commercial software suite that provides emergency information, patient and asset tracking, and visualization in near real time. During NSSEs, medical aid stations are placed at each venue to handle medical emergencies. Volunteers are assigned to staff each medical aid station and are responsible for entering data for each patient visit into handheld, electronic patient tracker devices (patient trackers). The patient trackers transmit data to HC Standard, which can then be securely accessed for review and analysis.

Examples of enhanced surveillance activities

THE 57TH PRESIDENTIAL INAUGURATION

The 57th Presidential Inauguration took place in DC on January 21, 2013. Members of the National Capital Region Collaborative, which included the Johns Hopkins University Applied Physics Laboratory and epidemiologists from DC, Maryland, and Virginia, worked collectively to perform enhanced surveillance activities for this event. The group developed a written protocol to describe procedures for communication among jurisdictions and the review and reporting of syndromic surveillance data by using ANCR ESSENCE. In addition to the predefined queries, a shared set of event-specific queries were created to

identify the incidence of meningitis; extreme (outdoor) environmental exposure or injury, including hypothermia and dehydration; symptoms indicating exposure to different viral and bacterial diseases, including, but not limited to, cholera, dengue, measles, pertussis, rubella, tuberculosis, typhoid, yellow fever, botulism, anthrax, plague, and tularemia; exposure to hazardous materials, including biohazardous materials; and ED records specific to inaugural-event attendees through the use of search criteria (e.g., inaug, downtown, parade, crowd, and outdoors). Data were reviewed once per day during the 2 weeks before and after inauguration day and twice on inauguration day. A flowchart of the data review process is shown in Figure 11.1.

Reports summarizing the data were posted on the newly developed ESSENCE reporting site, known as Pebble. This site was designed as a secure, Internet-based application to support information sharing among authorized public health ANCR ESSENCE users and non–public health partners, including emergency management, law enforcement, and the first-responder community. The Department of Defense, the Department of Health and Human Services, emergency medical

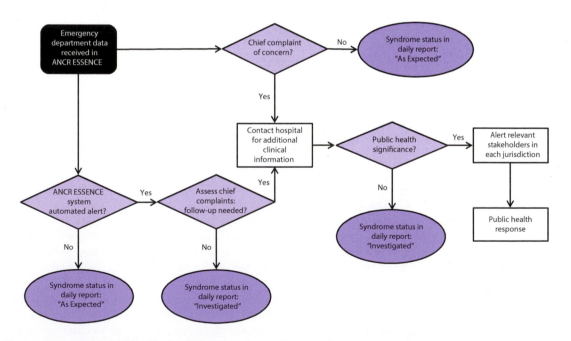

Figure 11.1 ANCR ESSENCE data review process during enhanced surveillance.

technicians, and DC DOH personnel used patient trackers to collect chief complaint data at medical aid stations located throughout the National Mall, along the inaugural parade route, and during inaugural balls.

Outcomes and lessons learned

No unusual patterns or increased frequency of a syndrome or subsyndrome were identified during the 57th Presidential Inauguration. No suspicious bioterrorism or injurious activity was detected. The Pebble site was further modified for this event to promote information exchange among public health and non–public health partners and improve situational awareness. Although posting information to the Pebble site was straightforward, the DC DOH, Maryland, and Virginia administrators did not use the site frequently during this event. The group agreed that sending an e-mail alert to notify users when a new report was posted might be helpful to increase the usefulness of this reporting method. Using HC Standard for the first time also presented certain challenges. Data collection on inauguration day was initially delayed because patient trackers were not predeployed at the medical aid stations and had to be delivered to

volunteers. The group recommended that patient trackers be given to volunteers ahead of time to avoid this problem in the future. Certain federal agencies did not use the patient trackers at the medical aid stations they operated but instead used their own electronic database. This made it challenging to obtain an accurate view of all patient visits, because we lacked access to all of the data. Figure 11.2 shows the types of chief complaints reported during the enhanced surveillance period. Among patients with specified or known chief complaints ($n = 184$), the chief complaint category with the greatest number of patients visits was hypothermia or cold exposure ($n = 41$).

UNITED STATES–AFRICA LEADERS SUMMIT

The United States hosted the United States–Africa Leaders Summit (ALS) on August 4–6, 2014. President Barack Obama invited leaders from 50 African countries and their delegations to participate in events that included a United States–Africa Business Forum, a Capitol Hill reception, a White House dinner, and Summit Leader Meetings (The White House 2014). African leaders from 50 countries attended this event, making it the largest event any U.S. president has ever held with African

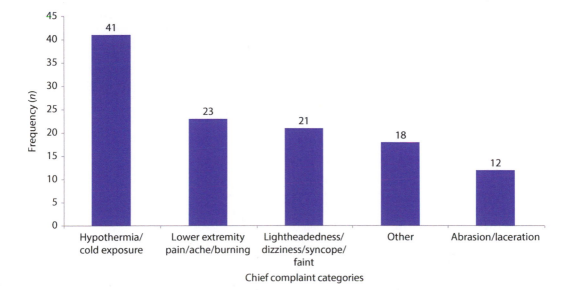

Figure 11.2 Five chief complaints reported at medical aid stations in DC during the 57th Presidential Inauguration by category—January 21, 2013.

heads of state and governments (Jarrett 2014). The protocol used to guide the review and reporting of ANCR ESSENCE data was based primarily on the program successfully implemented during the 57th Presidential Inauguration. However, certain modifications were made. The group sent by e-mail daily reports on query results in a Word® (Microsoft Corporation, Redmond, WA) document, because the Pebble site was underutilized during the inauguration. A report template was developed to ensure a consistent format. The group decided not to send a notice to EDs to include the words "Africa Leaders Summit" in the chief complaint for patients who were ALS participants, because of the low rate of compliance during previous events, including the inauguration. However, the DC DOH still sent a notice to DC health-care providers to inform them that ALS was taking place. Multiple queries were added or modified so that they were relevant to ALS. Three event-specific queries were created to detect the potential cases of Middle East Respiratory Syndrome, Ebola, and hyperthermia or dehydration. Medical aid stations were placed at each ALS event venue and staffed by HEPRA volunteers. DC DOH epidemiologists worked with the HEPRA staff to add preset fields to the patient trackers so that the chief complaint was assigned to one or more general categories (e.g., GI or respiratory symptoms).

Outcomes and lessons learned

None of the syndrome or subsyndrome query results that were initially flagged as potentially unusual or suspicious during the review of the ANCR ESSENCE data were ultimately associated with ALS or considered to pose a public health threat. Three patients visited a medical aid station. Two patients had a headache and were treated and released. The third patient was transported to the hospital with a complaint of "pressure to the [face] later dizzy and numbness to both legs." The new, simplified format for the daily report was easily implemented, provided a concise data summary, and was well accepted. These daily reports, combined with the established communication protocols, resulted in rapid assessment and decision making among jurisdictions. One concern noted in the collection

of medical aid station data was that DC DOH epidemiologists and HEPRA staff frequently identified data entry errors when they reviewed the data. Although HEPRA staff quickly corrected the errors, this indicated that volunteers need additional training.

Discussion and conclusion

Effective and timely public health responses during NSSEs require surveillance tools that provide reliable and timely information. ANCR ESSENCE and HC Standard are valuable tools for rapidly acquiring and sharing health data. These tools are also flexible in that system settings can be adjusted to specifically tailor results to each event (e.g., addition of event-related user-defined queries in ANCR ESSENCE and new data fields in the forms used by the patient trackers). Our experiences with these two events demonstrate the utility of leveraging electronic tools to combine data into a central system and to facilitate communication and data sharing among various jurisdictions. As we continue to refine our strategies for using these electronic tools, we hope to be even more effective in fulfilling our mission to protect the health and safety of DC residents and visitors.

2014 MICRONESIAN GAMES

PAUL WHITE
Public Health Division
Secretariat of the Pacific Community
Noumea, New Caledonia

RICHARD WOJCIK
Johns Hopkins University Applied Physics Laboratory
Laurel, Maryland

Introduction: The 8th Micronesian Games

The 8th Micronesian Games took place in July 2014 in Pohnpei State, Federated States of

Micronesia (FSM). The Micronesian Games are a quadrennial international multisport event that takes place in the Micronesian region of Oceania, a region centered on the islands of the tropical Pacific Ocean. In the 2014 Games, participant countries and territories included the Marshall Islands, Kiribati, Nauru, Palau, the Northern Mariana Islands, Guam, and the four states of Pohnpei, Chuuk, Yap, and Kosrae that constitute the FSM.

Under the auspices of the Pacific Public Health Surveillance Network (PPHSN), the Secretariat of the Pacific Community (SPC) jointly undertook a mass gathering syndromic surveillance activity during the 2014 Micronesian Games to enhance the existing syndromic surveillance system. PPHSN was created in 1996 under the joint auspices of the SPC and the World Health Organization. It is a voluntary network of countries and organizations dedicated to the promotion of public health surveillance and appropriate response to the health challenges of 22 Pacific Island countries and territories. The population under surveillance during the Games was the population of Pohnpei, participating athletes, and international visitors to the Games. The enhanced mass gathering surveillance initiative was supported by the Pohnpei Department of Health, SPC, and the Johns Hopkins University Applied Physics Laboratory (JHU/APL).

PPHSN was aware of several disease outbreaks or public health incidents of importance occurring regionally during the Games: there was a measles outbreak in Kosrae and Pohnpei State, FSM, and one confirmed case of measles in Chuuk State, FSM, and Guam; dengue serotype-3 had been confirmed in Nauru; and there was an outbreak of chikungunya in American Samoa.* Disease outbreaks such as measles have the potential for severe impacts that could inundate and overwhelm health services' ability to effectively control and manage and could disrupt and negatively impact the Games themselves.

* http://www.wpro.who.int/southpacific/programmes/
communicable_diseases/disease_surveillance_
response/PSS-10-August-2014/en/

To mitigate these communicable disease risks, the purpose of the enhanced surveillance was to (1) provide a simple surveillance system for detecting and responding to disease outbreaks in a timely and effective manner, (2) disseminate epidemiological information through the Pacific region to assist in country preparedness, and (3) ensure durable disease surveillance improvements beyond the mass gathering event.

Technology used for surveillance during the Games

JHU/APL was approached by the Public Health Division of the Research Evidence and Information Programme of the SPC to explore the feasibility of using the Suite for Automated Global Electronic bioSurveillance (SAGES) disease surveillance toolkit for mass gathering surveillance during the Games. SAGES, developed by JHU/APL, is a collection of modular, open-source software tools designed to meet the challenges of electronic disease surveillance in resource-limited settings. SAGES uses mobile and web-based methods to collect structured data from SMS, Wi-Fi, and Internet-connected devices. The primary data analysis tool, OpenESSENCE, provides a web-based interface with data analysis, visualization, and reporting capabilities.

For the Games, OpenESSENCE was hosted remotely because of a very short deployment and testing window. The cloud-based storage architecture was advantageous in reducing local storage server costs. The SAGES and SPC teams worked together to customize the data entry forms and visualizations to meet the specific needs of the enhanced surveillance during the Games. Although SPC explored the feasibility of wireless tablet data entry at the sentinal sites, connectivity issues at several remote sites prompted the use of paper forms at all locations, with data entry into OpenESSENCE being done at a central location. The paper data entry form and OpenESSENCE web-based data entry form are on the next page.

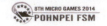 8TH MICRO GAMES 2014
POHNPEI FSM

STATE OF POHNPEI Department of Health Services
Public Health Surveillance Form

 SPC
Secretariat of the Pacific Community

Point of Care (name of dispensary/community health centre/private clinic/hospital/games village/venue):

Note: Please enter information into the rows below for each patient who has one or more of the eight syndromes listed.

VISIT DATE: ___ / ___ / 2014
mm / dd

First Name	Last Name	Date of birth	Age (Years)	Sex (M, F)	Country of residence	Village & Municipality of residence (for Pohnpei only)	Telephone/ Cell number	Current accommodation site (for visitors to Pohnpei)	Acute Fever and Rash Illness (AFR)	Watery Diarrhea	Non-watery Diarrhea	Influenza-like-illness (ILI)	Prolonged Fever	Fever and Jaundice	Food-borne disease outbreak syndrome	Heat-related illness	Onset date	Hospitalized?	Sample taken (and to be sent to lab)
				☐ M ☐ F	☐ Pohnpei ☐ Other (specify)				☐	☐	☐	☐	☐	☐	☐	☐		☐ Yes ☐ No	☐ Yes ☐ No
				☐ M ☐ F	☐ Pohnpei ☐ Other (specify)				☐	☐	☐	☐	☐	☐	☐	☐		☐ Yes ☐ No	☐ Yes ☐ No
				☐ M ☐ F	☐ Pohnpei ☐ Other (specify)				☐	☐	☐	☐	☐	☐	☐	☐		☐ Yes ☐ No	☐ Yes ☐ No
				☐ M ☐ F	☐ Pohnpei ☐ Other (specify)				☐	☐	☐	☐	☐	☐	☐	☐		☐ Yes ☐ No	☐ Yes ☐ No
				☐ M ☐ F	☐ Pohnpei ☐ Other (specify)				☐	☐	☐	☐	☐	☐	☐	☐		☐ Yes ☐ No	☐ Yes ☐ No
				☐ M ☐ F	☐ Pohnpei ☐ Other (specify)				☐	☐	☐	☐	☐	☐	☐	☐		☐ Yes ☐ No	☐ Yes ☐ No
				☐ M ☐ F	☐ Pohnpei ☐ Other (specify)				☐	☐	☐	☐	☐	☐	☐	☐		☐ Yes ☐ No	☐ Yes ☐ No
				☐ M ☐ F	☐ Pohnpei ☐ Other (specify)				☐	☐	☐	☐	☐	☐	☐	☐		☐ Yes ☐ No	☐ Yes ☐ No
				☐ M ☐ F	☐ Pohnpei ☐ Other (specify)				☐	☐	☐	☐	☐	☐	☐	☐		☐ Yes ☐ No	☐ Yes ☐ No
				☐ M ☐ F	☐ Pohnpei ☐ Other (specify)				☐	☐	☐	☐	☐	☐	☐	☐		☐ Yes ☐ No	☐ Yes ☐ No
				☐ M ☐ F	☐ Pohnpei ☐ Other (specify)				☐	☐	☐	☐	☐	☐	☐	☐		☐ Yes ☐ No	☐ Yes ☐ No
				☐ M ☐ F	☐ Pohnpei ☐ Other (specify)				☐	☐	☐	☐	☐	☐	☐	☐		☐ Yes ☐ No	☐ Yes ☐ No
				☐ M ☐ F	☐ Pohnpei ☐ Other (specify)				☐	☐	☐	☐	☐	☐	☐	☐		☐ Yes ☐ No	☐ Yes ☐ No
				☐ M ☐ F	☐ Pohnpei ☐ Other (specify)				☐	☐	☐	☐	☐	☐	☐	☐		☐ Yes ☐ No	☐ Yes ☐ No

Page __ / __   On the last page of each working day, please report on the following fields   Total number of encounters (all causes) for the day [____]   Total number of visits (syndromes only) for the day [____]

New... ✕

VisitDate:*	07-24-2014 🗓
PointOfCare:*	Select PointOfCare... ▾
First Name:*	
Last Name:*	
BirthDate:	07-24-2014 🗓
Age (years):*	Select Age (years)... ▾
Sex:*	Select Sex... ▾
Country of Residence:*	
Village (for people from Pohnpei only):	
Municipality (for people from Pohnpei only):	
Telephone/Cell Number:	
Current Accommodation site (for visitors to Pohnpei only):	
OnsetDate:	07-24-2014 🗓
Hospitalized?:*	Select Hospitalized?... ▾
Lab sample taken (and to be sent to lab):*	Select Lab sample taken (and to l ▾
Lab sample type:	
Lab result:	
Syndromes:*	Select Syndromes...

Save

Surveillance during the Games

The Games were held from July 19 to 29, 2014. The mass gathering surveillance activity enhanced the existing syndromic surveillance system. The existing surveillance consisted of weekly reporting of four syndromes from two sentinel sites in Pohnpei. During the Games, the enhanced mass gathering surveillance expanded daily reporting to include 8 syndromes from 11 sentinel sites around Pohnpei. The enhanced surveillance was in effect from July 17 to August 6, 2 days before the start of the Games and 8 days after the end of the Games. The four syndromes used in routine surveillance before and after the Games and the eight syndromes used in the enhanced surveillance system during the Games are given in Tables 11.1 and 11.2.

Table 11.1 Syndromes and case definitions used for routine surveillance

Syndrome	Case definition	Important diseases to consider
Acute fever and rash	Sudden onset of fever (>38°C) and acute nonblistering rash	Measles, dengue, rubella, meningitis, leptospirosis
Diarrhea	Three or more loose or watery stools in 24 hours	Cholera, viral or bacterial gastroenteritis, including food poisoning and ciguatera fish poisoning
Influenza-like illness	Sudden onset of fever (>38°C) and cough or sore throat	Influenza, other viral or bacterial respiratory infections
Prolonged fever	Any fever (>38°C) lasting 3 or more days	Typhoid fever, dengue, leptospirosis, malaria

Table 11.2 Syndrome and case definitions used for mass gathering surveillance during the Games

Syndrome	Case definition	Important diseases to consider
Acute fever and rash	Sudden onset of fever (>38°C) and acute nonblistering rash	Measles, dengue, rubella, meningitis, leptospirosis
Watery diarrhea	Three or more watery stools in 24 hours	Cholera
Nonwatery diarrhea	Three or more loose stools in 24 hours	Viral or bacterial gastroenteritis, including food poisoning and ciguatera fish poisoning
Influenza-like illness	Sudden onset of fever (>38°C) and cough or sore throat	Influenza, other viral or bacterial respiratory infections
Prolonged fever	Any fever (>38°C) lasting 3 or more days	Typhoid fever, dengue, leptospirosis, malaria
Fever and jaundice	Any fever (38°C) and jaundice	Hepatitis A
Heat-related illness	Dehydration due to heat, heavy sweating, paleness, muscle cramps, dizziness, headache, nausea or vomiting, fainting, extremely high body temperature (>40°C), rapid, strong pulse	Heat cramps, heat exhaustion, heat stroke
Food-borne disease outbreak	Clustering of at least two cases having gastrointestinal symptoms originating from some food outlet or catering site	Includes salmonella, staphylococcus, clostridium, campylobacter, and rotavirus infections

The 11 sentinel sites used for enhanced surveillance during the Games included 1 public hospital, 1 private hospital, 8 health clinics, and 1 high school, which was also a venue for the Games. Sentinel site staff recorded case numbers onto paper forms, which were collected daily by surveillance staff. The data from the paper forms were then entered into the OpenESSENCE web application at a central location. Using OpenESSENCE, the surveillance team generated epicurves that were integrated into a daily situation report ("sitrep"). The daily sitrep contained information on cases presenting the previous day, including a summary of key findings, case counts from each sentinel site for encounter cases and syndrome cases,* and epicurves showing the number of visits by date for the following:

- All encounter cases
- All syndrome cases
- All acute fever and rash cases
- All watery diarrhea cases
- All nonwatery diarrhea cases
- All influenza-like illness cases
- All prolonged fever cases
- All fever and jaundice cases
- All heat-related illness cases
- All food-borne disease outbreak cases

During the enhanced surveillance period, there were 5640 encounter cases and 408 syndrome cases reported from the 11 sentinel sites. Investigations were conducted when cases for each syndrome reached a set threshold level. Sitreps were distributed to Pohnpei State and key Games stakeholders and were also posted on PacNet (a network of Pacific region health professionals). After the period of enhanced surveillance, reporting reverted to weekly reporting of 4 syndromes, but the expanded coverage of 11 sentinel sites remained.

* Encounter cases represent all acute care cases visiting a clinic regardless of whether or not they have one or more of the eight syndromes. Syndrome cases represent all acute care cases visiting a clinic that have one or more of the eight syndromes.

Conclusion

SAGES OpenESSENCE augmented the enhanced syndromic surveillance system in place during the Games by providing a web-based data entry and analysis environment, enabling multiple data entry points and more timely processing of data. This in turn facilitated the accelerated preparation of the daily situation reports during the mass gathering, as multiple users could access the data simultaneously. The timeliness of the data reporting enhanced the ability to detect and respond to outbreaks early. Several other benefits were also apparent, including improved staff engagement with the surveillance system, improved transition from surveillance to response, and improved data quality, validity, and population coverage, providing an improved evidence base for surveillance and informed health planning and decision making.

For future mass gathering surveillance efforts, it is desirable to introduce the enhanced surveillance gradually with a longer lead time prior to the event in order to establish daily baselines. However, in practice, resource constraints may not permit a longer lead time (1 or 2 months versus 1 or 2 weeks). The lead time should also allow for training of all staff (including data entry staff) to ensure they are familiar with the enhanced surveillance system well in advance of the event.

Enhanced syndromic surveillance is an important mechanism for mass gathering surveillance; however, mass gatherings can also provide a unique chance to initiate or strengthen existing surveillance systems. In Pohnpei, web-based data entry has been sustained after the Games, and so have the expanded number of sentinel sites.

Acknowledgments

The author of this case study acknowledges Salanieta Saketa, Eliaser Johnson, Sameer V. Gopalani, Eliashib Edward, Charles Loney, Alize Mercier, Tebuka Toata, Christelle Lepers, Richard Wojcik, Sheri Lewis, Adam Roth, Yvan Souares, Onofre Edwin Merilles, Jr., Salanieta Duituturaga, Elise Benyon, Beryl Fulilaqi, and Damian Hoy for their assistance in this study.

GOING FOR GOLD: SYNDROMIC SURVEILLANCE PREPARATIONS FOR THE LONDON 2012 OLYMPIC AND PARALYMPIC GAMES

DAN TODKILL[1,2], GILLIAN SMITH[3], OBAGHE EDEGHERE[2,3], BRIAN McCLOSKEY[4], AND ALEX J. ELLIOT[3]

[1]Field Epidemiology Training Programme, Public Health England, U.K.; [2]Field Epidemiology Service, Public Health England, Birmingham, U.K.; [3]Real-time Syndromic Surveillance Team, Public Health England, Birmingham, U.K.; [4]Global Health, Public Health England, London, U.K.

Background

A mass gathering can be defined as "an organized or unplanned event (where) the number of people attending is sufficient to strain the planning and response resources of the community, state or nation hosting the event" and can include large sporting events (e.g., the Olympic Games), religious gatherings (e.g., the Hajj or Papal visits), and geopolitical meetings (e.g., the G8 Summit) (World Health Organization 2008).

Mass gatherings can not only generate considerable socioeconomic benefits for the host population but also have the potential to negatively impact the health of the population. Such negative effects may include the following:

- An increased risk of importation of infectious diseases (in particular those diseases to which the host population have naive immunity)
- Exposure of international visitors to endemic diseases in the host country
- Increased opportunity for transmission of infectious disease (due to close contact, increases in the pool of susceptible people, and/or pressures on existing infrastructure)
- An increased risk of bioterrorist activity
- Increased demand on health services
- Possible efflux of resident population and challenges to existing transport, communication, and social infrastructure that may disrupt usual health-care seeking behaviors

The use of disease surveillance systems during mass gatherings can support the timely identification and quantification of any impact (or reassure on the absence of impact) on public health and support prevention and control activities.

England hosted the 2012 Olympic and Paralympic Games. The London Olympic Games attracted over 10,000 athletes from 204 competing countries; had over 200,000 officials, volunteers, and workers; and sold over 8.1 million tickets (International Olympic Committee 2015). The London 2012 Paralympic Games hosted a further 4,237 athletes, 2.7 million spectators, and 70,000 volunteers (International Paralympic Committee 2015). The event was considered a huge success in terms of the sport displayed, the spectacle, and the organization. Hosting the Olympic and Paralympic Games represents a significant challenge to the health infrastructure of the host country (Tsouros and Efstathiou 2007). The Health Protection Agency (HPA, which became part of Public Health England [PHE] on April 1, 2013) played a key role in the provision of public health intelligence, using both preexisting and newly developed local and national surveillance systems. The surveillance systems and public health response were generally considered a success, with the Chief Medical Officer of the Games, Dr. Richard Budgett, reporting "the HPA have set a new benchmark for comprehensive surveillance and reporting" (Health Protection Agency 2013).

Surveillance activities during Olympic Games

Starting in 2009, the HPA worked in collaboration with partner organizations, including the National Health Service (NHS), DOH, and the International Olympic Committee, to develop and implement systems and processes for daily review of surveillance information and production of a daily situation report (SitRep) during the Games, coordinated by the HPA Olympics Coordinating Centre (OCC). Preexisting surveillance systems were "enhanced" to provide daily updates and new surveillance systems introduced. Surveillance activities planned for Olympic Games were described as "enhanced business as usual," meaning essentially that existing systems were used but processes were introduced for more frequent and/or more comprehensive reporting from the systems (Severi et al. 2012). A review of the surveillance and epidemiology services and an overview of international surveillance have been previously published (Jones et al. 2013; McCloskey et al. 2014). In summary, the changes made to traditional surveillance systems included the following:

- *Laboratory surveillance*: During the Games, routine national laboratory surveillance based on a network of HPA and NHS microbiology laboratories was coordinated by an Olympic national operational cell, which analyzed ongoing laboratory activity and reported on a daily basis. In addition, two laboratories were designated to process samples from athletes and visitors suspected of an infectious disease, new multiplex polymerase chain reaction assays were developed to support rapid testing, and statistical "exceedance" algorithms compared daily laboratory reports with reports from the previous 5 years to detect any increases in incidence above expected levels (Severi et al. 2012).
- *Notifications*: In England, medical practitioners have a statutory duty to inform the local health officer responsible of cases of infectious diseases of public health interest through a notification of infectious diseases (NOIDs) system. During the Olympic period, the system that was modified to allow medical practitioners included information on possible Olympic- and Paralympic-related exposures (e.g., notifications of food poisoning linked to an Olympic venue). In addition, 24-hour escalation procedures were put in place and visiting medical teams had notifications as a compulsory part of their temporary UK General Medical Council registration (Severi et al. 2012).
- *Undiagnosed serious infectious illness*: A sentinel surveillance system designed to identify new or emerging infections that might present as undiagnosed serious infectious illness (USII) was introduced. This system relied on trained clinicians in pediatric and adult intensive care units to report suspected USII using an online reporting tool, or to report weekly nil returns

(Heinsbroek et al. 2011). This system was decommissioned after Olympic Games (Dabrera et al. 2014).

- *Mortality*: During Olympic Games, the UK General Register Office provided daily information on the number of deaths (corrected for reporting delays) to support the monitoring of excess mortality (Severi et al. 2012).
- *Syndromic surveillance*: The syndromic surveillance systems operated during Olympic Games (Elliot et al. 2013) are described in detail next.

Syndromic surveillance during the London 2012 Olympic and Paralympic Games

SYNDROMIC SURVEILLANCE IN ENGLAND PRIOR TO THE LONDON 2012 GAMES

Syndromic surveillance is the real-time (or near-real-time) collection, analysis, interpretation, and dissemination of health-related data to enable the early identification of the impact (or absence of impact) of potential human or veterinary public health threats that require effective public health action (Triple S Project 2011).

A key feature of syndromic surveillance is that it is based on the presence of signs, symptoms, or proxy measures that constitute a provisional diagnosis or syndrome in (or near to) real-time, rather than markers of diagnostic confirmation such as laboratory confirmations. As such, adverse health effects or impact may be detected earlier than traditional methods enabling timely public health action (Lawson and Kleinman 2005). Syndromic surveillance systems have been demonstrated to provide early warning of increasing disease activity, for example, identifying rises in seasonal influenza (Cooper et al. 2009) and norovirus (Edge et al. 2006) or monitoring pandemic influenza (Smith et al. 2010).

A major role of syndromic surveillance systems is to provide reassurance to decision makers during incidents or events that there is no associated undetected morbidity in the community exemplified during the London 2012 Games (Health Protection Agency 2013). There is a growing evidence base for this role, for example, during incidents such as the Eyjafjallajökull volcano eruption

(Elliot et al. 2010) and extreme weather events (Hughes et al. 2014). In addition, when outbreaks or incidents are identified, there is potential to provide situational awareness in near real-time (Smith et al. 2010).

Within England, the PHE Real-time Syndromic Surveillance Team (ReSST) coordinates a national program of syndromic surveillance. This syndromic surveillance service has been operated by PHE or its predecessor organizations since 1999.

A feature of syndromic surveillance systems is that they are "passive"; they generally utilize health data that are already collected for other purposes, thus not placing additional data collection burdens on other organizations. Prior to the London 2012 Games, ReSST coordinated two national syndromic surveillance systems, the first monitoring general practitioner consultations within a network of general practitioners across the United Kingdom covering approximately 38% of the population (Harcourt et al. 2012). The second, the NHS Direct telehealth surveillance system, monitored calls reported to the national NHS Direct telephone health advice service, which provided information on the presenting symptoms and basic (anonymized) demographic data (Cooper et. al. 2009). The coverage of this system exceeded 90% of the population of England and Wales.

ENHANCED SYNDROMIC SURVEILLANCE DURING OLYMPIC GAMES

Syndromic surveillance preparations for the London 2012 Games began in 2010. ReSST undertook a risk assessment and gap analysis of the syndromic surveillance systems and service in operation at the time. This identified several areas that needed to be enhanced or developed in order to meet the surveillance requirements for the Games:

1. Monitoring of primary care (general practitioner) activity during "out of hours" (OOH) including evenings, weekends, and public holidays
2. Monitoring attendances at EDs to provide a proxy for severe presentation of disease
3. Enhanced statistical methodologies to provide assurance that unusual activity would be identified

4. Reporting mechanisms to the Olympic coordinating center to ensure that key information and messages were relayed in a timely fashion.

DEVELOPMENT OF GP OUT OF HOURS AND EMERGENCY DEPARTMENT SYNDROMIC SURVEILLANCE SYSTEMS

In order to meet the surveillance requirements for the Games, two new syndromic surveillance systems were developed and added to the existing HPA suite of systems.

These complemented the existing syndromic surveillance systems by offering the opportunity to monitor trends in clinical consultations in primary care settings outside normal daytime opening hours, and, potentially, presentations for the more severe end of the disease spectrum as would attend at EDs. It was anticipated that should urgent public health issues arise during the Games, these new systems covering unscheduled health-care provision would provide useful insight into their onset and evolution.

The development of each new syndromic surveillance system involved initially establishing a steering group that included surveillance and public health experts and clinical leads from each specialist field. Part of the remit of the steering group was to focus on aims and objectives for the new surveillance systems, identifying the public health value that each system would add. This was followed by the development of data specifications (including the development of a range of syndromic indicators) and data extraction and transfer procedures. The focus of these systems was initially centered on London, given its importance as the hub of the Games, and recruitment of data providers in London was prioritized to ensure the systems had maximal coverage in this area.

By May 2012, 46 individual providers of GP OOH service across England had been recruited to the GP OOH syndromic surveillance system, providing coverage in 30 of the 31 administrative districts in London. A range of syndromic indicators, based upon the clinical coding system used by GP OOH services, were developed, including indicators to support the monitoring of public health issues like the impact of respiratory pathogens (both seasonal and novel/emerging), environmental hazards (including the impact of extreme heat), potential chemical incidents including fires, and intentional release of chemical agents (Harcourt et al. 2012).

The ED surveillance system (EDSSS) is a sentinel syndromic surveillance system that collects anonymized attendance data from a network of EDs across England and Northern Ireland. It was established in July 2010, and by November 2014, 36 EDs were established across England. A key partner in setting up the system was the UK Royal College of Emergency Medicine (RCEM) (Royal College of Emergency Medicine 2015), which appointed a representative senior ED clinician to provide clinical expertise to the steering group and liaise with EDs during the process of recruiting EDs to the system (Elliot et al. 2012). In addition, the RCEM assisted in developing a minimum data set for reporting to the EDSSS, enabling a range of indicators designed to detect a broad range of public health problems (Elliot et al. 2012). Alongside the indicators (based upon the clinical diagnosis code assigned on discharge), information on urgency of presentation (triage), demographic details (age grouping, gender), and time of presentation was also collected.

ENHANCED STATISTICAL METHODOLOGIES

In preparation for the London 2012 Games, a program of development was initiated to improve the statistical analysis of existing syndromic surveillance data and to develop new methodologies for the new systems. Statistical algorithms were implemented in the syndromic surveillance systems to provide automated signals of unusual activity. Unusual activity may represent clinical consultations above expected levels (e.g., a statistically significantly higher daily GP consultations for diarrhea in London compared to the same day from previous weeks or years).

During the 2012 Games, these statistical algorithms were applied to all systems and automated to enable the PHE ReSST detect and review all statistical alarms with a further step involving the epidemiological assessment of those alarms to determine whether they were of public health significance that was undertaken by senior public health staff.

Key to the success of the statistical alarms was the availability of historical data from each syndromic surveillance system. This work emphasized the importance of establishing new systems well in advance of the mass gathering, or at least ensuring that historical data were available retrospectively for new systems, to enable statistical algorithms to compare observed data with historically expected values.

DAILY SYNDROMIC SURVEILLANCE REPORTING DURING THE OLYMPIC GAMES

Prior to Olympic Games, a combination of daily and weekly analyses of syndromic surveillance data and weekly dissemination of surveillance reports was undertaken by the ReSST. During Olympic Games, there was a requirement to increase the frequency of data analysis and reporting to daily (including weekends and public holidays) in support of the national OCC. The OCC was tasked with producing a national Games SitRep, which included key information from syndromic and other surveillance sources. To this end, the syndromic surveillance Olympic Games activities had to operate to very tight deadlines driven by an agreed "battle rhythm." Where necessary, data providers were requested to increase the frequency of data reporting and to ensure that daily data extracts were received by the ReSST as early as possible in the day. The ReSST developed a series of standard operating procedures to standardize and improve the efficiency of daily operations and also minimize errors.

A key component of the successful delivery of a national syndromic surveillance service during the Games was preparation. Three months in advance of the Games, the PHE ReSST initiated the daily Olympic battle rhythm, delivering an Olympic report each day (in addition to routine surveillance outputs) and resolving any structural process- and output-related issues ahead of the Games. This planning and preparedness phase enabled a smooth transition when the Games began as it enabled the team to normalize these new arrangements. The daily battle rhythm continued throughout the period of the Olympic and Paralympic Games and was discontinued after the Closing Ceremony.

HOW WAS THE TEAM STRUCTURED TO COPE WITH THE OLYMPIC WORK SCHEDULE?

To ensure the daily delivery of enhanced national syndromic surveillance services for the Games, the resources within the ReSST had to be carefully managed to cover these enhanced working requirements. The ReSST was split into two separate reporting teams to provide a 7-day cover, with each team including a varied skill mix consisting of senior scientists, information officers, and a consultant epidemiologist. Daily data analysis and interpretation was undertaken by the scientists and information officers, with the senior scientists taking the role of "Team Lead" and providing the daily lead for the team duties and the outputs and being the single point of contact for the consultant epidemiologist. The consultants provided a high-level strategic support for the team and the public health interpretation and were the single point of contact for national Olympic coordination teams.

In order for the service to be delivered 7 days a week for 3 months, a rota was developed. Each surveillance team was rostered to work a "4 days on 4 days off" pattern that ensured the continuous delivery of a syndromic surveillance service during weekdays, weekends, and public holidays while also providing the staff with a manageable working pattern over the duration of the Olympic reporting period.

To also ensure the delivery of a continuous service, the teams adhered to a structured handover process including a record of all outstanding actions, key messages on incident alarms/alerts, enquiries (internal/external), and any technical problems with IT systems.

Recommendations for future mass gathering events

After a review of the syndromic surveillance service delivered during Olympic Games, there were a number of key lessons and recommendations:

- *Wider and senior organizational support*: Syndromic surveillance covers a wide spectrum of syndromes, ranging from seasonal increases in respiratory symptoms to GI syndromes during environmental incidents such as flooding. It is important to seek the input of relevant subject matter experts, particularly those who also understand the principles that underpin syndromic surveillance activities when supporting the response to these events.
- *Adequate planning and preparation*: The development of effective syndromic surveillance systems takes time and investment as evidenced by more than 4 years of preparation for Olympic Games by ReSST and partners.
- *Internal and external stakeholder involvement*: Syndromic surveillance systems work best when developed and implemented through close collaboration between the operating team, data providers, and end users.
- *Never underestimate the value of your team*: Much resource is focused on developing complex data systems and automation of processes; however, one of the most valuable assets is the team of scientists and epidemiologist who operate these systems and bring with them a wealth of knowledge and experience.
- *The surveillance outputs need to be simple and have clear key messages*. The outputs and reports may be presented to politicians, ministers, and the public and therefore should have clear, concise messages and interpretation and actions for public health.
- *Do not underestimate the value of reassurance*: Often saying that nothing is happening is as important as reporting an event.
- Syndromic surveillance systems should not be used as a stand-alone system to other public health surveillance. Syndromic surveillance should complement and support the response to mass gatherings and should be integrated into the overall surveillance response.
- *Access to historical data is key*: Identifying deviations from normal (which could represent emergent public health problems) requires knowledge of background incidence. We would recommend at least 1 year worth of historical surveillance data where possible.
- It is recommended that a risk assessment of existing systems be undertaken to identify gaps in disease surveillance activities and an assessment of the potential for syndromic surveillance opportunities to address these gaps.

Olympics legacy for syndromic surveillance

The real-time syndromic surveillance systems have been described as a legacy of the 2012 Olympic Games (Elliot et al. 2013). The systems and processes developed for Olympic Games have continued to operate as an Olympic legacy and have been subsequently used to complement seasonal public health surveillance programs and support the response to public health incidents:

- Enhancing seasonal influenza and respiratory surveillance during the winter using ED and OOH surveillance systems to triangulate intelligence
- Improving the ability to support national heat wave and cold weather plans by monitoring ED attendances for heat/sun stroke in the summer and falls and sprains during periods of extreme cold weather
- Using new systems in the impact assessment programs of the new live attenuated influenza vaccine and rotavirus vaccines
- Providing situational awareness during national air pollution incidents
- Using ED data to monitor the occurrence of incidents of thunderstorm asthma (Elliot et al. 2014)

The PHE ReSST team is also in the process of evaluating the usefulness of other data feeds for use in syndromic surveillance: social media data, for example, Twitter, for potential early warning over existing systems; over-the-counter pharmacy sales for potential early warning and better estimates of patient self-treating behavior; and near-real-time ambulance dispatch data for better understanding the impact of environmental incidents, for example, heat waves, cold weather, and air pollution.

Preparing for and delivering a national syndromic surveillance service for the 2012 Olympics have provided a key set of skills and experiences that can be applied to other mass gatherings. As such, PHE provides experiences and advice to other countries who are preparing for mass gatherings, for example, the Rio 2016 Olympic and Paralympic Games.

Acknowledgments

The authors acknowledge support from NHS Direct; RCEM, EDs participating in the ED system (EDSSS), Ascribe Ltd. and L2S2 Ltd.; OOH providers submitting data to the GP OOHSS and Advanced Heath & Care; TPP and participating SystmOne practices and University of Nottingham, ClinRisk, EMIS, and EMIS practices submitting data to the QSurveillance database. The authors also thank the PHE ReSST and Dr. Ioannis Karagiannis, Field Epidemiology Training Programme fellow supervisor, for reviewing the manuscript.

PARTICIPATORY SURVEILLANCE FOR MASS GATHERINGS

JULIANA PERAZZO FERREIRA

Informatics Center

Centro de Informática da Universidade Federal de Pernambuco

Epitrack, Brazil

ONICIO B. LEAL-NETO

Aggeu Magalhães Research Center

Oswaldo Cruz Foundation

Epitrack, Brazil

DAMIAN HOY

Secretariat of the Pacific Community

Noumea, New Caledonia

ALIZE MERCIER

Secretariat of the Pacific Community

Noumea, New Caledonia

SALANIETA SAKETA

Secretariat of the Pacific Community

Noumea, New Caledonia

Introduction

Mass gatherings (MGs) are events that move large populations to a common location, usually related to a definite cause, motivated by leisure (e.g., sports events, carnival, and shows), religion (Hajj, World Youth Day), politics (marches, protests, presidential inauguration), or other situations. A mass gathering in a location brings an increased expectation for local tourism and investment, thereby generating an improvement or acceleration in all government-provided services to the population. The opportunity to provide a legacy of improved urban infrastructure, social facilities, and health services is attractive to the public and private sectors and society in general. In addition, the opportunities and risks are framed by possible changes in the business environment, media exposure, and health status. Focusing on this last element, it is necessary to undertake extensive planning and preparation within the public health sector to ensure preparedness for any events involving increased public health risks. For this, the systematization of methods is needed, and this case study will discuss some of the main features of MG preparedness undertaken within Brazil.

A brief history

Brazil is known worldwide for its numerous MGs that attract tens of millions of tourists from around the world, such as the yearly Carnivale and the Federation Internationale de Football Association (FIFA) World Cup in 2014. In order to meet the demand on several key services during these large events, the public sector must undertake extensive planning activities. Many cities in the country have organizational strategies during these events, focusing on the need to acquire information for the best crisis management. With the election of Brazil as the host country for the FIFA World Cup 2014, particular attention was paid to the public health sector and past experiences to understand the risks that could arise during the event. Historically, to date no MGs have ever experienced a crisis except for the 1972 Munich terrorist attacks and the 2013 Boston Marathon bombing. However, there have been a number of public health events associated with MGs, including an acute febrile disease outbreak during the Eco-Challenge-Sabah (Borneo, 2000), pertussis outbreak in Hajj (Saudi Arabia, 2002), leptospirosis outbreak during a triathlon event (Germany, 2006), mumps outbreak during Youth Festival Easter (Austria, 2006), influenza outbreak during World Youth Day (Sydney, 2008), and measles outbreak at a religious event (Germany, 2010).

A national forum, known as Health Theme Chambers, was established as a result of Brazil's decision to host the World Cup. This forum provided opportunities for discussion among the 12 host cities, promoting an understanding about sharing of information and other successful experiences that could be adopted to improve the public health infrastructure during the World Cup. In 2012, Brazil invested in national and regional strategies for improvement in data collection and in carrying out active surveillance. For example, the state of Pernambuco adopted mobile devices to collect field data with real-time transmission to situation rooms. This experience proved invaluable to situation rooms. The structure of the situation rooms was adopted for the Confederations Cup and World Cup, known as Integrated Centers for Health Joint Operations (CIOCS). The CIOCS made up a decentralized network, where each unit (state and/or host city) had decision-making autonomy and was coordinated by the national CIOCS based in the Ministry of Health.

In order to improve the sensitivity of the national system of health surveillance, after the Confederations Cup a movement was initiated with the purpose of implementing participatory surveillance as a complementary data source to traditional systems, providing greater proximity to the user. This strategy has materialized in both web and mobile platforms, generating the *Saúde na Copa* application, the world's first experience using participatory surveillance and MGs.

Impact on health systems of mass gatherings

There are two key public health challenges that a local healthcare system faces during mass gatherings. The first arises from the possibility of the spread of diseases by simple contact between travelers (tourists, athletes, workers, volunteers, media, authorities, etc.) and the local population. This can promote the spread of diseases by the visitors and expose visitors to existing endemic diseases while they are in a particular area. The second is the transient increase in the population within the same space and time. With an increase in population, density within living spaces naturally increases the demand for even the most routine of all public services, especially security, transportation, and health.

As noted previously in this book, the new version of the International Health Regulations in

2005 sought to develop, strengthen, and maintain the capabilities to detect, evaluate, notify, and report international public health risk events, including situations arising from MGs. Additionally, the IHR also developed a set of evaluation parameters and event notification processes that must be followed when it has been determined that a public health emergency of international concern has taken place. This stipulation made possible the use of unofficial mechanisms, including the use of technology for streamlining communication for event detection, monitoring and response to health problems, and reducing the damage caused by them. Participatory monitoring functions within the existing traditional structure of surveillance and health-care services.

Participatory surveillance system features for mass gatherings

Participatory surveillance is rooted in crowdsourcing methods that produce information and feed back that information to society in the form of collective knowledge. With the spread of digital social networks and knowledge platforms such as wiki style and web forums, the participation of users adding information led to a very favorable ecosystem for adopting a social control model of information. Data mining on social networks could be considered a type of participatory monitoring if the content published has data relevant to health. The big difference between this and participatory surveillance is the conscious user action in wanting to join a community, reporting symptoms in several cases that will compose the epidemiological scenarios.

One cannot forget that for the implementation and development of such a strategy, it is necessary to have strategic partners and then make concrete outcome of actions. In the case of *Saúde na Copa*, an integrated project involving public service, private businesses, and third sector services, provided good results and demonstrated that the integration between the various layers, when well-coordinated, can solve the problem of modernization of public health.

During the execution of the strategy, the *Saúde na Copa* was divided into components that facilitated its implementation: (1) planning, content production, and analysis; (2) financing;

and (3) development. The planning, content production, and analysis of the data were done by the Ministry of Health of Brazil. The application of the concept was to use the syndromic approach for the identification of clusters and the early detection of possible outbreaks, promoting rapid intervention. From a list of symptoms self-reported by users, it was possible to identify infectious diseases that were related to syndromes. If some clusters were detected, a risk mitigation action and epidemiological research are articulated through the Ministry of Health, along with the health departments of the states and cities hosting the Games. After the end of the Football World Cup, the strategy remained active for 30 days, allowing the identification of disease outbreaks with features of longer incubation periods.

The financing strategy was supported by the Skoll Global Threats Fund, promoting the development and ensuring that the strategy was launched in time for the World Cup, which would not happen by traditional means because of red tape in the public service. The development was carried out by a start-up innovative health tool called EpiTrack, and the partnership between the three organizations led to the reality of *Saúde na Copa*. The platform was developed in an open-source format, ruled by Creative Commons BY-NC, and is available at https://github.com/Epitrack/SaudeNaCopa so that any developer can adapt it to other situations.

The first point to be considered for the strategy is how it will be delivered. What will be the means by which the end user will be able to contribute information, what will be the setting for crowdsourcing in public health? In this scenario, the application was developed in three languages (Portuguese, English, and Spanish), for Android (native) and iOS platforms, and as a web app (both in HTML5). The app's multilingual feature served both the Brazilian population as well as foreigners present during the World Cup. In addition to the app, an open monitoring panel was created to allow users to monitor the distribution of others conducting participatory surveillance, thus emphasizing the collective nature of this type of surveillance. A more comprehensive version of the dashboard was used by the analysts of the Ministry of Health because they required more technical and epidemiological functionality that would help to rapidly visualize what was going on in the field.

The application was released weeks before the event and publicized via institutional communication channels as well as spontaneous media, assisting in the dissemination to new users. Recruitment was also done by push notifications on match days, encouraging existing users to disseminate the application during the Games to the people around them. To ensure continued participation during the Games, the engagement model implemented a gamefication functionality that encouraged users to update daily, their health status in exchange for points to develop their avatar until the last stage. Gamefication strategies have been a trend in online platforms where competition can drive greater participation, especially in the context of a competitive sporting event such as the World Cup.

An important aspect to highlight is the validation of the data collected and the metrics to be used. Due to the characteristics of crowdsourcing, in spite of the app being user-friendly, problems inherent to these factors may occur. For example, the deliberate inclusion of nonexistent situations generates "dirt" in the database; the team of analysts needs to be careful in identifying such a pattern. The users who post answers at short intervals or repeatedly brand all symptoms are considered spammers and are not part of the final accounting data.

The metrics for the analysis and construction of indicators was based on basic aspects such as descriptive statistics of demographic and health data and analytical aspects such as spatial analysis of the occurrence and concentration of users and syndromes.

The *Saúde na Copa* strategy for the incorporation of participatory surveillance in Brazil achieved excellent performance with over 9,000 downloads and 4,706 active members (i.e., participation more than once during the period) and 47,361 reports of their health status, where 11.3% had at least one symptom. Only 54.8% of the reported diseases occurred in the host cities, indicating that the participatory surveillance app was used even in regions that did not have World Cup games. This demonstrates the effectiveness of the dissemination strategy throughout the country. Use of the app by foreigners was low, however, representing only 1.4% of the total users.

Headache was the most reported symptom, followed by cough, sore throat, and fever. However, there was no detection of syndromic clusters, which was validated by the Ministry of Health, which also did not detect any concentrate cases or outbreaks in the same period.

Conclusion

Participatory surveillance through community engagement can bring improvement in public health. Features such as lower cost for data acquisition, timeliness of information, platform scalability, and integration of population and public health services provide positive features to improve the sensitivity and specificity of participatory surveillance indicators. Lessons learned from our experience indicate that it is necessary to make an investment in communications, marketing, and advertising to reach more users among various social strata. Just relying on traditional media and press conferences limited to specific consumer groups will not be sufficient. Investment in digital media can be a great opportunity to not only leverage the number of users but also enhance their participation. Another important aspect of participatory surveillance is the need for transparency with the participating citizens and the public writ large. The user feels motivated to participate if he or she receives something in return, and this participatory monitoring strategy offers greater details of how diseases are behaving. This ensures that the information reaches the user through maps or specific screens in the application and promotes bilateral confidence, resulting in the continuous and systematic participation of the population as a primary source of information.

REFERENCES

Role of mass gathering surveillance

Arbon, P., F.H. Bridgewater, and C. Smith. 2001. Mass gathering medicine: A predictive model for patient presentation and transport rates. *Prehosp. Disaster Med.* 16(3): 109–116.

Centers for Disease Control and Prevention. 2006. Surveillance for early detection of disease outbreaks at an outdoor mass gathering—Virginia, 2005. *Morb. Mortal. Wkly. Rep.* 55(3): 71–74.

National special security events: Enhanced disease surveillance in the District of Columbia

Federal Emergency Management Agency Emergency Management Institute. 2014. Incident command center resources, glossary of related terms. Last Modified May 2008. Accessed May 18, 2015. http://training.fema.gov/EMIWeb/is/ICSResource/Glossary.htm#S.

Global Emergency Resources (GER). 2014. HC standard patient tracking. Accessed May 19, 2015. http://www.ger911.com/hc-suite/hc-patient-tracking/.

Henning, K.J. 2004. What is syndromic surveillance? *Morb. Mortal. Wkly. Rep.* 53 (Suppl.): 5–11 (September 17, 2014).

Jarrett, V. 2014. U.S.-Africa Leaders Summit: President Obama Welcomes an historic gathering to Washington. The White House Blog. Accessed May 18, 2015. http://www.whitehouse.gov/blog/2014/08/04/us-africa-leaders-summit-president-obama-welcomes-historic-gathering-washington.

The White House. 2014. US-Africa Leaders Summit. Accessed May 18, 2015. http://www.whitehouse.gov/us-africa-leaders-summit#section-program-of-events.

United States Secret Service. 2014. National special security events. Accessed May 18, 2015. http://www.secretservice.gov/nsse.shtml.

Going for gold: Syndromic surveillance preparations for the London 2012 Olympic and Paralympic games

Cooper, D.L., N.Q. Verlander, A.J. Elliot, C.A. Joseph, and G.E. Smith. 2009. Can syndromic thresholds provide early warning of national influenza outbreaks? *J. Public Health* 31: 17–25.

Dabrera, G., B. Said, H. Kirkbride, and USII Collaborating Group. 2014. Evaluation of the surveillance system for undiagnosed serious infectious illness (USII) in intensive care units, England, 2011 to 2013. *Euro Surveill.* 19: pii: 20961.

Edge, V.L., F. Pollari, L.K. Ng et al. 2006. Syndromic surveillance of Norovirus using over-the-counter sales of medications related to gastrointestinal illness. *Can. J. Infect. Dis. Med. Microbiol.* 17: 235–241.

Elliot, A., R. Morbey, H. Hughes et al. 2013. Syndromic surveillance—A public health legacy of the London 2012 Olympic and Paralympic Games. *Public Health* 127: 777–781.

Elliot, A.J., H.E. Hughes, T.C. Hughes et al. 2012. Establishing an emergency department syndromic surveillance system to support the London 2012 Olympic and Paralympic Games. *Emerg. Med. J.* 29: 954–960.

Elliot, A.J., H.E. Hughes, T.C. Hughes et al. 2014. The impact of thunderstorm asthma on emergency department attendances across London during July 2013. *Emerg. Med. J.* 31: 675–678.

Elliot, A.J., N. Singh, P. Loveridge et al. 2010. Syndromic surveillance to assess the potential public health impact of the Icelandic volcanic ash plume across the United Kingdom, April 2010. *Euro Surveill.* 15: pii: 19583.

Harcourt, S.E., J. Fletcher, P. Loveridge et al. 2012. Developing a new syndromic surveillance system for the London 2012 Olympic and Paralympic Games. *Epidemiol. Infect.* 140: 2152–2156.

Health Protection Agency. 2013. London 2012 Olympic and Paralympic Games, summary report of the Health Protection Agency's Games Time Activities. https://www.gov.uk/government/uploads/system/uploads/attachment_data/file/398937/London_2012_Olympic_and_Paralympic_Games_summary_report.pdf.

Heinsbroek, E., B. Said, and H. Kirkbride. 2011. A new surveillance system for undiagnosed serious infectious illness for the London 2012 Olympic and Paralympic Games. *Euro Surveill.* 17: 471–476.

Hughes, H.E., R. Morbey, T.C. Hughes et al. 2014. Using an Emergency Department Syndromic Surveillance System to investigate the impact of extreme cold weather events. *Public Health* 128: 628–635.

International Olympic Committee. 2015. Official website of the Olympic Movement. Accessed January, 2015. http://www.olympic.org/london-2012-summer-olympics.

International Paralympic Committee. 2015. Official website of the Paralympic Movement. Accessed January, 2015. www.paralympic.org.

Jones, J., J. Lawrence, L.P. Hallström et al. 2013. International infectious disease surveillance during the London Olympic and Paralympic Games 2012: Process and outcomes. *Euro Surveill.* 18(32): 20554.

Lawson, A.B. and K. Kleinman. 2005. Introduction: Spatial and syndromic surveillance for public health. In *Spatial and Syndromic Surveillance for Public Health*. A.B. Lawson and K. Kleinman (eds.), Chichester, U.K.: John Wiley & Sons, Ltd.

McCloskey, B., T. Endericks, M. Catchpole et al. 2014. London 2012 Olympic and Paralympic Games: Public health surveillance and epidemiology. *Lancet* 383: 2083–2089.

Royal College of Emergency Medicine. 2015. College of Emergency Medicine. Accessed January, 2015. http://www.collemergencymed.ac.uk/.

Severi, E., E. Heinsbroek, C. Watson, M. Catchpole, and HPA Olympics Surveillance Work Group. 2012. Infectious disease surveillance for the London 2012 Olympic and Paralympic Games. *Euro Surveill.* 17: 20232.

Smith, S., A.J. Elliot, C. Mallaghan et al. 2010. Value of syndromic surveillance in monitoring a focal waterborne outbreak due to an unusual Cryptosporidium genotype in Northamptonshire, United Kingdom, June–July 2008. *Euro Surveill.* 15: 19643.

Smith, S., G. Smith, B. Olowokure et al. 2010. Early spread of the 2009 influenza A (H1N1) pandemic in the United Kingdom—Use of local syndromic data, May–August 2009. *Euro Surveill.* 16: 221–228.

Triple S. Project. 2011. Assessment of syndromic surveillance in Europe. *Lancet* 378: 1833–1834.

Tsouros, A.D. and P.A. Efstathiou. 2007. Mass gatherings and public health—The experience of the Athens 2004 Olympic Games. Accessed January, 2015. http://www.euro.who.int/document/e90712.pdf.

World Health Organization. 2008. Communicable disease alert and response for mass gatherings. Accessed January, 2015. http://www.who.int/csr/Mass_gatherings2.pdf.

Participatory surveillance for mass gatherings

Abubakar, I., P. Gautret, G. Brunette, L. Blumberg, D. Johnson, G. Poumerol, Z.A. Memish, M. Barbeschi, and A. Skan. 2012. Global perspectives for prevention of infectious disease associated with mass gatherings. *Lancet Infect. Dis.* 12: 66–74.

Blyth, C.C., H. Foo, S.J. van Hal et al. 2010. Influenza outbreak during World Youth Day 2008 mass gathering. *Emerg. Infect. Dis.* 16(5): 809–815.

Bogich, T.L., R. Chunara, D. Scales, E. Chan, L.C. Pinheiro, A.A. Chmura, D. Carroll, P. Daszak, and J.S. Brownstein. 2012. Preventing pandemics via international development: A systems approach. *PLoS Med.* 9(12): e1001354.

Brockmann, S., I. Piechotowski, O. Bock-Hensley et al. 2010. Outbreak of leptospirosis among triathlon participants in Germany, 2006. *BMC Infect. Dis.* 10: 91.

Centers for Disease Control and Prevention. 2001. Update: Outbreak of acute febrile illness among athletes participating in Eco-Challenge-Sabah 2000—Borneo, Malaysia, 2000. *Morb. Mortal. Wkly. Rep.* 50: 21–24.

Chan, E.H., T.F. Brewer, L.C. Madoff, M.P. Pollack, A.L. Sonricker, M. Keller, C.C. Freifeld, M. Blench, A. Mawudeku, and J.S. Brownstein. 2010. Global capacity for emerging infectious disease detection. *Proc. Natl. Acad. Sci. U.S.A.* 107(50): 21701–21706.

Chunara, R., C.C. Freifeld, and J.S. Brownstein. 2012. New technologies for reporting real-time emergent infections. *Parasitology* 1(1): 1–9.

Chunara, R., M.S. Smolinski, and J.S. Brownstein. 2013. Why we need crowdsourced data in infectious disease surveillance. *Curr. Infect. Dis. Rep.* 15(4): 316–319.

Debin, M., C. Turbelin, T. Blanchon, I. Bonmarin, A. Falchi, T. Hanslik, D. Levy-Bruhl, C. Poletto, and V. Colizza. 2013. Evaluating the feasibility and participants representativeness of an online nationwide surveillance system for influenza in France. *PLOS ONE* 8: e73675.

Deris, Z.Z., H. Hasan, A.S. Sulaiman, M.S. Wahab, N.N. Ning, and N.H. Othman. 2010. The prevalence of acute respiratory symptoms and role of prospective measures among Malaysian Hajj pilgrims. *J. Travel Med.* 17(2): 82–88.

Johansson, A., M. Batty, K. Hayashi, O. Al Bar, D. Marcozzi, and A.Z. Memish. 2012. Crowd and environmental management during mass gatherings. *Lancet Infect. Dis.* 12: 150–156.

Jost, C.C., J.C. Mariner, P.L. Roeder, E. Sawitri, and G.J. Macgregor-Skinner. 2007. Participatory epidemiology in disease surveillance and research. *Rev. Scient. Tech.* 26(3): 537–547.

Memish, A.Z., G.M. Stephens, R. Steffen, and Q.A. Ahmed. 2012a. Emergence of medicine for mass gatherings: Lessons from the Hajj. *Lancet Infect. Dis.* 12: 56–65.

Memish, Z.A., G.M. Stephens, and A. Al Rabeeah. 2012b. Mass gatherings health. *Lancet Infect. Dis.* 12: 10.

Oliveira, W., G.S. Dimech, O.B.L.N. Leal-Neto, M. Libel, and M. Smolinski. 2014. The world's first application of participatory surveillance at a mass gathering: FIFA World Cup 2014, Brazil. In *International Meeting on Emerging Diseases and Surveillance 2014*, p. 44.

Paolotti, D., A. Carnahan, V. Colizza et al. 2014. Web-based participatory surveillance of infectious diseases: The Influenzanet participatory surveillance experience. *Clin. Microbiol. Infect.* 20: 17–21.

Patterson-Lomba, O., S. Van Noort, B.J. Cowling, J. Wallinga, M.G.M. Gomes, M. Lipsitch, and E. Goldstein. 2014. Utilizing syndromic surveillance data for estimating levels of influenza circulation. *Am. J. Epidemiol.* 179: 1394–1401.

Pfaff, G., D. Lohr, S. Santibanez, A. Mankertz, U.V. Treeck, K. Schonberger, and W. Hautmann. 2010. Spotlight on measles 2010: Measles outbreak among travellers returning from a mass gathering, Germany, September to October 2010. *Eurosurveillance* 15(50): pii= 19750.

Schmid, D., H. Holzmann, C. Alfery, H. Wallenko, T.H. Popow-Kraupp, and F. Allerberger. 2008. Mumps outbreak in Young adults following a festival in Austria, 2006. *Eurosurveillance* 13(7).

Wilder-Smith, A., A. Earnest, S. Ravindran, and N.I. Paton. 2003. High incidence of pertussis among Hajj pilgrims. *Clin. Infect. Dis.* 37(9): 1270–1272.

Wójcik, O.P., J.S. Brownstein, R. Chunara, and M.A. Johansson. 2014. Public health for the people: Participatory infectious disease surveillance in the digital age. *Emerg. Themes Epidemiol.* 11: 1–7.

12

Promising advances in surveillance technology for global health security

SHERI H. LEWIS, HOWARD S. BURKOM, STEVE BABIN, AND DAVID L. BLAZES

The previous chapters have provided a comprehensive survey of current disease detection solutions for public health surveillance, both in terms of policy and practice. The theory and principles underlying why and how these technologies are being used, as well as how they are being applied to real-world surveillance situations, are presented. Several case studies describe overcoming challenges in developing settings, which underscore how technology can be used to leapfrog other less useful or outdated ones. However, we recognize that novel technologies are constantly being developed, and their application to disease surveillance is inevitable. Identifying which of these technologies will ultimately be useful, cost-effective, and sustainable is difficult. In this chapter, we discuss research areas and public health trends that hold promise to further revolutionize public health surveillance.

INFORMATION AND COMMUNICATIONS TECHNOLOGY

As information and communications technologies (ICTs) continue to evolve and penetrate the global marketplace, public health surveillance and, in particular, population-based surveillance need to be agile and able to quickly adapt to incorporate new innovations. This is a very daunting proposition in the field of public health that is often very slow to change and adapt to technology, but this reticence has improved in recent years out of necessity, as evidenced by the contributions throughout this book.

Cell phone usage and Internet penetration are rapidly increasing every year. As of the end of 2014, the International Telecommunication Union (ITU) reported the Internet as having nearly 3 billion users (International Telecommunication Union 2015). The efforts initiated by the World Bank to lay underwater fiber-optic cables on the western coast of Africa greatly improved speed and access to that part of the world when it became operational in mid-2010 (World Bank 2013). The Eastern African Submarine Cable System (EASSy) is a consortium of shareholders, predominantly African, and is the highest capacity system serving Sub-Saharan Africa and the first to provide connectivity from Eastern Africa to Europe and North America (EASSy 2010). EASSy is just one example of consortiums that are working hard to lay fiber-optic cables and expand the Internet's reach on the African continent.

It is estimated that by the end of 2014, mobile broadband penetration was up to 32% globally; however, this came down to 84% of the developed world and just 21% of the developing world. In Africa alone, the mobile broadband penetration was 20%, which was up from 2% in 2010. Of mobile cellular subscriptions, over 75% are from people living in the developing world (International Telecommunication Unit 2014).

Now that there are so many interconnected users, there has been much speculation over the value of new potential data derived from the increased use of ICTs to include social media sources, crowdsourcing applications, etc. However, it remains to be seen how useful these data truly are to the public health community. While there are research that shows there is correlation between overall population health and social media data, it has yet to be proven in an operational disease surveillance system. For example, it was shown that in the Philippines there was statistically significant correlation between dengue diagnosis data and Twitter data reporting on medically relevant "fever" (Coberly et al. 2014). However, to date these analyses, while promising, have yet to be proven out prospectively with epidemiologists acting on the information they learn from these data. As with all novel data sources, the epidemiologists who use this system will be the ones to provide this validation as only they can fully assess a data source's ability to add value to their surveillance activities.

WORKFORCE

In addition to the need for user validation for novel social media data sources, the overall acceptance of this type of data may likely increase as a more tech savvy workforce begins to evolve in the field of public health. Initial trepidation about entering data into web forms or via cell phones met the most resistance from those who had been practicing in the public health field for many years and were accustomed to using pencil and paper for their data collection and reporting.

Along the lines of ICT acceptance, in the early 2000s, as electronic disease surveillance systems were in their infancy in the United States, many public health professionals were skeptical about the increased reliance on electronic data, regardless of how it was created. Not only were they concerned about the possibility of electronic data being more error prone, but they had a real apprehension over how they would possibly respond to all the statistical alerts they would now be aware of. Given these types of systems are now readily accepted by the public health workforce in many industrialized nations, there are no longer the same types of concerns. Similarly, as more and more people become familiar with new technologies in their day-to-day lives, there is less resistance with relying on data transmitted this way, and potentially, in time, there may be less hesitancy to trust data sources such as social media. However, there will always be concerns over if and how one can validate data received by the general public as opposed to those in a clinical setting.

Regardless of the growing acceptance of ICTs within health departments around the world, research shows that even in developed countries, the number of public health informatics personnel still woefully lags the number needed to implement such technologies as electronic health records, health information exchanges, and electronic disease surveillance systems in a sustainable, meaningful way. In the United States, for example, researchers using data collected by the National Association for City and County Health Officials concluded that health departments can be grouped into low, mid, and high informatics capacity health departments, which tended to coincide with the breadth of public health services they provide to the citizens they serve. This also identified great disparities in the types of informatics employed in various health departments, with the high capacity health departments having the ability to collect and analyze more data thereby improving their overall ability to serve as an information broker within their jurisdiction (McCullough and Goodin 2014).

Similarly, while the data support the concept that the use of informatics improves the quality and safety of health-care delivery in developed economies, there are currently only specific applications versus robust data to prove the same point in developing economies. However, based upon the evidence, the value of informatics and the associated informatics workforce in any economy can be derived (Hersh et al. 2010).

So what is being done or what should be done to further the development of the public health informatics workforce globally? While the past 15 years have seen many individuals either learning informatics on the job or becoming more comfortable overall with the use of technologies in their personal lives, much more needs to be done in terms of formal education. While the number of public health informatics certificate or degree programs is increasing, both in the United States and overseas, the number of schools with these opportunities is still small. As of 2012, only 15 institutions had programs in health informatics, of which 14 were in the United States, and of the programs identified, more than half were in private institutions and therefore could be considered cost prohibitive (Joshi and Perin 2012). While today that number is certainly far greater than just a few years ago, particularly in non-United States locations, the number of programs and their limited accessibility, both physically and financially, will do little to help grow the global workforce at the degree to which it needs to expand.

The solution with the most promise is online or just-in-time education. As noted previously, Internet penetration is increasing exponentially every year. When schools offer online courses, they are able to transcend physical and national boundaries. Additionally, the cost associated with online programs is significantly lower than other programs (Joshi and Perin 2012). However, even more accessible are free open-access courses offered through many major universities as well as through entities such as Coursera. These courses can be accessed anytime, anywhere, and from any device, thereby allowing a public health professional in a remote village just as much access to education as one in a major global city.

Additional solutions, albeit more costly and labor intensive, include partnerships between donor organizations and local universities as well as relationships between international universities with vast experience in informatics and local universities in targeted areas. This approach enables a more intensive capacity to be developed in a given area which should, in theory, enable greater, more unified capacity for the long term as opposed to online education in which individuals are seeking training in a one-on-one fashion. That said, when curriculums are either not locally developed or largely influenced by nonlocal expertise, care must be taken to account for the differences in culture, practice, and local need.

CLOUD COMPUTING

One of the great difficulties public health departments face today, no matter where they are located, is the cost of information technology services. In the United States, for example, some health departments must pay over $200,000 to maintain a single server for a year, with many sophisticated electronic surveillance systems needing numerous servers to function efficiently. These costs add up quickly for often under-funded agencies such as public health. As a result of these costs, combined with shrinking public health budgets, they are being forced to think of new strategies to improve IT efficiencies.

As a result, many are turning to cloud computing as a reliable, scalable, and cost-effective alternative to purchasing and maintaining physical servers. While cloud computing can take on many meanings, in the context of running a disease surveillance system we are referring to the use of virtual computers that can be allocated dynamically (Loschen et al. 2014). As one can imagine, there are many associated benefits and challenges associated with the movement to this environment.

The benefits of cloud computing include efficiency, scalability, and reliability. Unlike physical servers that may not be utilized for more than a small number of minutes every day but still require maintenance, applications running in the cloud require machines to only be utilized for a brief period of time before those assets are released into the pool for others to use. This significantly lowers the cost to the health departments who would not require significant physical hardware. From the scalability standpoint, many organizations, particularly those who are just starting to become familiar with disease surveillance systems, may choose to only pilot the system in a select number of clinics, for example. By utilizing the cloud, they can quickly scale up to include many more data points without needing to buy additional equipment. And finally, cloud environments have the potential to be more reliable in which multiple backups exist.

However, there are also downsides, particularly when it comes to the use of the cloud in resource-limited areas. Protecting personal health information is extremely critical to public health authorities, so hosting this type of information on servers in someone else's data center may be concerning. Additionally, since a single machine used in cloud computing may be running multiple virtual servers, there is no physical separation between different systems that presents additional security concerns (Loschen et al. 2014).

Cloud computing is rapidly gaining popularity. As long as the benefits and risks are appropriately weighed by the end user, cloud utilization may be a viable alternative to physical hardware, which can be challenging from a financial and environmental standpoint.

THE QUANTIFIED LIFE

The amount of data that is currently collected is almost impossible to fathom, and it increases exponentially as technology reaches every corner of the world. It is estimated that every day 2.5 billion gigabytes of data are created, and much of these are in the health realm. People are increasingly collecting, analyzing, and acting upon data related to their bodily functions and health, to include biometric information (weight, heart rate), nutritional information (amount and type of food, where it is eaten), physiologic functions (number of hours of sleep, quantity of exercise), and even psychological status (mood) (Almalki et al. 2015). The utility of these data for individuals has been variably demonstrated in weight loss programs and other self-improvement areas. More difficult to extract from population-based health meta-data is the usefulness for the public's overall health. Further, there will likely need to be numerous validation steps that must be accomplished to assure the fidelity of these data.

People investing in the research field of global health security and disease surveillance need to think about how they can benefit from this greater interconnectedness in order to provide an earlier detection of an emerging infectious disease threat. This goes hand in hand with the concept of crowdsourcing, which is the process of soliciting content from a large group. For example, there are currently numerous websites that encourage people to provide health-related information regarding illness, so it can be determined if a given area is experiencing more than one type of illness than another area. These apps hold great potential, but again the issue continues to come back to validation. If we put this in the context of the Ebola epidemic, the very general case definition of elevated fever, malaise, body aches, vomiting, and diarrhea could be a multitude of conditions; however, when left in the hands of the untrained general population, people with conditions with similar symptomatology may unwittingly start to panic if they posted to a crowdsourcing site. This is reminiscent of the initial concerns of public health officials in the early days of electronic disease surveillance and their question as to how many alerts did they really need to act upon. Considering the lack of validation when the general public is reporting, the question quickly arises whether public health authorities should act upon a report of symptoms that are similar to highly infectious disease.

One could also imagine health data or behaviors being used to prioritize limited funding for preventive programs. Incentives might be automatically delivered to those who exercise regularly or lose a prescribed amount of weight. And educational programs might be better targeted to areas where there is less exercise across a population or a higher prevalence of obese patients.

The use of this type of information has great potential, but there is also a dark side. Privacy issues related to health conditions can affect potential employability or the ability to obtain health insurance. Biometric data can also be hacked in order to gain access to computer or other systems such as banking or databases. And just as our online search signature is considered unique, so are our biometrics. Unlike computer passwords though, our biometric properties are mostly impossible to change. Further, this space is evolving so quickly that there are no widely accepted guidelines to help regulate what is appropriate behavior and who should have access to raw or even processed data. The only constant is the understanding that data are valuable and will continue to be exploited unless they are protected and curated in a responsible manner.

INTERNET OF THINGS

In the same way in which we discussed the ubiquity with which cell phones and the Internet have permeated into peoples' everyday lives, there is another concept known as the "Internet of Things." The Internet of Things refers to the increasing number of technologies or platforms by which devices can "speak" to one another in an attempt to optimize performance or improve interoperability. Many pieces of routine equipment or appliances are now connected to the Internet and can be controlled remotely to optimize function—not only alarm systems but also thermostats and window blinds. It is not difficult to imagine how this might be applied to health and disease surveillance. The accelerated use of certain health supplies or medications may presage an outbreak of disease, and if a medication cabinet is able to monitor how many pills are used, these data may be useful to the local health department. The other possible link between Internet-connected equipment and disease surveillance is point-of-care testing. Several apps have already been developed, which allow smartphones to diagnose parasitic infections such as malaria, African eye worms (*Loa loa*), and lymphatic filariasis (elephantiasis) (D'Ambrosio et al. 2015). If these data are collected in the field, they can theoretically be automatically uploaded to the web and disseminated to public health officials, pharma companies, or funding agencies.

There are certainly ethical challenges related to putting personal level health data on the web. There are potential repercussions and legal concerns about drug use, as well as certain behaviors or medical conditions that predispose one to illness or untimely death. Obviously, this information is not only very personal and thus sensitive, but it is also potentially valuable to commercial entities whose job is to monetize opportunities wherever they can be identified. More and more data are collected without the knowledge of the individual, and fully informed consent will be important as data acquisition continues to be a lucrative endeavor.

PROMISING ADVANCES IN PREDICTIVE ANALYTICS

Once population-based surveillance is in place and data are routinely being collected, the question then turns to whether one can predict the outbreak of an endemic disease. For example, if health authorities could predict that there would be an outbreak of dengue in a particular part of a city, they would be able to tune their public health response accordingly. If they utilize targeted public health interventions, they could minimize the expenditure by only focusing on the area where the outbreak was likely to occur.

However, it is important to note that disease prediction differs from disease surveillance in several important ways. Detection uses information available today to determine whether a specific event or condition is currently present. Early disease outbreak detection presumes that the outbreak has already begun but is not obvious, perhaps because of small numbers of cases, or because the disease is only in its prodromal stage, or because something else is happening that obscures it. The important distinction is that detection is determining whether an outbreak is present and an immediate threat, whereas prediction is determining whether an outbreak may begin to occur at some point in the future. For example, a prediction model may use data available today to provide quantitative indications that a certain disease incidence will exceed a predefined threshold in a specific geographic area within a predefined time period in the future (e.g., weeks in advance).

Historically, disease prediction models have relied upon different types of determinations of high correlations of the disease with current or lagged values of various variables. However, one can generally slide timescales for different variables in ways that make them appear to correlate very well when, in fact, there is no causal mechanism. While there are numerous papers describing such models, it is now recognized that they rarely offer operational predictive value when provided with new data not used in the original analysis. Because of such disappointing results, more rigorous methods are now employed to discern truer measures of operational predictability (e.g., Chretien et al. 2014). Still, there have been questions raised over whether the so-called predictor variables were in any way causal or not (e.g., Kleinberg and Hripcsak 2011). This is due to the fact that there are many ways in which variable A may be predictive other than A occurs and causes C to happen. For example, A might not be sufficient alone but does cause C whenever A and B occur together. Alternatively, A might be sufficient to cause C but does not do so when A and B occur together, so B negates the effect of A. Also, it is possible that B causes C while A does not, yet A always occurs with B and B is not available for measurement. In this case, A is a predictor variable even though it does not cause C. As you might imagine, consideration of every logically possible combination escalates as the number of predictor variables increases. Fortunately, predictive analytics using automated methods can take into account many of the sundry complexities of such relationships. Methods in predictive analytics range from mathematically complex techniques to less mathematically, yet logically complicated, techniques such as process tracing of case studies.

Newer mathematical techniques applied to disease prediction include data mining of disparate data sets, such as climatological, socioeconomic, and disease case data. Fuzzy class association rules can be determined, where "fuzzification" is used to convert nonbinary data into quantitatively determined, yet overlapping, classes. Automated techniques often find thousands of fuzzy class association rules, which are then pruned to those most significant for prediction based upon predetermined criteria. The resulting classifiers may then be used in a final disease prediction model (e.g., Buczak et al. 2014). This data-driven approach not only takes into account the very complex interrelationships that may exist among large numbers of variables, but also avoids the common problem of model overfitting using autocorrelation techniques. Keeping the data used in model development separate from that used in model testing provides a realistic assessment of the accuracy of the predictive model (e.g., Chretien et al. 2014). To provide a model that is operationally useful, consideration also needs to be given to the fact that all data are not always immediately available to the model on the date of collection. Finally, new disease prediction models that involve user feedback in their development can now provide a timely advance notice of a disease outbreak for a region while minimizing false positives, which may result in alarm fatigue and unnecessary preparation of limited resources, and false negatives, which may lead the users to question whether the predictive model is really helpful (e.g., Corley et al. 2014). Predictive analytics may, therefore, provide the public health professional with a model that is robust, rigorous, and operationally useful (e.g., Chretien et al. 2014).

The hope would be that once disease surveillance systems are in place in many parts of the world, the information they provide can be a potentially valuable data source for prediction methods and increase the confidence of endemic disease predictions. These predictions could potentially prove invaluable as public health authorities allocate resources for response to include public education campaigns and other interventions.

FUSION ANALYTICS

While advances in medical informatics and database and network technologies are providing more data streams of increasing detail for population health monitoring worldwide, the growing wealth of information will not improve overall public health investigation and response capabilities unless analytical and visualization tools are available to reap the benefits of this multivariate, often disparate information. Even with single-source data streams, such as emergency department patient records, multivariate analysis needs arise. For example, surveillance by separate facilities, facility groups, health regions, or political subdivisions is commonly required. Also, the need to monitor for separate outcomes or outbreak types may require that records be stratified and monitored separately by syndrome or product group. Applying the univariate methods of Chapter 5 without regard to correlation or corroboration among separate data streams may discard valuable information that could be useful for improving sensitivity or for explaining away random anomalies in a single syndromic data stream.

Heuristically, the advantage of multiple data sources is that a combination of evidence types offers improved sensitivity to health events of interest. For example, in surveillance for waterborne disease outbreaks, a combination of a spike in the number of ED patients with gastrointestinal symptoms, with a drop in free chlorine concentration in drinking water, is a clearer cause for concern than either anomaly alone (Burkom et al. 2011). Furthermore, the combined evidence may improve the characterization of the spatial and temporal spread of disease, the identification of the population at risk, and the identification of effective interventions. In practice, however, multiple data sources can give contradictory indications and may potentially add confusion rather than clarity (Rolka et al. 2007).

Challenges

Along with the putative advantages in the analysis of multiple evidence sources, the challenges noted in Chapter 5 involved with cleaning, filtering, analyzing, and communicating become more complex as the number of evidence sources increases:

- *Required type of combination of evidence*: Practical interpretation terms such as "integration" and "fusion" vary widely among users. In some contexts, the requirement may be a convenient data dashboard, possibly with the ability to drill down to more specific visualizations but without algorithmic alerting (Cheng et al. 2011). For data streams with similar organization, multivariate alerting algorithms have been published (Kulldorff et al. 2007; Fricker et al. 2008). Other applications require higher-level decision aids combining disparate evidence types (Burkom et al. 2011; Dawson et al. 2015).

- *Data issues arising from multiplicity*: Along with the issues of data cleaning, preconditioning, and syndromic filtering extended to additional data types and streams within a data type, the management of multiple data sources poses additional challenges:
  - *Rate of acquisition*: Some streams may be available in near real time while others may be daily or weekly. How should analytic methods account for different acquisition rates in prospective monitoring?
  - *Clinical specificity*: For example, how should methods weight high-volume and timely syndromic evidence with sparse but more specific evidence such as presumptive diagnoses?
  - *Correlation among data streams*: Statistical methods of multivariate statistical process control depend on a stable variance–covariance matrix among included data streams. Other methods also rely on relationships among component streams. Both initial correlation analysis and occasional maintenance analysis are important to ensure that methods are applicable given inter-stream relationships.
  - *Management of data when only a subset of data streams is available*: In routine data acquisition and monitoring, dropouts of individual data streams are not uncommon, for reasons ranging from local system outages to changes in participation. Methods must be tested on data stream subsets and on changing availability as well as on the full complement of data streams.
  - *Validation*: Gaining acceptance of multivariate methods also poses challenges.

An alert in a combination of data streams may be harder to visualize and justify than an alert in a single stream. For example, an unusual rise in a diagnostic data stream may legitimately trigger investigation though the underlying event may be masked in accompanying syndromic data. Proper management of the aforementioned issues of evidence-weighting, inter-stream relationships, and visualization is essential. Another key validation challenge is the paucity of authentic benchmark data. There are few real-life training data sets labeled with outbreak dates and far fewer for multivariate data. Simulated signals have been widely used to test and validate methods in single data streams, but modelers of realistic simulated signals in multiple streams must answer additional questions: What is the expected delay between outbreak effects in different data streams? How do the magnitudes and durations of these effects vary? Assuming that an event affects separate data streams simultaneously and proportionally may produce unrealistic detection performance expectations (Frisen 2010).

Approaches

Authors have proposed multiple frameworks for outbreak detection and situational awareness using multivariate data. These efforts have focused on particular time series methods applied in other fields, disease types, population models of disease spread, spatiotemporal risk estimation techniques, and combinations of these. Most of them are restricted to specific disease scenarios and to the analysis of similar data from multiple regions, and few have been applied in an operational setting.

Published approaches and future approaches may be considered in terms of two prototype monitoring problems (Burkom et al. 2005; Frisen 2010). The *parallel monitoring* problem is the monitoring of parallel data streams representing different physical locations, such as counties or treatment facilities, possibly stratified by other covariates such as syndrome type or age group. The issue is how to maintain sensitivity while limiting the number of alerts that arise from testing the numerous resulting time series. A number of authors have applied the false discovery rate concept to reduce alerting caused by multiple testing (Marshall et al. 2004; Catelan and Biggeri 2010).

Additionally, the *consensus monitoring* problem is the testing of a single hypothesis using multiple sources of evidence. For example, suppose that the null hypothesis is that there is no current outbreak of gastrointestinal disease in the monitored population. Data streams available to test this hypothesis are syndromic counts of emergency department visits, outpatient clinic office appointments, and sales of over-the-counter remedies. Should decision-making be based on results of tests applied to the individual time series, or should a surveillance system apply a multivariate algorithm to the collection of visits, appointments, sales, etc.? To answer this question, the designer or monitor should consider the number and type of data streams available, the range of outcomes that must be monitored, required guidance for investigation and response, the available analytic expertise for system maintenance, and the documented evidence supporting the methods in question.

BIOSURVEILLANCE

Biosurveillance is a term that is being used more and more frequently, particularly by the international security community. The concept of biosurveillance is meant to be more encompassing than just "disease surveillance" as it defines a space in which information is gathered and analyzed for human, plant, and animal domains for the purposes of improved decision makers at all levels of authority—from local to global. The systems that fall under this overarching title are those developed not only for traditional public health surveillance but also for intentional attacks that would constitute bioterrorism (Margevicius et al. 2014).

While this terminology includes disease surveillance and the concepts and methods that we have devoted this book to describing, it is a much broader term that often lacks consensus when discussed across the various disciplines. This lack of common understanding often leads to challenges when starting to assess the usefulness of systems, particularly because they are systems that are often trying to serve the needs of many individuals at various levels of expertise, authority, and across multiple domains.

Biosurveillance systems struggle with the identification, acquisition, and analysis of disparate data sources given that they are often trying to meet the needs of many levels of decision-makers. Given this fundamental challenge, these types of systems run the risk of trying to be useful to many but, in reality, are useful to none. More thought needs to be given to how to collect and analyze actionable information from expert systems to effectively fuse data at appropriate levels while maintaining the integrity of the individual domain expertise.

To that end, while the concept of biosurveillance is extremely important and valuable, we caution public health authorities to stay true to their needs when developing a system. Systems can and should be scalable and adaptable over time, but first and foremost, they must do the job they were initially intended to do exceptionally well. Only then can a system be expanded to serve additional purposes.

CONCLUSIONS

As has hopefully been evident throughout this book, technology, combined with astute public health professionals, is truly the first line of defense in global health security moving forward. With the increasing availability of data, derived from a wide variety of sources, a growing lists of emerging threats, and the rapidity of disease spread enabled by globalization, epidemiologists are being asked to do more without the luxury of increased time or manpower.

Nations have long used health as a diplomatic tool. Improving the overall health of a given population has far-reaching effects on the economy and stability of a population, whether it is as small as a village or as large as an entire country. Indeed, improving the health of one population has effects on populations worldwide. Through the efforts of many government and nongovernment agencies around the world, some of which have been tackling this problem long before the Global Health Security Agenda (GHSA), the face of global health is slowly changing. Partner nations, now more than ever, are strongly committed to Global Health Security as a means to improve not only health but also global economic and political stability. We firmly believe that a "public health emergency anywhere is a public health emergency everywhere."

REFERENCES

Almalki, M., K. Gray, and F.M. Sanchez. February 24, 2015. The use of self-quantification systems for personal health information: Big data management activities and prospects. *Health Inform. Sci. Syst.* 3 (Suppl. 1): S1.

Buczak, A., B. Baugher, S. Babin et al. 2014. Prediction of high incidence of dengue in the Philippines. *PLoS Negl. Trop. Dis.* 8(4): e2771.

Burkom, H., L. Ramac-Thomas, S. Babin, R. Holtry, Z. Mnatsakanyan, and C. Yund. 2011. An integrated approach for fusion of environmental and human health data for disease surveillance. *Stat. Med.* 30(5): 470–479.

Burkom, H.S., S. Murphy, J. Coberly, and K. Hurt-Mullen. 2005. Public health monitoring tools for multiple data streams. *Morb. Mortal. Wkly. Rep.* 54(Suppl.): 55–62.

Catelan, D. and A. Biggeri. 2010. Multiple testing in disease mapping and descriptive epidemiology. *Geospat. Health* 4(2):219–229.

Cheng, C.K., D.K. Ip, B.J. Cowling, L.M. Ho, G.M. Leung, and E.H. Lau. 2011. Digital dashboard design using multiple data streams for disease surveillance with influenza surveillance as an example. *J. Med. Internet Res.* 3(4): 1658.

Chretien, J., D. George, J. Shaman, and R.A. Chitale. 2014. Influenza forecasting in human populations: A scoping review. *PLOS ONE* 9(4): e94130.

Coberly, J.S., C.R. Fink, Y. Elbert et al. 2014. Tweeting fever: Can twitter be used to monitor the incidence of dengue-like illness in the Philippines? *JHU/APL Tech. Dig.* 32(4): 714–725.

Corley, C.D., L.L. Pullum, D.M. Hartley, C. Benedum, C. Noonan, and P.M. Rabinowitz. 2014. Disease prediction models and operational readiness. *PLOS ONE* 9(3): e91989.

D'Ambrosio, M.V., M. Bakalar, and S. Bennuru. 2015. Point-of-care quantification of blood-borne filarial parasites with a mobile phone microscope. *Sci. Transl. Med.* 7(286): 286re4.

Dawson, P., R. Gailis, and A. Meehan. 2015. Detecting disease outbreaks using a combined Bayesian network and particle filter approach. *J. Theor. Biol.* 370: 171–183.

EASSy. January 1, 2010. About EASSy. Retrieved March 31, 2015. http://www.eassy.org/about.html.

Fricker, R.D., Jr., M.C. Knitt, and C.X. Hu. 2008. Comparing directionally sensitive MCUSUM and MEWMA procedures with application to biosurveillance. *Qual. Eng.* [Online]. Retrieved May 31, 2015. http://calhoun.nps.edu/bitstream/handle/10945/38753/MCUSUM-MEWMA_Comparison_Paper.pdf?sequence=1&isAllowed=y.

Frisen, M. 2010. Principles for multivariate surveillance. In H.J. Lenz, P.T. Wilrich, and W. Schmid (eds.), *Frontiers in Statistical Quality Control*, Vol. 9. New York: Springer, pp. 133–144.

Hersh, W., A. Margolis, F. Quiros, and P. Otero. 2010. Building a health informatics workforce in developing countries. *Health Aff. (Millwood)* 29(2): 274–277.

International Telecommunication Union. January 1, 2015. ITU Homepage. Retrieved May 31, 2015. http://www.itu.int/en/Pages/default.aspx.

International Telecommunication Unit. April 1, 2014. ICT facts and figures. Retrieved May 31, 2015. http://www.itu.int/en/ITU-D/Statistics/Documents/facts/ICTFactsFigures2014-e.pdf.

Joshi, A. and D.M. Perin. 2012. Gaps in the existing public health informatics training programs: A challenge to the development of a skilled global workforce. *Perspect. Health Inform. Manage.* (Fall 12) 1–13.

Kleinberg, S. and G. Hripcsak. 2011. A review of causal inference for biomedical informatics. *J. Biomed. Inform.* 44(6): 1102–1112.

Kulldorff, M., F. Mostashari, W.K. Duczmal, K. Yih, K. Kleinman, and R. Platt. 2007. Multivariate scan statistics for disease surveillance. *Stat. Med.* 26(8): 1824–1833.

Loschen, W.A., M.A. Stewart, and J.S. Lombardo. 2014. Public health applications in the cloud. *JHUAPL Tech. Dig.* 32(4): 745–750.

Margevicius, K.J., N. Generous, K.J. Taylor-McCabe et al. 2014. Advancing a framework to enable characterization and evaluation of data streams useful for biosurveillance. *PLOS ONE* 9(1): e83730.

Marshall, C., N. Best, A. Bottle, and P. Aylin. 2004. Statistical issues in the prospective monitoring of health outcomes across multiple units. *J. Roy. Stat. Soc. A* 167(3): 541–559.

McCullough, M.J. and K. Goodin. 2014. Patterns and correlates of public health informatics capacity among local health departments: An empirical typology. *Online J. Public Health Inform.* 6(3): e199.

Rolka, H., H. Burkom, G.F. Cooper, M. Kulldorff, D. Madigan, and W.K. Wong. 2007. Issues in applied statistics for public health bioterrorism surveillance using multiple data streams: Research needs. *Stat. Med.* 26(8): 1834–1856.

World Bank. January 1, 2013. Easter African Submarine Cable System (EASSy). Retrieved May 30, 2015. http://web.world-bank.org/WBSITE/EXTERNAL/TOPICS/EXTINFORMATIONANDCOMMUNICATIONANDTECHNOLOGIES/0,,contentMDK:21525831~isCURL:Y~pagePK:210058~piPK:210062~theSitePK:282823~isCURL:Y,00.html.

Index